AF702246

# SARS from East to West

# SARS from East to West

Edited by Eva-Karin Olsson and Lan Xue

LEXINGTON BOOKS
*Lanham • Boulder • New York • Toronto • Plymouth, UK*

Published in cooperation with
The Center for Crisis Management Research and Training (CRISMART)

Published by Lexington Books
A wholly owned subsidiary of The Rowman & Littlefield Publishing Group, Inc.
4501 Forbes Boulevard, Suite 200, Lanham, Maryland 20706
http://www.lexingtonbooks.com

Estover Road, Plymouth PL6 7PY, United Kingdom

Published in cooperation with The Center for Crisis Management Research and Training (CRISMART)

Copyright © 2012 by Lexington Books

*All rights reserved.* No part of this book may be reproduced in any form or by any electronic or mechanical means, including information storage and retrieval systems, without written permission from the publisher, except by a reviewer who may quote passages in a review.

British Library Cataloguing in Publication Information Available

**Library of Congress Cataloging-in-Publication Data**
Olsson, Eva-Karin.
SARS from East to West / edited by Eva-Karin Olsson and Lan Xue.
p. ; cm.
Includes bibliographical references and index.
Summary: "SARS from East to West is the production of international collaboration investigating the first major pandemic in the new millennium, SARS. As the only major outbreak of a deadly infectious disease in modern times, the SARS case is an excellent example of an emerging contagious disease in an interdependent and interconnected world and provided the bases for how subsequent pandemics, like the bird flu and swine flu, are viewed and managed." —Provided by publisher.
ISBN 978-0-7391-4755-9 (cloth : alk. paper) — ISBN 978-0-7391-4756-6 (pbk. )
I. Xue, Lan, 1959– II. Title.
[DNLM: 1. Severe Acute Respiratory Syndrome. 2. Communicable Diseases, Emerging--prevention & control. 3. Disease Outbreaks--prevention & control. 4. International Cooperation. 5. Mass Media. WC 505]
LC classification not assigned
616.2—dc23 2011028706

Printed in the United States of America

# Contents

# Acknowledgments

The editors and authors of this volume wish to thank a number of organizations and individuals for their support. Initial funding for the Swedish-Chinese collaboration was provided by the Swedish Research Council in collaboration with the Swedish International Development Agency (SIDA). Supplementary funding was provided by the Swedish Civil Contingencies Agency (and its predecessor, the Swedish Emergency Planning Agency) and the Swedish National Defense College. Additional support was provided by Uppsala University. Several Chinese institutions have directly or indirectly supported the project including the School of Public Policy and Management in Tsinghua University (particularly the Centre for Crisis Management Research), the Chinese Academy of Governance, Chinese University Hong Kong, the Ministry of Health of China, the Chinese Center for Disease Control and Prevention, and the Beijing Municipal Government.

A number of individuals have played important roles behind the scenes. Zongchao Peng and Kaibin Zhong have played an important role in helping to organize meetings of the Swedish and Chinese teams. Kaibin Zhong, Stephanie Young, and Greg Simons have coordinated the editing and copy-editing process patiently. Xia Liu and Qiang Zhang actively took part in this project and provided some advice and assistance for the Chinese cases.

Special thanks to Peg Hermann of the Maxwell School, Syracuse University who was an important facilitator and "matchmaker" of this project as well as a longtime friend and source of inspiration for many of us. We are also grateful to Stephanie Buus for her networking skills and editorial assistance in the initial phase of the project.

Original versions of this volume were first published in *The Journal of Contingencies and Crisis Management* and therefore we would like to thank the editorial staff for their comments and suggestions in improving these manuscripts. Likewise, previous published study reports made by the School of Public Policy and Management (SPPM) at Tsinghua University were also used in this volume.

*Eva-Karin Olsson and Xue Lan*

Stockholm and Beijing, June 2011

# Abbreviations

| | |
|---|---|
| CAP | Working Group on Severe Community-acquired Pneumonia |
| CCP | Communist Party of China |
| CDS | Department of Communicable Disease Surveillance and Response |
| CESC | Chief Executive's Steering Committee |
| CIPHS | Canadian Integrated Public Health Surveillance |
| CMOH | Chief Medical Officer of Health |
| CNISP | Canadian Nosocomial Infection Surveillance Program |
| CPHO | Chief Public Health Officer |
| CPIP | Canadian Pandemic Influenza Plan |
| CRISMART | Center for Crisis Management Research and Training in Stockholm, Sweden |
| DH | Department of Health |
| EMAT | Emergency Medical Assistance Team |
| FEHD | Food and Environmental Hygiene Department |
| GOARN | Global Outbreak Alert and Response Network |
| GTA | Greater Toronto Area |
| HA | Hospital Authority |
| HKSAR | Hong Kong Special Administrative Region |
| HKSARG | Hong Kong Special Administrative Region Government |
| HWFB | Health, Welfare and Food Bureau |
| IACC | Inter-departmental Action Coordinating Committee |
| IHR | International Health Regulations |
| MIIDSS | Major Incident Investigation and Disaster Support System |
| MoH | Ministry of Health |
| NACSPH | National Advisory Committee on SARS and Public Health |
| NCC | National Collaborating Centers for Public Health |
| NPC | National People's Congress |
| NPPCC | National Committee of the Chinese People's Political Consultative Conference |
| OMHLTC | Ontario Ministry of Health and Long Term Care |
| PERC | Political and Economic Risk Consultancy |
| PHAC | Public Health Agency of Canada |
| PSEPC | Public Safety and Emergency Preparedness Canada |
| PTAC | The Provincial Transfer Authorization Centre |
| SARS | Severe Acute Respiratory Syndrome |
| SHWF | Secretary for Health, Welfare and Food |

| | |
|---|---|
| SMI | Swedish Institute for Infectious Disease Control |
| SPPM | School of Public Policy and Management, Tsinghua University in Beijing |
| WHO | World Health Organization |
| WHO RC | WHO Representative in China |
| WPRO | WHO Western Pacific Regional Office |
| WTO | World Trade Organization |

# Chapter 1

# SARS: Meeting an Epidemic Head-On

Eva-Karin Olsson, Eric K. Stern, and Lan Xue [1]

The Severe Acute Respiratory Syndrome (SARS) epidemic, which is believed to have originated in southern China in the closing weeks of 2002 and subsequently spread to many other countries, proved to be one of the first severe and readily transmissible disease of the twenty-first century, a tremendous challenge that was faced not only by China, but the whole planet. Today's global society is facing an ancient threat in a new form, and therefore it is crucial to understand the processes and procedures that were utilized to combat SARS. According to the World Health Organization (WHO), the SARS virus eventually infected individuals in some 37 countries around the world, with 8,098 people infected and 774 deaths worldwide before it was brought under control in June 2003 (WHO, 26 September 2003).

SARS seemingly came from nowhere and rapidly spread across borders, catching officials off-guard while they were trying to ascertain what the exact nature of the threat was and stop it from spreading. Initially the mystery of SARS was compounded by the secrecy of Chinese officials who sought to keep a lid on the disease information to prevent potential panic, in a hope for the "best." The underestimation of the disease and lack of cooperation gave SARS a window of opportunity with which to spread across China and beyond the national borders, seriously affecting public health and welfare far from China, including Canada.

SARS demonstrated the potential of a newly emergent pandemic which can wreak havoc upon an unprepared and unprotected society. These effects on modern global society proved to be rather devastating, due to its highly interconnected and integrated nature. In this respect, SARS can be viewed as being a form of crisis. According to the CRISMART definition of crisis, there are three criteria or sets of circumstances that need to be met, either actual or in the perception of the crisis actors: 1) a threat to basic values, 2) urgency and 3) uncertainty (Stern, 1999; Stern, 2009).

Crises tend to follow a certain path in their tendencies and progression. Understanding how crises develop in a theoretical sense provides the practitioner, policymaker and researcher with a tool in which to take a proactive stance and avoid a number of "surprises" associated with the development of the crisis event. Ogrizek and Guillery (1999: xii) offer a series or progression of steps that a crisis can take from a more general point of view (the broader perspective).

- *Outbreak or serious accident*—the outbreak of a crisis.
- *Awareness*—the public become aware of a major risk.
- *Media*—media begin to focus on the event.
- *Scapegoating*—open or implied accusations of unethical behavior and so forth.

A lot is at stake; reputations (national and personal), international trade and commerce, financial concerns (potentially big losses or expenses), the effective functioning of society and last but certainly not least human lives. Some of these concerns may carry greater weight than other factors, which influences decisions that are made and taken. "Luckily" SARS did not prove to be as deadly as the post-World War One Spanish Flu epidemic, which killed millions of people. In spite of this (plus the advances in medical science and technology), there is clearly no room for complacency and sitting on one's laurels.

Other newly emerging diseases, viruses and bacteria are constantly coming to light. The contemporary Bird Flu (H5N1 strain) and A/H1N1 pandemic highlight the need to maintain a constant vigilance and to prepare society (locally, regionally, nationally and internationally) to meet these new challenges as they occur. This is not only in terms of advances in medical science and technology, but the equally important fine tuning of the processes and operating procedures of the relevant agencies responsible for protecting society. The Assistant Director General of the WHO, Margaret Chan, stated "the [H5N1] virus[2] was mutating to spread to humans and could cause global economic losses of US$800 billion in the first year of the pandemic alone" (Novosti, 17 July 2006). As a RAND report noted in 2003, in the post-cold war era, new amorphous challenges which do not stem from the actions of clearly defined individual states but from diffuse issues that transcend sovereign borders and bear directly off the effects of increasing globalization (such as the threats posed by new and reemerging infectious diseases on human populations), are redefining the nature and understanding of global stability, challenging policymakers to develop new, non-state-centered paradigms of security (Brower and Chalk, 2003). In order to boost preparedness and increase operational capabilities, it is necessary to examine and understand what has happened in the past, to ask a tough series of questions and to engage in critical self-evaluation and reflection.

- Were safeguards and/or procedures in place prior to the incident—if so were they effective?
- What was the nature of the threat?
- How quickly was the threat evaluated and were measures taken to combat this threat?
- Were those measures effective?
- What can be improved?

In summing up the results of the impact of SARS, it might be tempting to dismiss it as a minor threat not worthy of much attention, as the number of humans affected and killed is relatively low when compared with other human health concerns. However, it would be a grave mistake to allow complacency to set in at this stage. Instead the SARS outbreak(s) should be viewed in terms of a learning opportunity to dissect, analyze, draw conclusions and apply new knowledge to the area of managing new health threats, so we are better prepared to cope with the negative consequences they may bring and minimize the damage and disruption they may create.

## *SARS Research to Date*

Although a number of publications have emerged on the SARS pandemic since this rapidly spreading infectious disease occurred and was transmitted in late 2002 and early 2003, many of these publications are focusing on a relatively narrow section of the SARS problem. Thus a significant knowledge base has been formed on the issue of SARS from a medical and public health perspective. A variation of the public health/medical research has been to place SARS among other plagues and epidemics that have affected mankind over time, such as the Spanish Flu, Bubonic Plague, Yellow Fever and so on. Publications on the SARS phenomenon often have a specific geographic focus too, many limiting the scope of the study to one country. For example, *Learning from SARS: Preparing for the Next Disease Outbreak* (Washington, D.C.: The National Academies Press, 2004) edited by Stacey Knobler, Adel Mahmoud, Stanley Lemon, Alison Mack, Laura Sivitz, and Katherine Oberholtzer, part of the Pandemic Influenza Special Collection, a ten-book series, examines status of preparations, implementation strategies, and other aspects of the U.S. response to the threat of pandemic influenza.

In *SARS War: Combating the Disease* (Singapore: River Edge, New Jersey: World Scientific, 2003) edited by P. C. Leung and E. E. Ooi, the global SARS outbreak is traced and described, with a focus on the regions where the most infections have been identified. An overview of the whole saga is presented: how the disease spreads; how governments react; how societies and people cope and how health experts work fervently to identify the virus and search for a cure. The 2004 *Plagues and Poxes: The Impact of Human History on Epidemic Disease* by Alfred Bollet was published in New York by Demos Medical Publishing. This publication covers a number of epidemics and pandemics that have occurred throughout human history, including yellow fever, malaria, syphilis, cholera, the Spanish Flu and SARS. It seeks to place the SARS experience in the context of the experiences of the past diseases and epidemics. Edwin Torrey and Robert Yolken's *Beasts of the Earth: Animals, Humans and Disease* (New Brunswick, New Jersey: Rutgers University Press, 2005) puts the

SARS pandemic through a similar form of analysis. They look at a series of relationships and crises that have been faced by mankind over time. A significant question posed here being, is it possible to draw valuable lessons solely via this means of analysis given the significant changes that have taken place in global human society (the steady integration of local, regional and national communities and economies into an international/global network for example)?

A selection of other publications within this field has been provided by organizations, such as the World Health Organization's *SARS: How a Global Epidemic was Stopped*, published in 2006. Other recent publications with a public health/medical emphasis include: an edited volume by Malik Peiris, Larry J. Anderson, Albert DME Osterhaus, Klaus Stohr, Kwok-yung Yuen, *Severe Acute Respiratory Syndrome* (Malden, Mass.: Blackwell, 2005), which provides a comprehensive, authoritative reference guide for everyone in the medical and scientific community engaged in the fight against SARS; a book by Thomas Abraham, *Twenty First Century Plague: The Story of SARS* (Baltimore, Maryland: John Hopkins University Press, 2005), which traces the emergence of SARS, in the process examining the global politics and economics of disease, and provides the first behind-the-scenes account of how the global battle against SARS was fought and the incredible research efforts that finally led to identification of the virus; a comprehensive and up-to-date account of the clinical management of severe acute respiratory syndrome (SARS); *Severe Acute Respiratory Syndrome: From Benchtop to Bedside* (Hackensack, New Jersey: World Scientific, 2004), edited by Joseph J. Y. Sung, which covers the various aspects, from diagnosis, clinical presentation and therapeutic modalities to rehabilitation; *Viral Fitness: The Next SARS and West Nile in the Making* (New York: Oxford University Press, 2004), by Jaap Goudsmit, which presents a broad array of divergent virus systems in an understandable way.

Some other works seek to place SARS within the field of governance and management. One such publication is by David Fidler, *SARS: Governance and the Globalization of Disease* (New York: Palgrave MacMillan, 2004), which takes government policy, political aspects and society into consideration, and provides the first comprehensive analysis of the SARS outbreak and how it was successfully managed by the global effort led by the WHO. A similar approach is taken by John Wong and Zheng Yongnian in *The SARS Epidemic: Challenges to China's Crisis Management* (Singapore: World Scientific, 2004). By focusing on the extent of resilience of Mainland China and Hong Kong, the quality of their political leadership, the effectiveness of their political and institutional mobilization, the crisis-management capability of their respective bureaucracies, and the viability of their governance systems, this book examines how each of the two societies coped with this random external shock.

The reporting of SARS and an analysis of communications during the period of the SARS pandemic has also come under scrutiny. China's initial response to the crisis was to put it at best, negligent and at worst secretive. This has provided a rich source of material for researchers in the field of media/communications studies. One of the studies on the subject was written by S. Yu in 2003, *Lessons from SARS Coverage* appearing in Niemen Reports in winter 2003. There also have been some books about how SARS appeared in China in 2002 and spread across China and into Southeast Asia and North America in the winter and spring of 2003. For example, In *China Syndrome: The True Story of the Twenty First Century's First Great Epidemic* (New York: Harper Collins, 2006), Karl Taro Greenfeld provides a ground zero perspective on SARS—he was editing *Time Asia* when the first rumors of a virulent disease sweeping mainland Chinese hospitals hit his desk—and brings reportorial immediacy to this chronicle of how epidemiologists realized that the cases of "atypical pneumonia" scattered throughout Asia were the initial wave of severe acute respiratory syndrome, a new strain of avian flu.

This volume seeks to unite many of these rather diverse and dispersed subjects under the one cover. It touches upon most of the subject areas and aspects mentioned earlier; public health, governance, political aspects, societal aspects, media/communications under the umbrella of crisis management in Mainland China, Hong Kong and Canada during the time of the SARS pandemic. It thereby attempts to give the reader a more holistic and integrated view of this important event, and one that is more accessible given the fact that it can be found within this one publication.

## *Method*[3]

In several of the studies repeated in the volume, the analytical approach developed in Sundelius, Stern, with Bynander (1997) and refined in the research program *Crisis Management Baltic/Europe: National Crisis Management in an International Perspective* (e.g., Stern and Bynander, 1998; Stern, 1999) provides a point of departure. This methodology entails:

1. A detailed reconstruction of the crisis events using available government documents and reports, mass media sources (broadcast and print), previous scholarly investigations, and interviews with involved decision-makers, stakeholders, and citizens.
2. A dissection of the case into a series of crucial occasions for decision-making (a series of pressing "what do we do now?" problems which arise during the period of the crisis) which challenge the coping capacity of decision-makers. The selection criteria for identifying these decision occasions include:
   - the problems/dilemmas which most occupied the decision-makers,

- issues which were not emphasized by the crisis actors but which in retrospect had the potential to change the course of the crisis development, and
- episodes of particular pedagogical value—those which point to the "best" or "worst" practices and promise to point towards lessons of practical value.

3. Thematic analyses of phenomena pertinent to crisis management (see the following section on analytical themes and propositions).
4. Comparing and contrasting case findings with others documented in the CRISMART case bank and in international literature with the focus on processes rather than on structures.

This volume draws upon the work of researchers and practitioners in Mainland China, Hong Kong, Canada, the United States and Sweden and embraces a variety of methodological approaches. This variation adds value to the analysis of the various case studies. This allows the reader to look at the same problem from a variety of angles and perspectives, perhaps revealing some aspect that may otherwise remain hidden had a uniform approach been rigidly implemented. To use Lebow's analogy, a crisis is like a gem; that is, it should be viewed from a number of different angles in order to be able to truly appreciate it (Lebow, 1981).

## *Analytical Themes*[4]

The authors of the chapters in this volume were encouraged to explore a number of themes when analyzing their empirical findings. The themes are:

1. Crisis Preparedness, Prevention, and Mitigation
2. Leadership
3. Decision Units
4. Problem Perception and Framing
5. Value Conflict
6. Politico-Bureaucratic Cooperation and Conflict
7. Crisis Communication and Credibility
8. Transnationalization and Internationalization
9. Temporal Effects
10. Learning

*Preparedness, Prevention, and Mitigation*[5]: This theme focuses on the extent to which crisis managers and their organizations are prepared to respond to extraordinary events. Have they experienced serious crises before? Have they cultivated an "it can happen here" mentality and prepared themselves psychologically for the rigorous demands for crisis management? Do plans and infrastructure exist and are they adapted to the exigencies of the situation? Are decision-makers able to identify potential threats and quickly act to prevent them from escalating? Are windows of opportunity for limiting damage or making gains exploited?

*Leadership*: This theme focuses on the leadership styles and types exhibited by key actors in the crisis. Leadership may be operative—in the sense taking charge of the crisis management activities and coordination. It may also be symbolic—in the sense of showing through word and deed that the leading figures are participating in the crisis and empathizing with those who are at risk or who have already suffered losses. Leadership may be concrete and personal, or more abstract and distant. In deliberations, leaders may be directive/hierarchical or facilitative/collegial. Leadership should be seen as relational, inextricably linked to its followership and mediated by factors such as power, affect, culture, organizational structure, access to expertise and context. Finally, leaders vary in their propensities to micro-manage or delegate when it comes to critical decisions (see, e.g., Bass, 1997; Gardner, 1995; Hermann and Hagen, 1998).

*Decision Units*: This theme focuses on the question of how and where decisions are taken in the complex institutional systems which typically engage in crisis management. For example, crucial decisions can be taken by single individuals, tandems or dyads, small groups, organizational networks, etc. Similarly, decision units may be located and play various roles within a given political/administrative (or corporate) system. Decision units may be strategic or operative in nature and may be located at local, regional, national, or supranational (e.g., EU or UN) levels. Decision units may vary considerably in terms of their composition, mode of operation and placement across the course of a given crisis; it is not uncommon for upward (up-scaling) and downward (downscaling) shifts to occur in the complex politico-administrative escalation and de-escalation processes (see, e.g., Snyder, Bruck, and Sapin, 1963; Hermann, Hermann, and Hagen, 1987; Rosenthal, 't Hart, and Kouzmin, 1991; Stern, 1999). Finally, what are the criteria for determining which individuals and organizations will be included in (or excluded from) the decisional "loop" and the decision unit?

*Problem Perception and Framing*: This theme focuses on the subjective and socially constructed nature of crisis decision-making. Actors act not on uncontestable and objective knowledge of the situation but rather upon their perceptions and interpretations of what is happening (Snyder, Bruck and Sapin, 1963; Sylvan and Voss, 1998; Stern, 1999). While problem framing often takes place on a semi-conscious, intuitive level (especially by "naïve" decision-makers), problem-framing processes exert a profound influence upon the choices. In other words, once a problem has been framed, many possible lines of action have already been discarded and strong propensities for and constraints upon action created. Framing is heavily influenced by cognitive and social structures and processes such as (historical) analogical and metaphoric reasoning, culture, context, organization and information flow (Vertzberger, 1990; Larson, 1985; Khong, 1992). Why do particular actors perceive and frame problems as they do at various junctures of a crisis? Why do these problem images change (or remain stable) over the course of a crisis and its aftermath?

*Value Conflict*: This theme focuses on the potential for tension and conflict among the various values at stake in a crisis situation. An integral part of problem framing is identifying the values which are implicated in a given situation. This is often a demanding process and it is common for decision-makers to overlook values embedded in a complex issue, if they do not engage in rigorous critical deliberations (see, e.g., Steinbruner, 1974:16-17; Keeney, 1992). Crises, by definition, have profound implications for fundamental values such as preservation of human life, sovereignty/autonomy, economic well being, democracy, rule of law, and so forth. More parochial values—such as the personal and political fortunes of individual officials and parties—are also involved. Good crisis performances make careers—poor ones break them. It is common for multiple values to be at stake in crises and thus decision makers often face painful and stress-inducing dilemmas and tragic choices (Janis and Mann, 1977). Decision-makers may ignore or deny value conflict, which tends to generate unbalanced policy-making. They may recognize and accept value conflict—following Lenin's dictum that "You can't make an omelet without breaking eggs." They may choose to procrastinate and hope for the situation to improve. Alternatively, they may actively seek to resolve the conflict and find a transcendent solution which adequately protects the key values at stake.[6] How, then, do actors cope with the value conflicts which tend to emerge in crisis situations?

*Politico-Bureaucratic Cooperation and Conflict*: This theme focuses on the issue of patterns of convergence and divergence, parochialism and solidarity—among the actors and stakeholders engaged in a crisis. There are a number of documented dynamics which tend to create and exert certain pressures upon cooperation and solidarity in a crisis (e.g., the "rally around the flag" effect, leader attentiveness, and "groupthink").[7] However, there are also a number of countervailing tendencies. Crises often present particularistic risk which may induce political or bureaucratic actors to engage in defensive behaviors, which may in turn antagonize other actors and lead to conflict. For example, following failures or setbacks, it is common for actors to play a "blame game." Equally important, crises present opportunities as well as risks, and so actors may compete in seeking credit for their contribution (and denigrating that of others). Finally, situational and contextual factors tend to be moderated by the nature of personal relationships within policy communities and the strength of national cultural norms opposing opportunism in extraordinary situations (see, e.g., Rosenthal, 't Hart, and Kouzmin, 1991; Stern and Verbeek, 1998; Allison and Zelikow, 1999).

*Crisis Communication and Credibility*: This theme focuses on the relationship between crisis managers, the media, and the elite/mass public (see, e.g., Nohrstedt and Tassew, 1993; Nordlund, 1994; Pearce, 1995; Regester and Larkin, 1998; Henry, 2000). In democratic polities, maintaining credibility and legitimacy with the media and the public is an essential task of successful governance in crisis and more normal situations alike. According to Michael Granatt, communications expert in the United Kingdom, a progressive media response to a crisis consists of mayhem (finding out who, what, where and why), masterminding (background information and history sought), a manhunt, and an epilog (Harrison, 1999: 106). This progression of activity by mass media outlets needs to be taken into account and anticipated by crisis managers, and to ignore it at their peril. Crisis managers enter crises with varying degrees of credibility which they may gain or lose over the course of the crisis. Actors vary considerably in their approach to crisis communication. Some take a defensive/closed stance, which can easily antagonize the media and cost credibility. Others take a more proactive/open stance and seek to maintain the initiative in providing information and establishing friendly relations with the mass media. Actors vary considerably in the ways and the degree to which they coordinate crisis communication, the information strategies they choose, and the tactics they use. Similarly, some actors closely monitor how their messages are being received and act accordingly to correct problems, while others—focusing on other aspects of crisis management and distracted by stress—are oblivious to growing credibility problems. There are a number of recurring credibility "traps"—which involve creating gaps between words and deeds, expectations and performance—which can cost crisis management dearly, as can neglecting the symbolic aspects of crisis management (Stern, 1999:201-202; see also Hansén and Stern, 2001).

*Transnationalization and Internationalization:* This theme focuses on the tendency of crises to spill over national boundaries in an increasingly politically, economically, socially, and not least ecologically interdependent Europe. While some crisis-producing threats may arise within a single country, many actual and potential threats do not respect national borders. Infectious diseases, natural and technical disasters, financial turbulence, and terrorism are just a few examples of such threats. Similarly, coping with contemporary crises often requires transnational and international collaboration in order to deal with these cross-border threats (Buzan, 1991; 't Hart, Stern, and Sundelius, 1998; Buzan, Waever, and De Wilde, 1998; Steinbruner, 2000). Such cooperation may be either ad hoc or institutionalized, bilateral or multilateral. China is in this regard a transitional state insofar as it has elements of a number of systems (communist and capitalist) that exist simultaneously in the same political and economic space. This transitional or hybrid nature of the political and economic regime gets reflected in the manner in which the authorities seek to engage in crisis management. The international aspect is also examined within this work, giving cases of how the SARS problem was approached in Canada as well as China. This enables the reader to contrast and compare the methods used by the authorities in these two countries in attempting to contain and manage what had rapidly become a global problem.

*Temporal Effects*: This theme focuses upon sequencing and synchronicity—temporal effects which may have a profound effect on crisis management. Sequencing refers to the path-dependent nature of crisis decision-making. Choices made early in crises tend to constrain the possibilities for later action and steer the crisis management along a particular trajectory which may be difficult to change (see, e.g., Levy, 1991; Sundelius, Stern and Bynander, 1997; Billings and Hermann 1998). Often feedback, especially negative feedback, from early decisions will require further decisions—which together form a sequence. Synchronicity refers to the tendency of simultaneous events to influence each other via psychological and organizational mechanisms such as "availability," opportunity cost, cumulative stress, and distraction (Snyder, Bruck and Sapin, 1963; Haney, 1997; Stern, 1999). Synchronicity may appear within a single crisis (when multiple problems must be solved at the same time), between two simultaneous crises (as in the cases of Hungary/Suez in 1956, and Watergate/War in the Middle East in 1973), or between a crisis and other highly prioritized coincident activities such as elections, state visits, crucial legislative negotiations, and so on.

*Learning*: This theme focuses upon the extent to which actors are capable of analyzing their experiences and using the results as basis for change. As noted above in the discussion of problem framing, actors may attempt to use "lessons" from past experiences (encoded as historical analogies or as experientially-based "rules of thumb" as a guide for current action). Similarly, actors may respond to positive or negative feedback regarding their performance during a crisis by drawing lessons and by modifying their beliefs and practices. Actors commonly attempt to reflect upon crisis experiences after the fact, draw lessons for the future, and develop reform projects on the basis of interpretations of crisis experiences. Crises present considerable opportunities for learning, but post-crisis learning attempts are often distorted or derailed by a variety of typical social and psychological dynamics (see, e.g., Lebow, 1981; Levy, 1994; Breslauer and Tetlock, 1991; Lagadec, 1997; Stern, 1997).

## *Overview*

Lessons and ideas need to be drawn from previous experiences, in order to deal with the problems and issues of today. Findings teased out from past events can be integrated into the current knowledge and the formulation of standard operating procedures (SOPs) in order to improve crisis management practices. The ultimate test being: if we do understand and recognize the weaknesses and potential that come to light from previous experiences, do we actually integrate and make use of them?

This volume consists of eight different case studies relating to the SARS crisis, both in China (Mainland China and Hong Kong Special Administrative Region) and in the Greater Toronto Area. It was officially reported that in Mainland China alone, more than 5,300 people were sickened and 349 died of the disease. In chapter 2, the first case, *SARS in China: An Overview*, Kaibin Zhong analyzes SARS in China from a broad perspective. The SARS outbreak is broken down into periods, where its cycle and effects on the population and society are studied. He also looks at the effect SARS had on China in a time when it was witnessing structural changes and state reforms. This had the effect, as Zhong puts it, of fighting new wars with old procedures. The political and health infrastructure is examined, tracking the politicization of the SARS crisis in an attempt to turn a health crisis into a political opportunity.

Given the fact that SARS affected China most, Beijing became the hardest-hit city in the world, with more than half of Mainland China's cases occurring in the capital. In chapter 3, *SARS in Beijing: An Urban Response*, Qin Zhu covers the issue of tackling the problem in a large urban area, namely the capital city. The various stages of the SARS epidemic in Beijing are accounted for: from the outbreak and awareness stage to the responses and strategies aimed at neutralizing it. Details about the various challenges met by the authorities along the way in eventually defeating SARS are also given. Legitimacy, communication and the need to act quickly and decisively are key themes in this case.

The fourth chapter by Simon Shen, *The SARS Crisis and Crisis Management in Hong Kong*, explores how the crisis was tackled in the former British colony. A number of special circumstances in Hong Kong differentiated it from the rest of Mainland China; it is a special administrative region, former colony, high population density (over 6000 people per square kilometer), and its significant commercial importance. Issues concerning accountability, classifications, and the exercise of power are examined and tested.

Chapter 5 by Edward Deverell, *An Analytical Memoir of the WHO Operation in China,* gives a glimpse into the workings of the World Health Organization (WHO) in China during the SARS outbreak. The chapter is based on interviews with Peet Tüll, who spent time in Beijing during the SARS crisis assisting the WHO office. Thus this case has the aspect of an insider's perspective to the efforts that were needed in order to bring the situation under control, especially the aspect of relations between the Chinese authorities and the WHO during these trying times.

The geographical focus of attention then shifts to the Greater Toronto Area as Dan Markel and Christopher Stoney write on *Lessons Learned from the Greater Toronto Outbreak* in chapter 6. Canada was considered to be the hardest hit region by SARS outside of Asia. This chapter seeks to cover a number of issues: an overview of the SARS outbreak in the Greater Toronto Area, causes and mismanagement of the outbreak, key strengths and weaknesses in combating SARS, and lessons learned/reforms in the wake of the crisis.

Chapter 7 is by Logan Atkinson on *The Morality of Quarantine in Ontario, Canada*. In this chapter Atkinson broaches the sensitive issue of the use of quarantine as a means to stop the spread of an infectious disease. Just how effective is this mechanism in contemporary society, in an age where the issue of individual rights is viewed as being paramount? A certain aspect of moral dilemma enters into the equation when the use of quarantine is contemplated.

In chapter 8, *Early International News Flow About SARS: Interconnected or Unconnected?* Joan Deppa, Andrew Seaberg, and Grace Han Yao examine mass media reporting and how quickly (or otherwise) information on SARS was transmitted around the globe. They attempt to gauge how quickly and accurately information was spread, and delve into what the future may hold, in terms of the rapid transmission of accurate information on future health threats.

Stephanie Buus and Eva-Karin Olsson cover *China and SARS: Crisis Management in a Legitimacy Vacuum* in chapter 9. The mass media plays an essential role in the formation of opinions and the creation of a "reality" through the information and images that are transmitted. The news stories and headlines on SARS are examined to see what images or messages were conveyed to the public. Such images can either bestow or remove legitimacy from key actors involved in a crisis.

The volume ends with concluding observations by Eva-Karin Olsson and Kaibin Zhong. They also present suggestions for future crisis management research and practices.

## Notes

1. The authors would also like to thank Eva-Karin Olsson, Kaibin Zhong, Stephanie Buus, Greg Simons, and Stephanie Young for their valuable input and feedback on earlier versions of this chapter.

2. According to WHO (2010) and as of May 6, 2010, 294 people have been known to have died from the H5N1 virus since late 2003.

3. The following section builds upon Sundelius, Stern, and Bynander (1997: chapter 6) as well as Nohrstedt and Stern (1999).

4. The following section also builds upon Sundelius, Stern, and Bynander (1997: chapter 6) as well as Nohrstedt and Stern (1999).

5. For more information on crisis prevention and mitigation, see, e.g., Ender and Kim (1988), Waugh (1988) and Lund (1996). For more skeptical examinations of the potential for risk elimination and accident prevention, see Wildavsky (1988) and Perrow (1999).

6. For more about value conflict, see George (1980) and Farnham (1998:26-39).

7. See, for example, Rosati (1981) and Janis (1982).

## *References*

Allison, G., and P. Zelikow (1999) *Essence of Decision: Explaining the Cuban Missile Crisis.* (2nd ed.). New York: Longman.

Bass, B. M. (1997) *Transformational Leadership: Industrial, Military, and Educational Impact.* Hillsdale, NJ: Lawrence Erlbaum Associates.

Billings, R., and C. Hermann (1998) "Problem Identification in Sequential Policy Decision Making: The Re-representation of Problems." In *Problem Representation in Foreign Policy Decision Making,* edited by D. Sylvan and J. Voss. Cambridge: Cambridge University Press.

Breslauer, G., and P. Tetlock, Eds. (1991) *Learning in US and Soviet Foreign Policy.* Boulder: Westview.

Brower, J., and P. Chalk (2003) *The Global Threat of New and Reemerging Infectious Diseases: Reconciling U.S. National Security and Public Health Policy.* Santa Monica, CA: RAND.

Buzan, B. (1991) *People, States, and Fear: An Agenda for International Security Studies in the Post-Cold War Era.* Boulder: Rienner.

Buzan, B., O. Waever, and J. De Wilde (1998) *Security: A New Framework of Analysis.* Boulder: Rienner.

Ender, L.R., and J.C.K. Kim (1988) "The Design and Implementation of Disaster Mitigation Policy". In *Managing Disaster: Strategies and Policy Perspectives,* edited by L.K. Comfort. pp. 67-85. Durham: Duke University Press.

Farnham, B.R. (1998) *Roosevelt and the Munich Crisis: A Study of Political Decision-Making.* Princeton: Princeton University Press.

Gardner, H. (1995) *Leading Minds: An Anatomy of Leadership.* New York: BasicBooks.

George, A.L. (1980) *Presidential Decisionmaking in Foreign Policy: The Effective Use of Information and Advice.* Boulder: Westview Press.

Goudsmit, J. (2004) *Viral Fitness: The Next SARS and West Nile in the Making.* New York: Oxford University Press.

Greenfeld, K. T. (2006) *China Syndrome: The True Story of the Twenty First Century's First Great Epidemic.* New York: HarperCollins.

Haney, P.J. (1997) *Organizing for Foreign Policy Crises: Presidents, Advisers and the Management of Decision Making.* Ann Arbor: The University of Michigan Press.

Hansén, D., and E. Stern. (2001) "From Crisis to Trauma: The Palme Assassination Case." In *Managing Crises: Threats, Dilemmas, Opportunities,* edited by U. Rosenthal, R.A. Boin, and L.K. Comfort. pp. 177-199. Springfield: Charles C Thomas.

Harrison, S., Ed. (1999) *Disasters and the Media: Managing Crisis Communications.* London: MacMillan Press.

't Hart, P., E. Stern, and B. Sundelius (1998) "Crisis Management: An Agenda for Research and Training in Europe." *Cooperation and Conflict* 33(2): 207-224.

Henry, R.A. (2000) *The Complete Guide to Crisis and Risk Communications. . . . You'd Better Have a Hose If You Want to Put out the Fire: Professional Tips, Tactics, Dos, Don'ts and Case Histories.* Windsor, California: Gollywobbler Productions.

Hermann, M.G., and J.D. Hagen (1998) "International Decision Making: Leadership Matters." *Foreign Policy. Frontiers of Knowledge: The State of the Art in World Affairs.* (Special edition). Spring issue, pp. 124-137.

Hermann, M.G., C. Hermann, and J. Hagen. (1987) "How Decision Units Shape Foreign Policy Behavior." In *New Directions in the Study of Foreign Policy*, edited by C. Hermann, C. Kegley and J. Rosenau. pp. 309-338. Boston: Allen and Unwin.

Janis, I. (1982) *Groupthink: Psychological Studies of Policy Decisions and Fiascoes.* (2nd ed.) Boston: Houghton Mifflin.

Janis, I., and L. Mann. (1977) *Decision Making: A Psychological Analysis of Conflict, Choice, and Commitment.* New York: Free Press.

Keeney, R. (1992) *Value Focused Thinking*. Cambridge: Harvard University Press.

Khong Y.F. (1992) *Analogies at War*. Princeton: Princeton University Press.

Knobler, S., A. Mahmoud, S. Lemon, A. Mack, L. Sivitz, and K. Oberholtzer, Eds. (2004) *Learning from SARS: Preparing for the Next Disease Outbreak.* Washington, D.C.: The National Academies Press.

Lagadec, P. (1997) "Learning Processes for Crisis Management in Complex Organizations." *Journal of Contingencies and Crisis Management* 5(1): 24-31.

Larson, D.W. (1985) *The Origins of Containment: A Psychological Explanation*. Princeton: Princeton University Press.

Lebow, N. (1981) *Between Peace and War: The Nature of International Crises*. Baltimore: Johns Hopkins University Press.

Leung, P. C., and E. E. Ooi, Eds. (2003) *SARS War: Combating the Disease*. Singapore: River Edge, New Jersey: World Scientific.

Levy, J. (1991) "The Role of Crisis Management in the Outbreak of World War I." In *Avoiding War: Problems of Crisis Management,* edited by A.L. George. pp. 62-102. Boulder: Westview.

Levy, J. (1994) "Learning and Foreign Policy: Sweeping a Conceptual Minefield." *International Organization* 48(2): 279-312.

Lund, M.S. (1996) *Preventing Violent Conflicts: A Strategy for Preventive Diplomacy.* Washington DC: United States Institute of Peace.

Nohrstedt, D., and E. Stern (1999) "Conclusion: Patterns and Problems in Estonian Crisis Management." In *Crisis Management in Estonia: Case Studies and Comparative Perspectives* 3, edited by E. Stern and D. Nohrstedt.pp. 294-315. Stockholm: ÖCB [The Swedish Agency for Civil Emergency Planning].

Nohrstedt, S.A., and A. Tassew. (1993) "Communication and Crisis: An Inventory of Current Research." Psykologiskt försvar [Psychological Defense]. Rapport nr. [Report number] 163:1.

Nordlund, R. (1994) "A Triangle Drama: Authorities, Citizens and Media in Crisis." Psykologiskt försvar [Psychological Defense]. Meddelande nr. [Newsletter] 136:b.

Novosti: Russian News and Information Agency (17 July 2006) "Bird Flu Pandemic Could Claim $800bln in First Year Alone—WHO, RIA." Available at: http://en.rian.ru

Ogrizek, M., and J-M. Guillery (1999) *Communicating in Crisis*. Piscataway, NJ: Aldine Transaction.

Pearce, D.D. (1995) *Wary Partners: Diplomats and the Media*. Washington D.C.: Congressional Quarterly Inc.

Perrow, C. (1999) *Normal Accidents*. Princeton: Princeton University Press.

Regester, M., and J. Larkin. (1998) *Risk Issues and Crisis Management: A Casebook of Best Practice*. London: The Institute of Public Relations.

Rosati, J.A. (1981) "Developing a Systematic Decision-Making Framework: Bureaucratic Politics in Perspective." *World Politics* 33(2): 234-252.

Rosenthal, U., P. 't Hart, and A. Kouzmin (1991) "The Bureau-Politics of Crisis Management." *Public Administration Review* 69(1): 211-233.

Snyder, R.C., H. Bruck, and B. Sapin, Eds. (1963) *Foreign Policy Decision Making*. New York: The Free Press.

Steinbruner, J. (1974) *The Cybernetic Theory of Decision*. Princeton: Princeton University Press.

Steinbruner, J. (2000) *Principles of Global Security*. Brookings Institute.

Stern, E. (1997) "Crisis and Learning: A Conceptual Balance Sheet." *Journal of Contingencies and Crisis Management* 5(2): 69-86.

Stern, E. (1999) *Crisis Decisionmaking: A Cognitive-Institutional Approach*. Stockholm Studies in Politics 66. Dissertation. Stockholm University, Dept. of Political Science.

Stern, E. (2009) "Crisis Navigation: Lessons from History for the Crisis Manager in Chief." *Governance*. Vol. 22: no 2, p. 189-202.

Stern, E., and F. Bynander, Eds. (1998) *Crisis and Internationalization: Eight Crises Studied from a Cognitive-Institutional Perspective*. Vol. 2. Stockholm: ÖCB [The Swedish Agency for Civil Emergency Planning].

Stern, E., and B. Verbeek, Eds. (1998) "Whither the Study of Governmental Politics in Foreign Policymaking: A Symposium." *Mershon International Studies Review* 42: 205-255.

Sundelius, B., E. Stern, and F. Bynander. (1997) Krishantering på svenska—teori och praktik. [Crisis Management the Swedish Way: In Theory and Practice]. Stockholm: Nerenius and Santérus förlag.

Sung, Joseph J. Y., Ed. (2004) *Severe Acute Respiratory Syndrome: From Benchtop to Bedside*. Hackensack, New Jersey: World Scientific.

Sylvan, D., and J. Voss, Eds. (1998) *Problem Representation in Foreign Policy Decision Making*. Cambridge: Cambridge University Press.

Vertzberger, Yaacov Y.I. (1990) *The World in Their Minds: Information Processing, Cognition, and Perception in Foreign Policy Decisionmaking*. Stanford: Stanford University Press.

Waugh, W.L. (1988) "Current Policy and Implementation in Disaster Preparedness." In *Managing Disaster: Strategies and Policy Perspectives,* edited by L.K. Comfort. pp. 111-125. London: Duke University Press.

WHO (World Health Organization) (26 September 2003) "Summary of Probable SARS Cases with Onset of Illness from 1 November 2002 to 31 July 2003 (Revised 26

September 2003)," available at: www.who.int/csr/sars/country/table2003_09_23/en/index.html.

WHO (World Health Organization) (6 May 2010) "Cumulative Number of Confirmed Human Cases of Avian Influenza A/(H5N1) Reported to WHO," available at: www.who.int/csr/disease/avian_influenza/country/cases_table_2010_05_06/en/index.html.

Wildavsky, A. (1988) *Searching for Safety*. New Brunswick: Transaction.

# Chapter 2

# SARS in China: An Overview*

Kaibin Zhong**

## 1. Introduction

### 1.1 Research Question and Aim

After SARS was first detected on November 16, 2002, in South China's Guangdong Province, it spread to more than twenty provinces, autonomous regions and municipalities within a few months and infected thousands of people and claimed hundreds of lives. Prevention and monitoring became a "top priority," since the disease was "a sudden and severe disaster" and "a serious problem affecting us socially and economically" (People's Daily, 22 April 2003). The deadly SARS virus quickly spread worldwide to more than thirty countries and regions, and posed a tremendous threat to public health and safety in the context of accelerated globalization and economic diversification.

In this context China unintentionally became a leading actor in the first global public health crisis of the twenty first century. The crisis was also the first great challenge facing the new Chinese leadership and had an unpredictable impact upon it. After the devastating terror attacks of September 11 in the United States, the SARS outbreak was quickly recognized as a non-traditional security threat. Furthermore, it was understood that a public safety crisis of this magnitude could potentially affect China's future development. This is crucial in light of China's entry into the World Trade Organization (WTO) where there are stronger demands for balanced development and governance structural reforms (Yu, 2000; Hu, 2003a). The crisis forced the entire nation (everyone from the government to the ordinary people) to discuss the impacts the crisis had on China's reform process and to reflect upon the lessons learned.

This chapter offers an overview of the SARS crisis in China in 2003,[1] and focuses on the central and local governments' delay in responding. In addition, a chronology of the SARS crisis based on an epidemiological and impact analysis is included as well as a staged-model analysis of the local and central governments' responses and an institutional response analysis of the fight in combating SARS in China.

The key research questions in this chapter are how did the SARS virus spread in China and why did the local and central governments fail to stop the new disease? In other words, why did it take the system so long to detect and react to the new disease, thus inducing a crisis that may have been avoidable? In answering this, I argue that there was a significant time lag in the local and central governments' response to the disease in Mainland China. In the four stages of the SARS crisis, the government's delay in responding clearly resulted in the expansion of the deadly disease. This implies that the institutional forces (including institutional sensing and action) failed to effectively respond to a new kind of battle in an increasingly modernized and globalized environment. Hence, one can conclude that the SARS epidemic in China was a case of "fighting a new war with old weapons."

*1.2 The General Context of China's Public Health Emergency Response System*

China has maintained fast economic growth for more than twenty years since the outset of economic reform programs in the early 1980s. While greater attention has been paid to economic growth, less importance has been attached in dealing with the problems of the non-economic aspects of reform. The problem worsened with globalization and open conditions and a swiftly-changing and open society of information, especially after China's entry into the WTO in 2001 (Niu, 2001; Han, 2002; Hu, 2003b). In recent years public health emergencies occurred from time to time, which greatly damaged lives, public property, economic development, and social stability (Niu, 2001; Wei, 2002; Hu and Hu, 2003). The increasing transnational threat of infectious disease deserves special attention within the context of the involving definition of security in the Post Cold-War era. Along with the development of globalization, modern medical practices, urbanization, climatic change and changing social and behavioral patterns, the chances of a major public health emergency are much greater, and the difficulties and complexities in handling such emergencies increase with a large margin (Hsiao, 1995; Brower and Chalk, 2003; Xue and Zhu, 2003).

Why was the health system so prone to collapse when facing the SARS epidemic? It was argued that the design of the system was not well prepared for a public health emergency on such a large scale (People's Daily Online, 4 June 2003). Specific laws and regulations regarding public health emergencies were not available before the SARS outbreak, nor was an operation mechanism for dealing with public health emergencies in the government. The only legal basis the government could rely on were "Laws on Infectious Disease Prevention and Treatment" (1989) and "Implementation Measures for Infectious Disease Prevention and Control" (1991). The emergency response structure is a network of disease prevention and control at four levels: central, province, prefecture, and county. It is in charge of the Centers for Disease Control and Prevention (CDC) and health administrative departments at different levels and is coordinated by other departments. The State Council issued "Emergency Regulations on Sudden Outbreaks of Public Health Incidents" on May 9, 2003 (Xinhua News Agency, 13 May 2003). The regulation marked the inclusion of responses to public health emergencies into the legal system and the improvement of response mechanisms. The regulation stipulated the prevention, preparation, reporting, informing, responding and legal responsibility in handling public health emergencies.

Moreover, China does not have a well-trained rapid response team and lacks an appropriate regulation system, both of which severely impede the surge capacity of a timely response to public health emergencies and integrated disease prevention and control. China's traditional health emergency response system has shown some vulnerabilities and inabilities both in dealing with traditional and newly emergent diseases. In a study in 2003 by the Hong Kong-based Political and Economic Risk Consultancy (PERC), China ranked below the other Asian countries on the issue of addressing and dealing with various public health emergencies, and the difference was even more dramatic when China was compared to the non-Asian countries (Table 1).

**Table 1: National Capacities in Dealing with Public Health Emergencies**

| Country/Region | Score |
|---|---|
| Australia | 2.14 |
| China | 7.50 |
| England | 0.82 |
| Hong Kong | 4.21 |
| India | 8.00 |
| Indonesia | 9.14 |
| Japan | 4.00 |
| Malaysia | 5.33 |
| Philippines | 6.60 |
| Singapore | 2.33 |
| South Korea | 7.00 |
| Taiwan | 5.25 |
| Thailand | 5.25 |
| Vietnam | 7.38 |
| United States | 0.86 |

Note: A higher score indicates poorer performance.
Source: the Political and Economic Risk Consultancy (PERC, 2003).

*1.3 SARS: An Overview*

On November 16, 2002, an abnormal case was detected in Foshan City, Guangdong Province. The case was later called Severe Acute Respiratory Syndrome (SARS).[2] The first reported SARS patient was announced on December 15 in China (People's Daily Online, 26 March 2003). From January to March, the epidemic in Guangdong entered its peak, and the virus spread to other provinces and regions. On March 1, 2003, a Beijing hospital admitted its first patient with SARS, an imported case (People's Daily Online, 13 April 2003). On March 23, the Shangxi Province reported its first SARS cases (People's Daily Online, 1 April 2003). More cases were detected thereafter in other provinces, municipalities and autonomous regions.

Moreover, the virus began moving around the world in late February 2003, via international air travel. After fighting "a sudden and severe disaster" (People's Daily Online, 20 April 2003), the total number of SARS cases was contained and the number of new cases tapered off. On June 24, the World Health Organization (WHO) announced it was taking Beijing off the SARS list and lifting the travel advisory for Beijing since there were obvious disease mitigation measures in line with relevant standards set by the WHO (People's Daily Online, 24 June 2003).

After the first case was reported in the Guangdong Province in November 2002, SARS eventually spread to over 24 provinces, autonomous regions, and municipalities in China, and later affected over 32 countries/regions in Asia, America and Europe. According to China's Ministry of Health (MoH) and WTO, from November 11, 2002, to June 24, 2003, SARS had reached 24 provinces and municipalities, and 266 counties and districts of Mainland China. Of the 5,327 people who contracted SARS, 4,959 had recovered and 349 had died. Among them were 2,521 confirmed cases and 193 fatalities in Beijing with a mortality rate of ca 8 percent. In Beijing 399 medical workers (16 percent of them) had been infected of which 12 (3 percent of them) had died. Mainland China had to cope with the first and largest SARS outbreak. The second outbreak occurred in Hong Kong (1,755 cases and 300 deaths) and the third in Taiwan (665 cases and 180 deaths).

The global SARS outbreak developed quickly and dramatically, creating challenging and stressful conditions for the staff and health authorities with every incident. The containment of this epidemic required heroic efforts and extraordinary measures that were difficult to sustain over time. According to WTO, the global morbidity of the disease had reached 8,422 cases as of August 7, and according to the reports the average mortality among these cases was 9 percent (Zhong Nanshan et al., 2003).

## 2. Theoretical Framework

Crises involve situations where cherished national, organizational, and personal values are at stake, and such events often cast a long shadow in the sense that they may profoundly affect political perceptions and choices for years or decades to come (Stern, 1999: 3). During crisis situations, policymakers cannot afford to wait to tackle the crisis change until its consequences become painful, because by then they will already be committed to further change. Time lag means the period of time between when the functions are lost at an impact site and when those functions are replaced by mitigation. In general, the time lag varies by the type and timing of mitigation in relation to the impacts. There is no time lag if the mitigation fully offsets anticipated impacts prior to or at the time of impact.

Crisis prevention and preparedness are delicate and relatively thankless tasks for crisis managers facing a contingency. Early alerts permit managers to begin tracking and preparing for possible measures, but they are dependent upon good intelligence and prompt decisions. In the real world, the time lag between decision and outcome may preclude effective learning. Some decisions are too risky to try in the real world but can be explored in a simulation (Sterman, 2000). Moreover, Schmitt (1985) argues that the preference of liberal jurisprudence for fixed, codified general norms, along with a strict separation of powers, exacerbates the problem of a time lag within the structure of political and legal decision-making.

With the development of society, crisis occurs more often and is more changeable, extensive and dangerous. The increasing complexity of the threats facing the globe requires an integrated national security framework to address them. It is critical for the key security instruments to work together in a fully integrated way to address the security interests. All the components must come together as one integrated system within which all parts communicate in real time. Any time lag in system performance will immediately destroy the critical state of "suspension of belief" that is necessary for immersion into the scenario and to keep headquarters informed.

There is a lack of integration in China's public health emergency management system, and this was strongly demonstrated during the SARS outbreak. To closely examine and search for the cause of the time lag during the fight against SARS, this chapter firstly traces a detailed chronology of the events from November 2002 (when SARS, via back-tracking was first discovered) to July 2003 (when Beijing was removed from the list and the battle against SARS was declared over). Outbreaks in China and efforts to contain the disease are portrayed. By providing a somewhat quantitative analysis of the spread of SARS and investigating the three stages before, the time line can be divided into four periods. Then I examine the responsive steps taken by the central and local governments, and this provides an important framework for the "time lag" in each stage. Finally, based on an institutional response analysis, the vulnerability and incapability of the system to sense and react to such a new disease is discussed. Policy implications are also discussed by way of conclusion.

## *3. Analysis*

### 3.1 The Diffusion of SARS in China: An Epidemiological and Impact Analysis[3]

Since recognition of the first SARS case in Guangdong Province in November 2002, health care workers engaged in basic medicine, clinical medicine and preventive medicine have done much work and made encouraging progress in understanding the etiology, epidemiology, diagnosis, treatment and prevention of SARS. Using available data on SARS released by China's MoH and WHO, the characteristics of the SARS epidemic can be concluded, mainly evolving the distribution by region, time, population and mortality rate.

#### 3.1.1 Regional Distribution

WHO recorded 8,422 clinically diagnosed cases and 916 deaths by August 7, 2003. The SARS epidemic spread to thirty two countries and regions. The majority of cases occurred in Asia, Europe, and North America. In Asia, the primary affected countries were China (including Mainland China, Taiwan, Hong Kong, and Macao) and Singapore. There were 5,327 cases and 349 deaths in Mainland China. These cases were mainly concentrated in the regions of Beijing, Guangdong, Shanxi, Hebei, Inner Mongolia Autonomous Region, and Tianjin. In Beijing and Guangdong, the number of patients amounted to 4,033, representing ca. 76 percent of the total cases in China. The first case report came from Heyuan City in Guangdong, but after a retrospective investigation, it is now believed that an earlier case occurred in Foshan City of Guangdong on November 16, 2002, the first known case in the world. SARS was then transmitted to Shanxi, Sichuan and Beijing as a result of long distance travel. Subsequently, SARS spread to other regions.

#### 3.1.2 Time Distribution

The first reported case occurred in November 2002 and SARS became a global epidemic in February 2003. The greatest number of simultaneous cases occurred between mid March and mid May in 2003. In Mainland China, in the regions of Foshan City and Heyuan City in the Guangdong Province, and Hechi City in the Guangxi Autonomous Region, there were early primary SARS cases, but there is no evidence of mutual transmission. The onset peak of SARS in Guangdong was in February, and the epidemic affected other regions from the beginning of April to the middle of May, possibly reflecting the time of importation of the infection source. As the frequency curve of the new cases in the Guangdong Province, North China and nationwide demonstrates (figure 1), the outbreak of

SARS began to escalate in the beginning of February and mid-April following a lapse in infection control procedures, resulting in two outbreak peaks. The first peak occurred around February 5-10, in Guangdong, with the daily average of reported new cases soaring to over 100. The other peak was dated from April 20 to May 10 with most of the cases distributed in North China which had a daily average of 100 reported new cases. The very top of the peak curve appeared on April 27-28, with the daily average of 202 new cases.

**Figure 1: New Cases in Guangdong Province, North China and nationwide in Mainland China (Until May 30)**

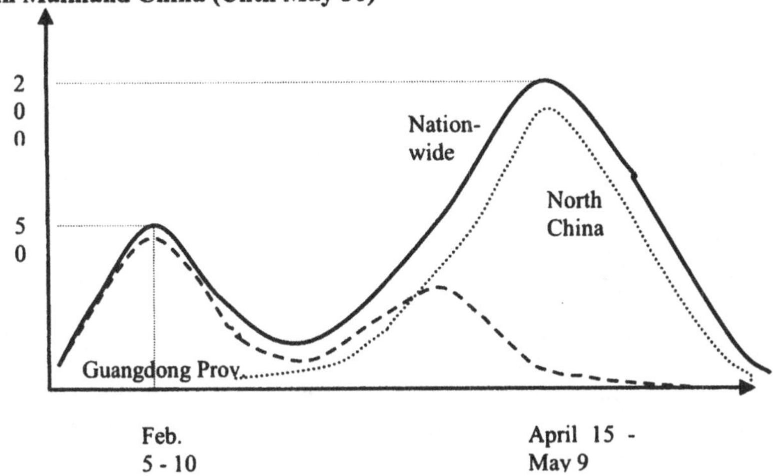


Source: China's MoH Press Release (2003) at www.moh.gov.cn

3.1.3 Population Distribution

The majority of SARS patients were young and middle-aged adults. According to the statistics from Mainland China, the age of onset was twenty to sixty years old, an age group accounting for 85 percent of all patients. Among these patients, about 30 percent were in their twenties which is the age group with the highest incidence rate. The incidence rate in the ten to fifteen year old age group was much lower than in adults, and the incidence rate of the age group under nine years old was the lowest. Although the case number among the elderly population was low overall, the mortality rate in this group was high. The difference in incidence rate was not statistically significant between males and females. A high incidence rate among medical workers was characteristic of the SARS distribution by occupation. Of all patients, the proportion of medical workers was about 20 percent (in some provinces, even as high as 50 percent). Students accounted for ca 9 percent of all patients, which were sporadic.

#### 3.1.4 Mortality Rate

As reported by WHO, the average SARS mortality rate worldwide was 9 percent from November 1, 2002, to May 31, 2003. The total mortality rate of SARS in Mainland China during the 2002-2003 epidemic season was 0.024/100,000 and the fatality rate among infected patients was 7 percent, below the average mortality rate worldwide. The majority of deaths occurred in the elderly (the fatality rate among patients older than sixty years old was 11 percent-14 percent, and accounted for about 44 percent of all deaths). The fatality rate increased with age, and was also high in patients suffering from other diseases, such as hypertension, diabetes, cardiac disease, emphysema, and neoplasms.

### *3.2 Combating SARS in China: A Staged-Model Analysis*

As the pattern of the epidemic demonstrates, the SARS outbreak in Mainland China initially grew slowly with just a few probable cases detected in the first three months in 2003, most of which were recorded in Guangdong Province.[4] However, the outbreak began to escalate in mid-April following a lapse in infection control procedures, which allowed the disease to spread rapidly within the hospital and then into the wider community. In dealing with the emergency that followed, health authorities rapidly introduced a series of sweeping measures. The life circle of the SARS crisis can be divided into four stages based on the number of SARS cases (including new cases and accumulated cases), death toll and mortality rate, infection rate of medical workers, among others. Notably, there was a "time lag" in each stage whenever responses were made by the local and central government and measures were taken.

#### 3.2.1 Stage I: Portent and Incubation (the end of 2002 to February 2003)

The first stage started at the end of 2002, when the first SARS case was detected, and lasted until February 2003, just before the major SARS outbreak in Guangdong Province. In the beginning SARS was detected in just a few areas and it appeared that few people had been affected. The main tasks of this stage were: identification of the disease, collection of important information, sorting out key information, real-time and dynamic surveillance, risk assessment, effective isolation of the disease, and creation of a firewall that could shield an organization from catastrophic losses.

Neither the Guangdong Provincial government nor the central government had been alert enough to the occurrence of the epidemic, partly because a new government was being installed.[5] The Chinese leadership did not seize the first favorable chance to curb SARS.

### 3.2.2 Stage II: Outbreak and Spread (from February to early May)

The second stage started in February 2003 when SARS broke out in the Guangdong province and lasted until early May when the average of new infections on a three-day basis reached a climax and the number of accumulated cases was rapidly increasing. Along with the spread of SARS in the Guangdong province, social panic increased, buying sprees frequently occurred and rumors were spread, all of which exacerbated the crisis. It was a second chance that the government missed. In the end of March and early April, the governments in the northern part of China (in particular, Beijing) remained passive despite the looming SARS threat and had not learned lessons from what had happened in the Guangdong province. Hospitals in Beijing belong to four separated parts: central government, local government, the army, and the armed police, which do not have jurisdiction over each other. The divided information channels made it difficult to detect the causes of the epidemic, to clearly identify the channels of contamination, and to sum up the situation. The SARS epidemic shifted from Guangdong, where over 95 percent of the national SARS cases were recorded before early April, to Beijing and North China, which became the hardest-hit area by the end of April. Here was a third chance that was missed by the Chinese leadership.

April 20 witnessed the turning point of the Chinese leadership's attitude toward SARS (Xue et al., 2003a). From mid-April on, the Chinese leadership keenly realized the seriousness of the SARS crisis by taking responsibility and immediately adopting measures. In late April, the Chinese leadership removed the Minister of Health and Mayor of Beijing from office, demonstrating its dedication to speeding up the redevelopment of its public health and disease prevention system. The fact that Vice-Premier Wu Yi[6] was appointed as Minister of Health and the Hainan Party Secretary, and that Waung Qishan[7] was appointed acting Mayor of Beijing demonstrated the resolution and confidence of the Chinese leadership to fight SARS. Other strong measures were also taken by the Chinese leadership. For example, the virus was recognized as an epidemic disease by law in a very short time so that the SARS prevention work would have a legal basis. Likewise, the SARS virus was under emergent research by the country's scientific research organizations.

### 3.2.3 Stage III: Fastigium and Stability (May)

The three-day average of new infections in the first ten days of May reached a climax and then dropped off. The daily average of new infections was 32 between May 10 and May 30. Due to an increase in discharged patients, the actual number of cases reached its highest point in mid-May and began to decline the end of May. During this period the accumulated number of cases slowly increased. The death toll and mortality rate also increased but were lower than the world average rate. This was the utmost critical stage.

At this stage, the measures adopted by the Chinese leadership in mid-April began to take effect because of a "policy time lag." The leadership used the crisis management system to generate rapid response to the emergency. It also actively cooperated with the media by releasing reports on the situation of the epidemic to the public. It provided favorable policies as a means of compensation for industries hit hard by SARS and medical aid was provided for impoverished SARS patients. For example, a large-scale public health plan was launched nationwide, including all the cities, provinces and regions (People's Daily Online, 1 May 2003). In south China's Guangdong Province, where the country's first SARS case was reported, more than eighty million residents were mobilized to clean private residences, wash public facilities, and attend lectures on public health (Xinhua News Agency, 2 May 2003). As a result, the public quickly stepped out of the shadow of panic, and social and economic order was restored. The negative influences of SARS began to fade.

#### 3.2.4 Stage IV: Recession and Recovery (June)

On June 13, the WHO announced that China's northern province of Hebei, Tianjin Municipality, and Inner Mongolia Autonomous Region had been removed from its "recommendation against non-essential travel to the area" list (People's Daily Online, 15 June 2003). On June 25, the WHO removed Beijing from its list of SARS-infected areas and lifted its travel advisory on the city, saying the risk to travelers visiting Beijing "is now minimal" (People's Daily Online, 24 June 2003). Experts said the "double removal" could be interpreted as the country's victory over the epidemic under China's newly-elected leadership (Xinhua News Agency, 24 June 2003).

Chinese Premier Wen Jiabao said at the China-ASEAN leaders' meeting on the fight against SARS that the Chinese leadership and Chinese people were doing their best to transform a crisis into an opportunity. Also the premier said that "what a nation loses to a disaster is compensated for in its progress."(Xinhua News Agency, 4 May 2003) As an old Chinese saying goes, "A disaster can be converted to good fortune at the right time." China began to recover and learn from the SARS crisis. At this stage, the SARS crisis in China has passed its fastigium and entered a stage of recession and recovery. The SARS situation at this stage was: few or no new infections, large increase in discharged patients and decrease in actual patients, steady accumulated cases, and few deaths. The main tasks of this stage were to properly deal with the problems arising from the SARS crisis, recharge the public's spirit, recover and rebuild hard-hit areas and industries, gain experience and extract lessons from the crisis, promote reform in the structure of public management, and coordinate comprehensive development in society.

### *3.3 Combating SARS in China: An Institutional Analysis*

SARS seriously threatened public health and safety and had a significant impact upon the development of social economy and international communication. The CCP and government took every possible measure to fight SARS, and finally won the battle. Thus, the key question of the SARS response in Mainland China was, "Why did the system take so long both to detect and react to the new disease thus inducing a crisis that may have been unnecessary?"

#### 3.3.1 Institutional Sensing: Fighting a New War with Old Weapons

SARS is a new infectious disease in human beings so there is still quite a bit of uncertainty. The infectious source, pathology and early diagnosis of SARS, as well as the management of SARS (especially the development of a new vaccine) are still being examined.[8] The fight against SARS in China is a story of "fighting a new war with old weapons." This contributed to the fact that the system took so long to detect and react the new disease, which in turn induced an unnecessary crisis.

Firstly, the public health system failed to give adequate warning. During China's fight against SARS, the biggest problem was not Chinese doctors' incomplete understanding of the newly-emerged virus, but the embarrassing situation of the country's traditional public health and disease prevention and control system, which was outdated and a new one had not been established yet. When challenged by the sudden SARS outbreak, China's disease prevention system, which had been praised by WHO several times, was described as "not prepared for a sudden public health crisis and did not effectively communicate with the public" (People's Daily Online, 4 June 2003).

As early as November 16, the first case was recorded and the SARS outbreak in Guangdong entered its peak February 3-14, but it was not until April that the Chinese authorities admitted the extent of the epidemic and began the necessary public health measures to contain the spread of the virus. At that point, however, the SARS virus had spread to dozens of countries, and international panic was spreading. The situation in Beijing also revealed the government's "time lag" in responding (Table 2). In comparing the SARS response in Beijing, Hong Kong and Singapore, it is clear that it took Beijing the longest time to implement measures to combat SARS.

**Table 2: Government Responses in Beijing, Hong Kong and Singapore**

| | Beijing | Hong Kong | Singapore |
|---|---|---|---|
| | **Date (Time lag from first case)** | **Date (Time lag from first case)** | **Date (Time lag from first case)** |
| Occurrence of the first case | March 1 | February 21 | March 13 |
| Release of the first case | March 26 (25 days) | March 10 (17 days) | March 13 |
| Legally recognized as epidemic | April 14 (44 days) | March 27 (34 days) | March 24 (11 days) |
| Hospital visitations limited | - | March 27 (34 days) | March 24 (11 days) |
| Enforcement of a quarantine policy | April 23 (53) | March 31 (38 days) | March 24 (11 days) |
| Closure of primary and middle schools | April 24 (54 days) | March 27 (34 days) | March 26 (13 days) |

Note: The "occurrence of the first case" refers to date of the first SARS patient of the affected areas, instead of the first carrier patients with the SARS virus (Hu Angang, 2003a: 284).

Secondly, there was a general lack of public communication in the early stages of the SARS episode. The Chinese leadership came under international fire for initially being slow to publicize information about the disease. Addicted to secrecy, censorship and manipulation, China's new/old rulers were anxious to contain news of the medical crisis to prevent damage to the country's image and, it would appear, ensure an uninterrupted flow of visitors and investors to the Canton Export Fair (Jin, 2000). As one survey conducted on February 12, 2003, revealed, nearly half of the people in Guangzhou (the city capital of Guangdong Province) got information from their friends and relatives, and the overseas media (including the internet) served as very important information sources for the public.[9] The four mainstream news agencies in China were analyzed: *People's Daily (Renmin Ribao)*, *Guangming Daily (Guangming Ribao)*, *Evening*

*News of China Central TV (CCTV)*, and *China Daily (Zhongguo Ribao)*. It was observed that they had few reports[10] on SARS in the early stages of the crisis (i.e., before the end of April). In addition, the government failed to provide transparent information. This intensified the influence the other information sources had on the public and made the government more vulnerable to criticism. Thus reports in the non-mainstream media gained more attention, but the news was usually inaccurate and incomplete and resulted in panic in some regions.

Thirdly, the traditional "internal vigilance and outward calm" approach to crisis management was unable to deal with SARS as a non-traditional crisis. Before the end of April, the local and central governments combated SARS with more traditional propaganda, which can be called "internal vigilance and outward calm". However, globalization has diversified information technology and the dissemination of information. When the public's information channels were limited in the past, the government's propaganda policies of "internal vigilance and outward calm" could to some extent prevent the unnecessary panic caused by crisis information. However, now a great number of informal information channels have been set up and are not under the government's full control: such as telephones (including cell phones), and the Internet (especially the forum and the BBS). In the beginning of a crisis, the public is often faced with delayed, incomplete and asymmetrical information and knowledge. With the presence of alternative information sources, it became increasingly difficult for the Chinese authorities to maintain the stance that SARS was a small problem which they had under control.

### 3.3.2 Institutional Action: The Inadequate Emergency Response System

The SARS epidemic constituted a greater threat than both the Asian financial crisis of 1997 and the flood disaster of 1998 in China. It was the first major test for China's new leadership. The "time lag" in the response efforts demonstrated that China's legislative and administrative bodies as well as its medical and scientific departments had failed to keep up with the spread of the SARS disease.

Firstly, the current crisis management system in China clearly demonstrated its weakness in addressing contingencies and crises such as SARS. On the one hand, the current countermeasures to deal with public emergencies and critical situations in China are relatively sporadic. The existing laws are characterized by a strong tendency for independence and strongly tainted by separate management of different agencies.[11] Therefore problems regarding numerous aspects, such as coordination in responding to crises, have appeared to come out of the blue. On the other hand, since China currently lacks a unified national contingency management institution, it is unable to incorporate the process of early crisis control into long term strategic goals, planning, and the daily management of the government. In fact, the government has yet to work out counter-terrorism strategies from the more general goals of national security and national interests, which leads to difficulties in the management process once a crisis breaks out. The government often acts impromptu, or "sharpens its spears at the last moment" (Xue et al., 2003b: 120-132). And as it hastily goes into battle, it falls into a reactive and reflexive mode characterized by collisions. At the same time, the rapid response mechanisms this nation currently employs cannot fully adjust themselves to the requirements of crisis management. This is demonstrated by the interagency independence and unilateralism, which leads to the relatively strong abilities of the government to respond quickly to single crises.

Secondly, the political/administrative mobilization system shares a big cost in dealing with different sorts of crises. Actually the structure of political and social mobilization in China has remained almost unchanged amidst economic development. SARS information and preventive mobilization in China, however, is still basically based on China's already existing units,[12] which had become an integral part of restructuring Chinese society (Liu, 1999; Yu, 2000; Wang, 2001). On April 17, the Standing Committee of the Political Bureau of the Chinese Communist Party (CCP) Central Committee held a meeting to discuss strengthening control over the SARS epidemic.[13] This meeting stressed establishing a monitoring system with an increased sense of personal responsibility and accountability in order to ensure that every task was properly completed. The chief leaders of the CCP and government organizations at all levels were urged to personally oversee the monitoring of the SARS outbreak, since they would be held accountable for the overall situation in their respective jurisdictions, thus marking the beginning of political mobilization.[14] Soon after that, China's new leadership adopted a series of measures aimed at combating the contagious disease that proved to be quite effective: mobilizing large numbers of people to carry out monitoring work, establishing a sound monitoring network, removing incompetent officials, putting large numbers of suspect and probable SARS patients in quarantine, and preventing the spread of the disease to China's vast rural areas (Xinhua News Agency, 8 May 2003). All in all, the political system behaved in a traditional manner and consisted of huge costs.

Thirdly, conflicts among the different government agencies and different regions resulted in an uncoordinated effort. The national level lacked a comprehensive system with one office responsible for coordinating efforts and decision making. Mechanisms for coordinating different crises and managing multiple crises had not been established. Furthermore, the roles that different levels and different functional sectors of the government should play in managing crises were not defined or clarified in the legislation. The conflict between the different sectors and regions was a significant factor accounting for Beijing's failure to deal with SARS at the early stage. Because of the special status as China's political and cultural capital and its unique political/administrative structure, Beijing had to deal with various conflicts between Beijing Municipality and the central government. The CCP General Secretary Hu Jintao and Premier Wen Jiabao had many times given clear instructions requiring Beijing Municipality to set up unified control mechanisms for dealing with the epidemic; all medical resources should be unified and mobilized by the Beijing municipal government, and collected and reported information regarding the epidemic conditions should be integrated (Saich, 2003).

## *4. Conclusion*

Starting from the late 1970s, China effectively shifted from Mao's revolutionary principles to Deng's reforms, which were the most significant since the founding of the Peoples' Republic of China (Dittmer, 1994:199). During the SARS epidemic, China tried "fighting a new war with old weapons." The system took a long time to detect and react to the new disease thus inducing an unnecessary crisis. In each of the four crisis stages, it was revealed that the local and central governments were delayed in responding to the SARS crisis. This implies that institutional response (including institutional sensing and institutional action) failed to adjust itself to the conditions of the modern, globalized world in fighting a new war.

SARS was seen by hopeful observers as further evidence of China's desire to build and improve its crisis management system. China's new and reportedly reformist-inclined Communist leadership seems to have exerted its authority and used SARS as a catalyst for change. Soon after winning the "war on SARS" in June 2003, China's new leadership began to spare no effort to recover and learn from the unexpected crisis. On April 29, 2004, Premier Wen Jiabao said at the China-ASEAN leaders' conference on fighting SARS that the Chinese government and Chinese people were doing their best to transform a crisis into an opportunity. Also, the Premier said that "what a nation loses to a disaster, it will receive compensation in its progress"(Xinhua News Agency, 3 May 2003). However, it is unrealistic to think that something like SARS will lead to significant short-term changes in the way the Chinese political system works, but it has successfully revealed certain weaknesses in China's traditional style of crisis management. The advent of SARS revealed some of the key contradictions in China's development strategy, including balancing state security and secrecy with the need to appear open and accountable with the West, and balancing rapid economic growth with improved social infrastructure. The crisis also revealed that China's politico-administrative system has not kept pace with the country's increased integration into the international community.

Since experiencing an economic boom and its entry to WTO, balanced development and government structural reform are now needed in China.[15] According to various data, both the frequency and severity of major risks and crises have increased, and these crises demonstrate certain characteristics and trends about China's transition. The recent spread of HIV/AIDS and the SARS epidemic have placed enormous stress on the Chinese health care system, as would be the case for any health care system. It challenged China's new leadership and greatly provoked reflections on the public health and crisis management system, the governance framework, and new concept of development (Hu, 2003b). The new reform phase has made a shift from the government being the "parent" protecting and improving the economy to a government establishing a framework where competition is the driving force in improving the economy/business.

## Notes

* Some preliminary elements of this chapter appeared in reports made by the Tsinghua team (2003a, 2003b) during the SARS outbreak.

** I would like to express my gratitude to the many people that made this chapter possible. I owe many thanks to my colleagues at School of Public Policy and Management (SPPM) Tsinghua University and at CRISMART (Swedish National Defense College) for reading and providing valuable comments: in particular, Lan Xue, Hu Angang, Eric Stern, Zongchao Peng, and Greg Simons. For the remaining faults and errors in this chapter, I assume sole responsibility.

1. It should be noted that SARS broke out again in Beijing and in the Anhui Province in April 2004. For more details, please see the appendix "Chronology of SARS in China (2002-2004)."

2. If not specially mentioned, the statistics in this chapter were taken from press releases made by China's MOH and WTO during the SARS outbreak.

3. This part has drawn much insightful information from Zhong Nanshan et al. (2003). To sum up the recent experiences in SARS prevention and management in China and to make full preparation for controlling SARS if it were to recur this winter or next spring, the Ministry of Health of China has entrusted the Chinese Medical Association (CMA) with organizing a nationwide compilation, a "Consensus for the management of severe acute respiratory syndrome," which is to describe SARS in terms of etiology, epidemiology, pathology, laboratory investigation and imaging technology, and put emphasis on the diagnosis and treatment of SARS.

4. One possible explanation for the few cases reported in the first three months may be that the government tried to cover up the situation in the beginning.

5. China was undergoing a major leadership transition that started formally in November 2002 at the Sixteenth Party Congress and did not end until March 2003 with the Tenth National People's Congress.

6. Ms. Wu is an experienced politician in China with good connections and a reputation for getting things done. She has worked with former Premier Zhu on WTO-entry terms and is considered not only well versed in Beijing politics but also trusted by the foreign community.

7. Wang is the son-in-law of Yao Yilin. He has a significant reform track record, dating back to 1980, in the rural and financial sectors as well as provincial leadership (Saich, 2003).

8. Chinese President Hu Jintao and Premier Wen Jiabao had just taken up their positions when SARS exploded in China. The real transfer of power took place at the Communist Party of China's 16th National Congress in 2002. The National People's Congress (NPC) and the Chinese People's Political Consultative Conference (CPPCC) convened earlier in 2003 and were seen only as providing the formal endorsement of that transfer. Beginning in 2002, talks about a fourth period of ideological liberation started to emerge.

9. This survey was conducted by the Guangzhou Social Situation & Poll Survey Center (Guangzhou Shequn Minyi Zhongxin) with a sampling of 525 citizens. See Yang Cheng Evening News (14 February 2003).

10. The electronic versions of these four mainstream news organizations were analyzed.

11. Speaking at the fifth Sino-Germany law forum, Cao Kangtai (Director of the Legislative Affairs Office of the State Council) said China had made remarkable progress in emergency-related legislation, setting up 35 laws, 36 administrative regulations, 55 department rules and 111 documents for handling emergencies (People's Daily Online, 18 April 2004).

12. "Unit" is an important concept for anyone wanting to understand China, and the concrete effects of the unit are much more far-reaching (Lu, 1989; Li, 1994; Yang and Zhou, 1994).

13. It was pointed out that SARS control was having a significant impact on the health and lives of the people as well as China's overall situation, and that control mechanisms were key to cutting off the epidemic's transmission route (People's Daily Online, 18 April 2003).

14. The national mobilization system had evolved from so-called defense mobilization, which plays a significant role in times of war or severe natural disasters. In 1994, China established a national committee on defense mobilization (Xinhua News Agency, 26 October 2003).

15. The economic impact of SARS caused concern over decreased consumption which would be exacerbated by the concerns of foreign investors and the cancellation of the May Day holiday. Thus, SARS was linked to the need to maintain economic development (Xinhua News Agency, 10 May 2003; People's Daily, 17 May 2003; Saich, 2003).

## *References*

Brower, Jennifer and Peter Chalk (2003) *The Global Threat of New and Reemerging Infectious Diseases: Reconciling U.S. National Security and Public Health Policy.* California: RAND Corp.

China's Ministry of Health (MoH) Press Release. Available at: www.moh.gov.cn

Han Li (2001). "Informal Regulation in China's Legislative Process", *Strategy and Management,* Vol. 5, 2001.

Henderson, Gail E. (2003). "Myths and Realities: The Context of Emerging Pathogens in China." Testimony before The Congressional-Executive Commission on China,

May 12, Washington DC Roundtable on, "Dangerous Secrets: SARS and China's Health Care System." Available at: www.cecc.gov.

Hsiao, William. (1995) "The Chinese Health Care System: Lessons for Other Countries." *Social Science and Medicine*. Vol. 41, No. 8, pp. 1047-1055.

Hu Angang (2003a). *China: A New Concept for Development*. Hangzhou: Zhejiang People's Press.

Hu Angang, Ed. (2003b). *Looking through SARS: Health and Development*. Beijing: Tsinghua University Press.

Hu Linlin and Hu Angang. "From Disparities to Equal Health Development: Analysis of the Rural-Urban Disease Model Difference." *Management World*, Vol. 1, 2003, pp. 78-87.

Jin, Xin. (2000). *Problems in China: Severe Challenges Facing China in the New Century*. Beijing: Chinese Social Science Press.

Li, Hanlin et al. (1994). "Unit Phenomena and System Reform in China." *China Social Science Quarterly*. Vol. 5, pp.5-16.

Liu, Zhifeng, Ed. (1999). *Report on the Reforms of China's Political System*. Beijing: China Cinema Press.

Lowell, Dittmer (1994). *China under Reform*. Boulder, Colorado: Westview Press, Inc.

Lu, Feng (1989) "Unit: A Special Organizational Form." *China Social Science*. Vol.1, pp.71-73.

Niu, Wenyuan (2001) "Social Burning Theory and China's Social Security Precaution System (outline)." Discussion sketch of "Management of Emergencies in Social Transformation." Symposium jointly organized by SPPM, Tsinghua University and Chinese Association of Administrative Management. Beijing, November 26, 2001.

People's Daily Online (1 April 2003) "China 'Safe' Despite SARS Epidemic: FM Spokesman."

People's Daily Online (18 March 2005) "China, ASEAN to Improve Co-Op on Epidemic Prevention."

People's Daily Online (1 May 2003) "Chronology of China's Fight against SARS since April 20."

People's Daily Online (18 April 2004) "Enactment of Emergency Law Urgent: Official."

People's Daily Online (13 April 2003) "First SARS Patient in Beijing Reports Recovery."

People's Daily Online (26 March 2003) "Guangdong Reports Progress in Combating Atypical Pneumonia."

People's Daily Online (15 June 2003) "Inner Mongolia celebrates lifting of travel advisory."

People's Daily Online (20 April 2003) "Official Explains Rise of SARS Cases in Beijing."

People's Daily Online (4 June 2003) "SARS Costly for China: Vice Health Minister."

People's Daily Online (18 April 2003) "Senior Chinese Leaders Meet to Discuss SARS Control."

People's Daily Online (24 June 2003) "WHO Removes Beijing from SARS List, Lifts Travel Advisory."

People's Daily (27 November 2001) "Editorial: A Major, Historic Event in China's Reform and Opening Process."

People's Daily (22 April 2003) "SARS: A Task We Should Give Top Priority to."

People's Daily (17 May 2003) "Unswervingly Carry out Development, the Foremost Important Task."

People's Daily (18 August 2003) "China Urges Continuous Alert on SARS Resurgence."

Saich, Tony (2003) "SARS: China's Chernobyl or Much Ado about nothing?" *China Public Administration*. Vol. 1, pp. 1-15.

Schmitt, Carl (1985). *The Crisis of Parliamentary Democracy*. Ellen Kennedy trans.

Sterman, J.D. (2000) *Business Dynamics: Systems Thinking and Modeling for a Complex World.* Boston: McGraw-Hill.

Stern, E. (1999) *Crisis Decision-Making: A Cognitive-Institutional Approach*. Stockholm: Stockholm University.

Tsinghua team (2003a) *Studies on Crisis Management: SARS Special Publication*. Crisis Management Research Center, Tsinghua University.

Tsinghua team (2003b) *Study Reports on China's Situation: SARS Special Publication*. Center for China Studies, Tsinghua University.

Wang, Xu (2001). "On Centralization of Jurisdiction." *Strategy and Management*. Vol. 5, pp. 28-36.

Wei, Bo et al. (2002). "Prevention and Control for Public Health Emergencies." *Guangxi Preventative Medicine*. Vol. 2, pp. 106-110.

WHO Press Release (2003) Available at: http://www.who.int/csr/sars/en/

WHO website (2003) "Update 95—SARS: Chronology of a Serial Killer." Available at: http://www.who.int/csr/don/2003_07_04/en/

Xinhua News Agency (8 May 2003) "China: Ministry Issues Circular on Controlling Spread of SARS to Rural Areas."

Xinhua News Agency (24 June 2003) "Liu Qi Points Out that the 'Double Removal' Marks the Great Triumph National Spirit."

Xinhua News Agency (3 May 2003) "SARS—An Opportunity China Reshuffles Public Health, Disease Prevention System."

Xinhua News Agency (26 October 2003) "University to Train Government Trouble Shooters."

Xinhua News Agency (10 May 2003) "We firmly Grasp Opportunities in the Time of Danger and Disaster."

Xinhua News Agency (13 May 2003) "Wen Jiabao's Speech at a Seminar on Implementation of 'Emergency Regulations on Sudden Outbreaks of Public Health Incidents'."

Xue, Lan and Qin Zhu (2003) "Public Health Emergency Response: The Case of the United States." *China Public Administration*. Vol. 8, pp. 51-56.

Xue, Lan, Qiang Zhang, and Kaibin Zhong (2003a) "Be on Your Guard and Restructure: Reviewing the Stages of Change in China's Crisis Management from the SARS Outbreak." *Reform*. No. 3, pp. 5-20.

Xue, Lan, Qiang Zhang, and Kaibin Zhong (2003b) *Crisis Management in China: The Challenge of the Transition*. Beijing: Tsinghua University Press.

Yan, Lan and Liu Xianshu (25 June 2003) *China's Youth Daily*.

Yang, Xiaomin and Yihu Zhou (1993) *China's Unit System*. Beijing: China Economic Press.

*Yangcheng Evening News (Yangcheng Wanbao)* (14 February 2003) "Survey: Half People Got Information from Their Friends and Relatives."

Yu, Keping, Ed. (2000) *Governance and Good Governance*. Beijing: Social Science Press.

Zhong, Nanshan et al. (2003). "Consensus for the Management of Severe Acute Respiratory Syndrome (Part 1)." *Chinese Medical Journal*. Vol. 116, No 14, pp. 1603-1635.

## *Chapter 2 Appendix*

## Chronology of SARS in China (2002-2004)

16 November 2002
—First known case of atypical pneumonia appears in Foshan City, Guangdong Province, China, but is not identified until much later.

10 February 2003
—The WHO Beijing office receives an email message describing a "strange contagious disease" that has "already left more than 100 people dead" in Guangdong Province in the space of one week. The message further describes "a sense of 'panic' where people are currently emptying pharmaceutical stocks of any medicine they think may protect them."

11 February 2003
—WHO receives reports from the Chinese Ministry of Health about an outbreak of acute respiratory syndrome which has resulted in 300 cases and five deaths in Guangdong Province.

12 February 2003
—Health officials from Guangdong Province report a total of 305 cases and five deaths of acute respiratory syndrome. The cases and deaths occurred from November 16, 2002 to February 9, 2003. Laboratory analyses for influenza viruses are negative.

14 February 2003
—The Chinese Ministry of Health informs WHO that the outbreak in Guangdong Province is clinically consistent with atypical pneumonia. The outbreak is said to be under control.

17 February 2003
—A 33 year old Hong Kong man, who had traveled with his family to Fujian Province, China in January, dies of unknown causes in Hong Kong. His eight year old daughter died, of unknown causes, while in mainland China. His nine year old son is hospitalized.

19 February 2003
—An outbreak of the "bird flu" in Hong Kong is reported to WHO following the detection of the A (H5N1) influenza virus in the nine year old boy.

—WHO activates its global influenza laboratory network and calls for heightened global surveillance.

20 February 2003
—The Department of Health in Hong Kong confirms that the boy's father was likewise infected with a strain of the influenza A (H5N1) virus.

21 February 2003
—A sixty-four year old medical doctor from Zhongshan University in Guangzhou (Guangdong Province) arrives in Hong Kong to attend a wedding. He checks into the ninth floor of the Metropole Hotel (room 911). Although he developed respiratory symptoms five days earlier, he feels well enough to sightsee and shop with his fifty-three year old brother-in-law, who resides in Hong Kong.

22 February 2003
—The Guangdong doctor seeks urgent care at the Kwong Wah Hospital in Hong Kong and is admitted to the intensive care unit with respiratory failure (he had previously treated patients with atypical pneumonia in Guangdong). He warns medical staff that he fears he has contracted a "very virulent disease." Health authorities in Hong Kong learn that his symptoms had developed on February 15, at which point he would have still been on the Chinese mainland.

23 February 2003
—A seventy-eight year old female tourist from Toronto, Canada checks out of the Metropole Hotel and begins her homeward journey. On arrival in Toronto she is reunited with her family.
—A team of WHO experts arrives in Beijing, but is only granted permission to work at the central level.

24 February 2003
—The Global Public Health Intelligence Network (GPHIN) picks up a report stating that over fifty hospital staff are infected with a "mysterious pneumonia" in the city of Guangzhou.
—In Hong Kong, a twenty-six year old local man develops a respiratory tract infection, but does not seek medical attention. From February 15 to 23, he had visited an acquaintance staying on the ninth floor of the Metropole Hotel.

25 February 2003
—The brother-in-law of the Guangdong doctor is admitted to Kwong Wah Hospital but later discharged.

26 February 2003
—A forty-eight year old Chinese-American businessman is admitted to the French Hospital in Hanoi with a three day history of fever and respiratory symptoms. His recent travel history includes a January trip to Shanghai, and a private trip from February 8 to 10 to Guangdong Province, and Macao. He traveled to Hong Kong on February 17, departed for Hanoi on February 23, and fell ill there. Shortly before his departure from Hong Kong, he had stayed on the ninth floor of the Metropole Hotel in a room across the hall from the Guangdong doctor.
—The businessman is visited by a WHO official, Dr Carlo Urbani, based in Vietnam.

28 February 2003
—Dr Urbani, alarmed by the unusual disease and concerned it might be a case of avian influenza, notifies the WHO office in Manila. The WHO headquarters moves into a heightened state of alert.

1 March 2003
—The brother-in-law of the Guangdong doctor is re-admitted to Kwong Wah Hospital.
—A twenty-six year old woman is admitted to a hospital in Singapore with respiratory symptoms. A resident of Singapore, she was a guest on the ninth floor of the Hotel Metropole in Hong Kong from February 21 to 25.

4 March 2003
—The Guangdong doctor dies of atypical pneumonia at Kwong Wah Hospital.

5 March 2003
—In Hanoi, the Chinese-American businessman, in a stable but critical condition, is air-med evacuated to the Princess Margaret Hospital in Hong Kong. Seven health care workers who had cared for him in Hanoi become ill. Dr Urbani continues to help hospital staff contain further contamination.
—The seventy-eight year old Toronto woman dies at Toronto's Scarborough Grace Hospital. Five members of her family are found to be infected and are admitted to the hospital.

7 March 2003
—Health care workers at Hong Kong's Prince of Wales Hospital complain of respiratory tract infection symptoms, which progress to pneumonia. All have an identifiable link with Ward 8A.

8 March 2003
—In Taiwan, a fifty-four year old businessman with a travel history to Guangdong Province is hospitalized with respiratory symptoms.

10 March 2003
—At least twenty-two staff members at the Hanoi hospital are ill with influenza-like symptoms. Twenty show signs of pneumonia, one requires breathing support, and another is in critical condition.
—The Ministry of Health in China asks WHO to provide technical and laboratory support in order to identify the cause of the Guangdong outbreak of atypical pneumonia.

11 March 2003
—Dr Urbani departs for Bangkok, on a Thai flight, where he is scheduled to give a presentation at a meeting on tropical diseases the following day. He is ill upon arrival and is immediately hospitalized.

12 March 2003
—WHO issues a global alert about cases of severe atypical pneumonia following mounting reports of contamination among hospital staff members in Hong Kong and Hanoi.
—At the French Hospital in Hanoi, twenty-six staff members are reported ill. Of these, twenty-five have either pneumonia or acute respiratory syndrome, and five are in critical condition. The hospital is closed for new admissions.
—Hong Kong health authorities formally report an outbreak of an unidentified flu-like illness among hospital staff. As of midnight on March 11, fifty health care workers had been screened: twenty-three were found to have febrile illness, and eight showed early signs of pneumonia on chest X-rays. An additional three health care workers present with febrile illness and two show signs of pneumonia.

13 March 2003
—WHO sends emergency alert to its partners in the Global Outbreak Alert and Response Network (GOARN).
—The Chinese-American businessman dies in isolation at the Princess Margaret Hospital in Hong Kong. No cases among hospital staff are reported.
—The Ministry of Health in Singapore reports three cases of atypical pneumonia in young women who had recently returned to Singapore after traveling to Hong Kong. All had stayed on the ninth floor of the Metropole Hotel in late February.
—The forty-four year old son of Toronto's first SARS case dies in Scarborough Grace Hospital.

14 March 2003

—In Hong Kong, thirty-nine staff members at three hospitals undergo treatment for flu-like symptoms. Twenty-four exhibit signs of pneumonia and are described as in "serious condition."

—Health authorities in Ontario, Canada take steps to alert doctors, hospitals, ambulance services, and public health units across the province that there are four cases of an atypical pneumonia in Toronto that have resulted in two deaths. All cases occurred within a single family.

—The first members of a WHO GOARN multidisciplinary outbreak control team arrive in Hanoi.

15 March 2003

—At 2:00 a.m., Singapore health authorities notify the WHO staff by urgent telecommunication that a thirty-two year old physician, who had treated the country's first two SARS cases, had boarded a flight from New York City to Singapore via Frankfurt, after having attended a media conference. Shortly before boarding the flight, he reported his symptoms to an alert medical colleague in Singapore, who then notified the health officials. WHO identifies the airline and flight number. The physician, his thirty year old pregnant wife and sixty-two year old mother-in-law are removed from the flight in Frankfurt and placed in isolation. They become Germany's first SARS cases.

—WHO issues a rare travel advisory as evidence mounts that SARS is spreading by air travel along international routes. WHO names the mysterious illness after its symptoms: severe acute respiratory syndrome (SARS) and declares it "a worldwide health threat."

—WHO issues its first definitions of suspect and probable SARS cases. WHO further calls on all travelers to be aware of the signs and symptoms and issues information to the airlines.

—Health Canada reports eight cases of atypical pneumonia, including two deaths.

—Four intensive care specialists arrive in Hanoi to reinforce the GOARN team there.

—The Singapore Ministry of Health reports sixteen cases of atypical pneumonia.

16 March 2003

—Over 150 suspect and probable cases of SARS are reported from around the world.

17 March 2003

—China provides a first brief report to WHO about the Guangdong outbreak. The outbreak is said to have tapered off.

—WHO sets up a network of eleven leading laboratories in nine countries to expedite detection of the causative agent and develop a robust and reliable diagnostic test. A similar network is set up to pool clinical knowledge on symptoms, diagnosis, and management. A third network is set up to study SARS epidemiology.

18 March 2003
—Cases are now being reported in Canada, Germany, Taiwan (China), Thailand, and the United Kingdom as well as in Hong Kong, Vietnam, and Singapore. The cumulative total of cases reported to WHO are 219 cases and four deaths.
—Hong Kong reports 123 cases, Hanoi fifty-seven, and Singapore twenty-three.
—Data indicate that the overwhelming majority of cases occur in health care workers, their family members, and others having close face-to-face contact with patients, supporting the view that SARS is spread by contact with droplets when patients cough or sneeze.

19 March 2003
—The brother-in-law of the Guangdong doctor dies in a Hong Kong hospital.

20 March 2003
—The USA reports its first cases.
—The cumulative total of cases climbs to 306, with ten deaths.

21 March 2003
—A WHO coordinating officer arrives in Singapore to assess the possible need for international assistance.
—WHO issues policy guidelines on hospital discharges and follow-up visits.

22 March 2003
—Hong Kong scientists devise first "hand-made" diagnostic test and announce isolation of a candidate causative agent. The exact identity of the virus remains elusive.
—Thirteen countries on three continents report a cumulative total of 386 cases and eleven deaths.

23 March 2003
—A five person WHO GOARN team arrives in Beijing and seeks permission to travel to the Guangdong Province.

24 March 2003
—The Singapore Ministry of Health announces home quarantine measures whe-

reby all contacts of SARS patients are required to stay home for ten days. More than 300 persons are affected.

25 March 2003
—Nine passengers linked to the March 15$^{th}$ flight from Hong Kong to Beijing develop SARS after returning to Hong Kong. The flight is eventually linked to SARS cases in twenty-two passengers and two flight attendants.
—Scarborough Grace Hospital in Toronto is closed to new patients and all visitors.

26 March 2003
—The first electronic "ground rounds" consultation on SARS symptoms, diagnosis, and management is held, bringing together in real time eighty clinicians from thirteen countries.
—China reports a cumulative total of 792 cases and thirty-one deaths in the Guangdong Province from November 16, 2002, to February 28, 2003. Officials had previously reported 305 cases and five deaths from mid-November to 9 February.
—The WHO team in China reviews the case definition used during the outbreak of the atypical pneumonia and concludes that the cases most likely represent the same disease now referred to as SARS.
—With the new data from China, world cumulative total of cases soars to 1,323, with forty-nine deaths.
—Ontario health officials warn of a possible health emergency.

27 March 2003
—Scientists in the WHO lab network report major progress in the identification of the causative agent, with results from several labs consistently pointing to a new member of the coronavirus family.
—Hong Kong announces the closure of schools until April 6 and places 1,080 people under quarantine.
—Chinese authorities report SARS cases in other parts of China.
—WHO issues more stringent advice to international travelers and airlines, including recommendations on screening at certain airports.

28 March 2003
—China joins WHO collaborative networks.
—Some airlines in the affected countries begin screening their outward bound travelers.
—Financial analysts assess effects on stock markets and predict significant economic consequences if the outbreak is not under control by June.

29 March 2003
—WHO infectious disease specialist, Dr Carlo Urbani, the first WHO officer to identify the outbreak of this new disease and who treated the earliest cases in Hanoi, dies of SARS in Thailand.

30 March 2003
—Canadian health officials close York Central Hospital to new patients and request hundreds of its employees to quarantine themselves. Thousands of Toronto residents face quarantine at home.
—Hong Kong health authorities announce that 213 residents of the Amoy Gardens housing estate have been hospitalized with SARS since reporting on the disease began. Of this total, 107 reside in a single wing of the thirty-five story Block E building. Most patients from Block E live in vertically-interrelated apartments.

31 March 2003
—Health authorities in Hong Kong issue an unprecedented isolation order in an attempt to prevent further spreading of SARS.
—In Singapore, a sixty-four year old man selling vegetables at a large wholesale market visits his brother in the Singapore General Hospital.

1 April 2003
—In Hong Kong, the number of cases linked to Amoy Gardens continues to grow and strongly suggests that the disease has spread beyond its initial focus in hospitals, with tertiary as well as secondary cases almost certainly occurring.
—WHO epidemiologists determine that, since March 19, nine residents of Beijing, Taiwan (China) and Singapore have developed SARS after being in Hong Kong.

2 April 2003
—WHO recommends that persons traveling to Hong Kong and the Guangdong Province consider postponing all but essential travel plans until further notice. This is the most stringent travel advisory issued by WHO in its fifty-five year history.
—Chinese authorities announce updated figures for the period from March 1 to 31: 361 new SARS cases and nine deaths in the Guangdong Province.
—Chinese government gives the WHO team permission to travel "immediately" to Guangdong.
—The cumulative world total of SARS cases passes the two thousand mark.

3 April 2003
—WHO team arrives in Guangdong and starts working immediately. Over the next days, the team visits Foshan City, where the first known case was reported in November, and Guangzhou City. All team requests for access to sites and interviews with health staff at all levels are readily granted.
—Chinese Minister of Health appears on national television to address SARS-related issues.

4 April 2003
—China begins daily electronically reporting SARS cases and related deaths, nationwide by province.
—The Singapore health authorities trace ninety-four SARS cases back to the country's index case, linked to the Metropole Hotel.

6 April 2003
—A fifty-three year old Finnish staff member of the International Labor Organization dies of SARS in Beijing. He had traveled to Beijing on the March 23rd flight from Hong Kong.

7 April 2003
—WHO reports that around-the-clock international collaborative efforts to develop a diagnostic test are proving more problematic than hoped. Of the three diagnostic tests available, all have limitations as tools for stemming the SARS epidemic.
—Morgan Stanley's chief economist, Stephan Roach, estimates the global economic impact of SARS at about US$ 30 billion.

8 April 2003
—In Singapore, the sixty-four year old vegetable seller is admitted to the emergency room of a hospital. He is not isolated until twelve hours later, when his symptoms indicate SARS.
—A cumulative total of 2,671 cases and 103 deaths are reported from seventeen countries.

9 April 2003
—The interim report of the WHO investigative team in China is presented to the Ministry of Health. The report notes that the health system in the Guangdong Province had responded well to the outbreak, but serious concerns are expressed about the capacity of other provinces, which lack the strong health system seen in Guangdong, to cope with the challenges posed by SARS.

—The WHO team further expresses concern about the situation in Beijing, where only a minority of hospitals makes daily reports of SARS cases. Contact tracing is not carried out systematically in Beijing, and health authorities fail to vigorously investigate rumors.

10 April 2003
—A growing number of investigative media reports suggest that the cases in Beijing military hospitals are not being frankly reported.

11 April 2003
—South Africa reports its first probable SARS case. Cases have now been reported in nineteen countries on four continents.

14 April 2003
—The WHO team in Beijing fails to secure permission to visit military hospitals.
—The cumulative number of worldwide cases passes the three thousand mark.

15 April 2003
—The Beijing team is given permission to visit military hospitals, but they do not receive authorization to report their findings. A first visit is made.
—Hong Kong reports nine SARS deaths, the largest number of deaths in one single day reported to date.

16 April 2003
—Exactly one month after its establishment, the WHO laboratory network announces conclusive identification of the SARS causative agent: an entirely new coronavirus, unlike any other human or animal member of the Coronavirus family.
—In Hong Kong, doctors report that SARS patients from the Amoy Gardens cluster are not responding to treatment as well as patients from other clusters.
—The WHO team in Beijing estimates that the number of cases in the city is in the range of one hundred to two hundred. The estimate contrasts sharply with the thirty-seven cases officially reported two days previously. The team is granted permission to visit one military hospital.

17 April 2003
—Economic analysts in the Far East estimate initial SARS-related damage to regional GDP growth at US$ 10.6–$15 billion.

—China's losses, at US$2.2 billion, are the highest, but Hong Kong, where the outbreak has already cost US$1.7 billion, is the biggest SARS-related economic casualty.
—In Hong Kong, retail sales have fallen by half since mid-March, the number of tourists from mainland China has decreased 75 percent to 80 percent, and the entertainment and restaurant industries have recorded an 80 percent drop in business.

18 April 2003
—The WHO team in Beijing expresses strong concern over inadequate reporting of SARS cases in military hospitals as rumors about undisclosed cases mount.
—Hong Kong officials release the findings of an extensive investigation into a possible environmental cause of the Amoy Gardens cluster of cases. Attention is focused on possible transmission via the sewage system, though many other routes of exposure were also investigated. An unusual observation is made; sixty-six percent of patients in the Amoy Gardens cluster suffered from diarrhea. In most other clusters of cases, diarrhea is typically seen in only two percent to seven percent of cases.

19 April 2003
—China's top leaders advise officials not to cover up cases of SARS.
—Toronto authorities investigate a cluster of thirty-one suspect and probable SARS cases in members of a charismatic religious group, the health care workers who treated them, and close family and social contacts. Concern centers on opportunities for widespread community transmission during two large gatherings of the religious group on March 28 and 29.
—The Vietnamese government considers closing its 1,130 km border with China.

20 April 2003
—Beijing authorities announce 339 previously undisclosed cases of SARS, bringing the cumulative total of SARS cases in China to 1,959. Chinese authorities further announce that the traditional week-long May Day holiday will be shortened.
—The mayor of Beijing and the Minister of Health, both of whom had downplayed the SARS threat, are removed from their Communist Party posts.
—Singaporean health officials close a large wholesale fruit and vegetable market following the detection of a cluster of three SARS cases linked to the market. Cases are traced back to the sixty-four year old vegetable hawker.

22 April 2003
—Chinese authorities report a cumulative total of 2,001 SARS cases with ninety-two deaths.

23 April 2003
—Beijing officials suspend all primary and secondary schools for a two-week period.
—Chinese authorities report a cumulative total of 2,305 probable cases of SARS and 106 deaths. The number of cases in Beijing is now 693.
—In Singapore, eight probable and fourteen suspect SARS cases are now linked to the vegetable hawker at the wholesale market.
—WHO advises travelers to Beijing and Shanxi Province, China, and Toronto, Canada to consider postponing all but essential travel plans.
—The cumulative number of probable SARS cases climbs to 4,288, with 251 deaths. China reports 106 of the deaths and Hong Kong reports 105.

25 April 2003
—Outbreaks in Hanoi, Hong Kong, Singapore, and Toronto show signs of peaking.

28 April 2003
—Vietnam is removed from the list of areas with recent local transmission, making it the first country to successfully contain its outbreak.
—The cumulative total number of cases surpasses five thousand.

30 April 2003
—WHO lifts its travel advice for Toronto.
—China, accounting for 3460 probable cases of the global total of 5,663, now has more cases than the rest of the world combined.

2 May 2003
—The cumulative total of cases surpasses six thousand.

3 May 2003
—WHO sends a team to Taiwan, which is now reporting a cumulative total of one hundred probable cases.

7 May 2003
—WHO estimates that the case fatality ratio of SARS ranges from 0 percent to 50 percent depending on the age group affected, with an overall estimate of case fatality of 14 percent to 15 percent.

8 May 2003
—Travel recommendations are extended to Tianjin and Inner Mongolia in China and to Taipei, Taiwan.

13 May 2003
—Outbreaks at the remaining initial sites show signs of coming under control, indicating that SARS can be contained.

14 May 2003
—Toronto is removed from the list of areas with recent local transmission.

17 May 2003
—The first global consultation on SARS epidemiology concludes its work. The consultation confirms that control measures recommended by WHO are supported by available evidence. The experts further confirm the consistent effectiveness of these measures, which include early identification and isolation of patients, vigorous contact tracing, management of close contacts, and public information and education to encourage prompt reporting of symptoms.
—Travel recommendations are extended to Hebei Province, China.

21 May 2003
—Travel recommendations are extended to all of Taiwan.

22 May 2003
—Health authorities in Canada inform WHO of a new hospital-based cluster and five cases of acute respiratory illness in Toronto.
- The cumulative global total of cases surpasses eight thousand.

23 May 2003
—Travel recommendations for Hong Kong and the Guangdong Province are removed.
—Research teams in Hong Kong and China announce the detection of a SARS-like virus in the masked palm civet and raccoon-dog. These and other wild animals are traditionally consumed as delicacies and sold for human consumption in markets throughout southern China.

26 May 2003
—Toronto returns to the list of areas with recent local transmission.

27 May 2003
—The World Health Assembly adopts a resolution on SARS recognizing the

severity of the threat posed by this new disease and call on all countries to report cases promptly and transparently. WHO's capacity to respond to outbreaks is strengthened in a second resolution.

31 May 2003
—Singapore is removed from the list of areas with recent local transmission.

3 June2003
—The number of newly reported probable cases in China declines to a weekly average of slightly more than two.

12 June 2003
—A team of senior WHO officials arrives in Beijing to assess the situation of SARS control in China.

13 June 2003
—Travel recommendations for the Hebei, Inner Mongolia, Shanxi and Tianjin provinces in China are removed. The Guangdong, Hebei, Hubei, Inner Mongolia, Jilin, Jiangsu, Shaanxi, Shanxi and Tianjin provinces are removed from the list of areas with recent local transmission.

17 June 2003
—A two-day global SARS conference opens in Kuala Lumpur, Malaysia, to assess the status of research on SARS and to compare national strategies used to contain the disease.

18 June 2003
—The global outbreak enters its hundredth day as the number of new cases reported daily dwindles to a handful.

23 June 2003
—Hong Kong is removed from the areas with recent local transmission.

24 June 2003
—Travel recommendations are removed for Beijing, the last remaining area subject to WHO travel advice. Beijing is also removed from the list of areas with recent local transmission.

2 July 2003
—Toronto is removed from the list of areas with recent local transmission.

5 July 2003
—Taiwan, the last area with recent local transmission, is removed from the list.
—WHO declares that SARS outbreaks have been contained worldwide, but calls for continued vigilance.

16 July 2003
—The national headquarters for SARS prevention and treatment holds a summing-up meeting in Beijing.

25 July 2003
—A commendation ceremony is held in Beijing for people who excelled in the hard fight against SARS.

18 January 2004
—The two suspected SARS patients in the southern Guangdong Province have been confirmed with contracting the disease.

22 April 2004
—The Chinese Ministry of Health reports one suspected case in Beijing.
—Beijing initiates its health warning system.
—Five other people who have had contact with SARS patients also report having fevers and are put in isolation at a hospital. Doctors keep under observation 171 other people, who also have had contact with the SARS casualty, to make sure they do not develop any symptoms.

23 April 2004
—The Chinese Ministry of Health reports one suspected case and one confirmed case in the Anhui Province.

24 April 2004
—Beijing releases the diagnosis process of the confirmed SARS case.

25 April 2004
—The Anhui Province releases related information regarding the train taken by the SARS patient Song.
—The Chinese Ministry of Health announces that four new suspected cases have been reported in Beijing.

26 April 2004
—All those who may have had contact with the affected areas in Chinese CDC are quarantined.

—International health officials blame a breach in lab security for China's latest emergence of SARS as Chinese authorities keep nearly five hundred people in quarantine in an attempt to contain the virus before a major holiday.

27 April 2004
—No new cases are reported on China's mainland.
—In Beijing two people who had contact with a SARS patient report having fevers.

28 April 2004
—The Anhui Province traces 154 people who have had contact with a SARS patient.
—The new SARS patient remains in critical condition.

29 April 2004
—Beijing reports two more confirmed cases, one in critical condition.

30 April 2004
—The suspected victim who had died in the Anhui Province is confirmed as a SARS case.
—WHO feels no travel restrictions are necessary.

1 May 2004
—Beijing confirms a SARS case.
—No cases are reported in the country's other regions.

3 May 2004
—Eighty-eight people in Beijing and forty-four people in the Anhui Province are released from medical observation.

4 May 2004
—Beijing confirms three suspected cases. They are the father and ward-mates of the confirmed case.

5 May 2004
—Beijing's first confirmed SARS patient (Li) has recovered and is discharged from hospital.

6 May 2004
—159 people in Beijing and 103 people in the Anhui Province are removed from medical observation.

7 May 2004
—161 people at the Virus Institute of Chinese CDC are removed from medical observation.
—Two Beijing hospitals used to isolate potential victims of the recent SARS outbreak resume to normal operations.
—More than 200 medical workers, in-patients and helpers are released from isolation at Jiangong Hospital and Renmin Hospital (affiliated to Beijing University).

8 May 2004
—115 people are released after being quarantined following contact with SARS patients in the Anhui Province.

21 May 2004
—The last SARS case in Beijing is discharged from Ditan Hospital.

23 May 2004
—All of the 747 people in Beijing who had had close contact with SARS patients are removed from isolation, marking the end of the outbreak.
—The prevention and control operation in Beijing and the Anhui Province is officially completed.
—The transmission of SARS has been eliminated.

1 June 2004
—The Chinese Ministry of Public Health announces that from today it has suspended daily surveillance reports on the SARS epidemic (the "zero report" mechanism) since the latest outbreak was effectively brought under control. However, surveillance and reports on SARS will be continued on a regular basis via nationwide computer network system in which all legally-reported communicable diseases are monitored.
—The Chinese Ministry of Health announces that Beijing has closed the Anti-SARS Headquarters.
—Beijing discontinues all SARS-related emergency control measures.
—A SARS case in Guangdong is confirmed.

25 June 2004
—People are no longer required to fill out a form reporting their health situation to the custom authorities upon departing China. However, incoming passengers to China still need to report their health situation to the custom authorities.
—A joint expert team from WHO and the Chinese Ministry of Public Health leave Beijing for east China's Anhui Province for a SARS investigation.

29 June 2004
—Vice Minister Wang Longde announces at a conference held at the state council news office that the SARS outbreak in Beijing and the Anhui Province was over and that a report would soon be released.
—The Chinese government gears up to launch a comprehensive disease prevention and control network that within three years covers both its urban and rural areas. At a morning press conference the Ministry of Health delivers a message on the prevention of HIV/AIDS and other communicable diseases.

1 July 2004
—The Chinese CDC assembly announces the cause and accountability of the 2004 SARS outbreak in Beijing and Anhui.
—The Chinese Executive Health Minister, Gao Qiang, confirms that the 2004 SARS outbreak in Beijing and Anhui came from the lab.
–Vice Premier Wu Yi stresses that lessons should be learned from the 2004 SARS outbreak and that measures should be taken to strengthen disease prevention and control work.

2 July 2004
—Senior officials at the China's Disease Control and Prevention Center take responsibility for negligence and resign. Director Li Liming steps down due to his poor crisis management of the SARS outbreak. Four of his colleagues are also removed from their posts.

# Chapter 3

# SARS in Beijing: An Urban Response[1]

Qin Zhu

## *1. Introduction*

On March 1, 2003, Beijing witnessed its first case of SARS. The SARS epidemic in Beijing reached its peak with more than one hundred new cases per day on average between the end of April and the beginning of May. The SARS crisis quickly evolved from a public health emergency in an individual region into a global compound crisis which had a great impact on various areas such as the economy, politics, and diplomatic relations.

Due to the severity of the epidemic and the special political status of Beijing, the SARS outbreak in Beijing became the national focus of attention. This crisis challenged the new government and greatly provoked reflections on the country's public health system, crisis management system, ongoing government reforms, and economic development. In this chapter, I present my analysis of the occurrence and spread of SARS from a crisis management perspective. It is my hope that we can learn from the experiences, draw important lessons, and offer some suggestions for improving a country's ability to meet an epidemic, establish a highly efficient crisis management system, and optimize its public governance framework.

## *2. General Context*

Beijing is the political and cultural center of China as well as an international metropolis covering a large geographic area (more than 16,800 square kilometers) with a population of over twenty million people. It is also a city undergoing rapid economic growth and urban development. In 2002, the GDP increased as much as 10 percent in Beijing. In the first quarter of 2003, the GDP had increased to 13 percent.

China's long-lasting rapid economic growth has been the focus of the world. However, the over-emphasis on the quantity of economic growth (GDP) by ignoring quality has resulted in a severe imbalance in China's development (Xue and Qin, 2003b).[2] Likewise the nation's imbalanced development has negatively affected Beijing. For example, there are severe defects and problems in the city's transportation and public health systems as well as in the environment, and these limit the city's capability to deal with an emergency or a crisis. These are the projecting expressions of the fragility of this metropolis. It's true that Beijing has preliminarily set up its public health system based upon disease prevention, medical treatment and emergency aid based on the three-leveled medical prevention health network which covers the entire city. However, the significance of public health in promoting economic growth and social progress has not been sufficiently recognized for a long time, and consequently the government has invested too few resources into the public health system. For example, in 2001 and 2002, the health expenses accounted for 5.4 percent and 5.5 percent, respectively, of the general budgetary financial expenditure. As a result, there are major problems in the public health system (Beijing's Statistics Annual, 2003; Sina, 2003).

At the same time, it should be pointed out that Beijing, as China's political and cultural capital, has special status and complex structures for meeting such challenges. Firstly, there are many multifarious institutions and organizations in Beijing. The Central Government (including many departments, committees, and agencies) are located here. The country's top leaders live here. Furthermore, many international institutes and foreign organizations have offices in Beijing. Secondly, Beijing's huge floating population is another big challenge, which presents many uncertainties about the actual population of the city. Finally, and above all, Beijing holds a special status in the political field since its governance and policy decisions are often directly influenced or controlled by the high-level national officials who live and work in Beijing.

## *3. Combating SARS in Beijing: A stage model analysis*

Beijing's response to the SARS crisis was closely connected with the development of epidemic. We first review the development of the situation in Beijing.

On November 26, 2002, the first SARS case was identified in Foshan City in Guangdong Province. In February 2003 a sharp peak in the SARS outbreak was visible in Guangzhou. At that time, SARS cases seemed to appear in clusters and had not yet spread nationwide.

On March 1, 2003, Beijing treated its first SARS case which was a person who had come from the Shanxi Province. Within just one month SARS rapidly spread in Beijing and with a peak in mid April, Beijing became the second most severely SARS affected city after Guangzhou. From March 1 to June 11, 2003, over 2,520 SARS cases were reported in Beijing, accounting for 47 percent of the total number of SARS cases on the mainland and 29 percent of the total cases in the world. During this period, nationwide transmission of SARS occurred. Beijing, in a broader sense the whole nation, went through a great crisis.

We can divide the process of Beijing's SARS crisis and its response to this crisis into three stages: 1. precautions and preparations before the crisis (from the end of 2002 to the end of February 2003), 2. responses and management during the crisis (from March 1 to June 24, 2003), and 3. post-processing and learning after the crisis (from June 25, 2003 to the present).

### *3.1 Precautions and preparations before the crisis*

During this period, the epidemic in China mainly occurred within the Guangdong Province, giving rise to panic and disorder in this area. In November 2002 when the first SARS case appeared in Guangdong and triggered large-scale infections, there were very few reports about SARS in the media. On February 11, 2003, SARS outbreaks were evident in Zhongshan and Guangzhou, and the Guangdong Provincial Bureau of Health held a press conference, acknowledging the presence of a new kind of infectious disease. Since then, the phrase "atypical pneumonia" became well-known.

The next day after this press conference (i.e., February 12), Beijing began to establish monitoring stations for "atypical pneumonia" in eleven top-class hospitals. This was the only measure reportedly taken by the authorities in Beijing against SARS at this stage according to the public documents I looked at. However, these efforts turned out to be in vain, as revealed by the occurrence of the epidemic. The key point of this problem lies in the fact that Beijing failed to foresee the potential of an epidemic, giving it very little consideration in their planning. Moreover, Beijing was too conceited to be vigilant and its confidence outweighed its cautious mentality. For example, I could hardly find any public documents that indicated that the Beijing authorities had even tried to inform the local hospitals and/or citizens of this disease and prevention methods. As a result, the Beijing authorities missed a great opportunity to implement effective measures to prevent the epidemic and/or to keep it under control when time allowed. Therefore, as far as the first stage of crisis management (i.e., precautions and preparations) was concerned, many of the dangers concerning the SARS outbreak in Beijing were concealed by the authorities.

### *3.2 Responses and management during the crisis*

From March 1 (when the first SARS case appeared) to June 24, 2003, Beijing experienced the full epidemiologic cycle of SARS: input, spreading, exploding, decline and termination. I have divided up this period into five significant stages in relation to crisis response and crisis management.

#### 3.2.1 March 1-March 22: Beijing's first SARS case reported and local transmission

On March 1, Beijing hospitalized its first SARS case: a female Shanxi resident, 27 years old. She had gone to Guangdong for business on February 18 and felt sick on February 21. She returned to Taiyuan (the capital of Shanxi) on February 23 and was diagnosed with pneumonia on February 26. On March 1, she came to the No. 301 Hospital in Beijing for treatment and was then transferred to the No. 302 Hospital. The second input SARS case was a male. He had returned to Beijing from Hong Kong and felt sick on March 14. He immediately went to the Dongzhimen Hospital for treatment, infecting nearly 50 people including medical workers, other patients, other passengers onboard the same flight with him, and his relatives. Local transmission in Beijing was now a fact.

During this period, the government was confronting a crucial problem, mainly how to make a correct prediction and judgment of the situation at hand and its probable consequences. On the premise of maintaining stability, two main questions arose. Whether or not to make the epidemic situation known to the public? How to implement resolute measures to prevent the epidemic from spreading? One possible choice for the government was to cut off the transmission channel for the virus by isolating the infected victims and to call upon the public and hospitals to take precautionary measures so that the epidemic could be controlled at a low cost and the crisis could be eliminated in its infancy. Unfortunately, the government chose to do nothing about it, thus missing a wonderful opportunity to resolve this crisis.

On March 12, WHO issued its first global SARS warning, but this was not reported by the domestic media. In fact, the domestic mainstream media reported very little on SARS. In addition, the central government and Beijing authorities underestimated the potential consequences of the epidemic. This can, in part, be explained by the fact that the annual plenary sessions of the National People's Congress (NPC) and the National Committee of the Chinese People's Political Consultative Conference (NPPCC) were being held at that time, so the government's attention was elsewhere. On the other hand, one could argue that the government intentionally suppressed information about the SARS epidemic in order to retain national stability.

### 3.2.2 March 23–April 3: Growing pressure from the international community and government passivity

The epidemic was still spreading at this stage. There was growing criticism and increasing pressure from the international community. For example, on March 23, WHO sent its expert team to Beijing to investigate the situation. Rumors and suspicion quickly spread throughout the city of Beijing.

Slowly but surely, the government began to understand the gravity of this event and its potential consequences. The key problem the government was confronted with was how to deal with international pressure, in order to preserve not only the image of Beijing but also the image of the entire country. A few solutions could have been to cooperate more closely with the international community, to report more openly about the epidemic in Beijing, or to implement concrete preventative measures faster in order to keep the epidemic under control. As a matter of fact, the central and Beijing government did adopt some measures. For example, on April 1, 2003, it started to issue daily SARS reports to WHO on the situation in Beijing. However, the accuracy of this information was disputed.

On March 24, 2003, WHO officials arrived in Beijing and the Beijing Municipal Bureau of Health circulated a notice concerning the SARS epidemic situation to all hospitals under its supervision. At that point, SARS cases had claimed two lives in Beijing. On March 26, the spokesman of the Beijing Municipal Bureau of Health stated that since the beginning of March, hospitals in Beijing had received and treated all together eight SARS patients, of which three had died. Two medical workers had reported having symptoms similar to SARS and had been put into isolation. No single SARS case had originated in Beijing; all reported SARS cases had been "imported" from elsewhere. This was the first public report about Beijing's epidemic situation. On April 1, the Ministry of Health started to report the number of SARS cases to WHO daily and published a status report of the domestic epidemic situation every five days. On April 3, the Ministry of Health held a press conference and claimed that up to March 31 there had been a total of twelve SARS cases in Beijing. The health minister Zhang Wenkang said that the epidemic situation on the mainland was under control. But in fact, according to the statistics made later, there had been fifty one SARS cases in Beijing by March 31; the epidemic situation of Beijing and the whole nation were far from being under control. Instead, the epidemic experienced a climax with a large-scale outbreak from mid April to early May.

At this stage the government reacted passively to international criticism and pressure by concealing the truth rather than trying to prevent SARS from spreading by educating the public and implementing resolute actions. Beijing once again missed the opportunity to prevent, or at least minimize, a crisis by failing to inform the public of the situation in an honest and timely manner, to implement prompt precautionary measures, and to cooperate with the international community.

### 3.2.3 April 4–April 19: Government faces a confidence crisis

This period of decision-making started when Jiang Yanyong (a retired military doctor) revealed the truth about the epidemic situation in Beijing to the foreign media during a press conference held by Ministry of Health on April 3, 2003. This event resulted in numerous news reports and criticism from the international media. The international community, thus, showed extreme distrust of the Chinese government, and Beijing's image was seriously damaged. On April 11, Beijing was again declared by WHO as a SARS-infected area. The image of the central and Beijing governments and their credibility were severely challenged both at home and abroad. During this period, the SARS outbreak was no longer a simple public health emergency, but a compound crisis with several values at stake: trust, diplomacy, and economy. At this time, the most critical problems the government was confronted with were how to deal with the international community's criticism and hostility, how to calm the public's fears, and how to reestablish its credibility.

Senior officials and leaders of the nation began to pay keen attention to the SARS situation in Beijing.[3] Likewise, the Beijing government also started to attach increased importance to the SARS situation and implemented additional measures to control the epidemic. In response to the increased attention given to SARS, people rushed to purchase medicines and prices were driven up. Beijing Drug Administration was forced to circulate an urgent notice on April 13, demanding medical suppliers to strictly observe the regulations on medicine prices by Commodity Prices Administration, strictly prohibiting hiking up prices.

On April 16, the municipal government decided to establish the aid mechanism for the low-income patients in order to make sure that all SARS patients in Beijing were treated in a timely and effective manner. This meant that the government would cover all of their medical fees for low-income SARS. This showed that the government had begun to understand the social problems the epidemic was causing and it made efforts to resolve these problems in an effort to control the situation.

Although the government had actively taken up a series of measures to address the SARS crisis at this stage, there was still evidence indicating that the government was concealing the truth about the actual epidemic situation in Beijing.

### 3.2.4 April 20–May 8: The turning point

The epidemic situation reached the stage of outbreak climax. In the face of overflowing criticism, distrust and even hostility from the international community as well as public disorder, the central and Beijing governments were confronted with a growing public health crisis.

April 20 was undoubtedly a turning point for China's battle against SARS, especially of Beijing's battle. On that day, the central government removed Zhang Wenkang (health minister) and Meng Xuenong (the mayor of Beijing Municipality) from their posts in the CCP (Communist Party of China), and dispatched supervision teams to areas of special concern. On April 20, in complying with the instructions of the CCP Central Committee, the senior officials in Beijing held a meeting in order to discuss appropriate measures to be taken. On April 21, six local hospitals were designated for treating SARS cases. On April 22, Waung Qishan took over as acting mayor to lead the Beijing's anti-SARS measures. At the same time, the municipal government also decided to designate the Xiaotangshan Hospital in Changping District as a "SARS-only" hospital and sending all SARS patients there. On April 23, the Beijing authorities decided to put the most seriously infected areas into isolation. The next day, the Attached People's Hospital of Beijing University was closed and isolated. It was the first key area which was seriously infected by SARS and put into isolation. On April 25, SARS was listed under the Law on Prevention and Cure of Infectious Diseases and thereafter was managed as an official infectious disease.

Therefore, certain appropriate measures were implemented against SARS and they soon had a positive effect.

Once the epidemic was made public, there was great panic and unrest among the citizens of Beijing. In addition to controlling the epidemic situation, a major issue for the government was to calm the citizens' fears and concerns in order to prevent social upheaval. On April 22, the spokesman of Beijing Municipal Government refuted the rumor of "blocking off the city." At the same time, a large amount of commodities for epidemic prevention arrived in Beijing in order to help build a defense for citizens.

By the end of April, Beijing had basically formed an effective system for combating SARS and controlling the epidemic. The system was continuously improved since the government attached great importance to it. It proved to be so effective that in just ten days the daily number of newly infected SARS patients reported dramatically declined.

In May, controlling the epidemic situation was still a major task for the Beijing authorities. Now that these measures had been operating in a good manner, the municipal government started to think about the social and economic consequences caused by the SARS crisis. The government needed to address the negative economic consequences caused by the SARS crisis and to meet the special needs of certain social groups hit hard by the crisis. Therefore, the Beijing government adopted a number of related measures. On April 2, the General Office of Beijing Municipal Committee of CCP and Beijing Municipal Government issued an Emergency Circular on Intensifying SARS Prevention and Control among Migrant Workers and on Construction Sites in an attempt to better protect migrant workers. On April 6, Workplace Injury Insurance Rules was promulgated, according to which, medical workers infected with SARS while treating patients would be defined as workplace injury. On May 6, Beijing Municipal Bureau of Finance and Local Taxation Bureau urgently drafted Preferential and Supporting Measures on Taxi Taxation of Beijing Municipality.

### 3.2.5 May 9–June 24: SARS epidemic declines and everyday activities resume

On May 9, the newly infected SARS cases declined to half the number the day before, reaching less than fifty for the first time. The epidemic situation in Beijing had entered the stage of decline, thus the corresponding crisis management reached the stage of recovery from the crisis. During this period of decision-making, one critical problem still remaining for the government was to keep the epidemic situation under control, to get Beijing removed from WHO's list of SARS-infected areas, and to lift the travel advisory against the city as soon as possible. Another troubling matter was how to walk out of the shadow of SARS and restore the city's normal social and economic activities. The government needed to terminate the state of emergency and resume its everyday activities as well as plan and implement reforms.

During this period, Beijing established a number of laws and regulations concerning SARS, and adopted a series of precautionary measures in order to prevent negligence during the period of decline. On May 13, some related departments such as the Beijing Municipal Commission of Commerce, the Commission of Economy, the Bureau of Finance, the Bureau of Health, the Drug Administration, the First Aid Center, and the Center of Disease Control formed the Material Ensuring Group under the Joint Working Team of SARS Prevention and Treatment to ensure the supply of medical protection goods in Beijing. On May 18, they started trying to put into operation the network system for monitoring epidemic situations in the Center of Disease Control. The epidemic situation in Beijing was effectively kept under control. On May 19, the reported number of newly confirmed SARS cases declined to seven. Ten days later, there were no newly confirmed SARS cases reported. On June 2, Beijing reported three "zeros" for the first time: no newly suspected patients, no newly confirmed patients, and no new SARS deaths.

SARS had negatively influenced people's private and professional lives, and there was a desperate need to return to normal activities (Crisis Management Research Group, 2003: No. 14). Thus, the government made attempts to resume and strengthen the city's ordinary social and economic activities, and implemented a series of macro-control measures to eliminate the negative economic impact caused by SARS.

On June 20, the last eighteen SARS patients recovered and left Xiaotangshan Hospital. On June 24, WHO announced that Beijing's epidemic situation had been mitigated, complying with WHO's standards. WHO decided to remove Beijing from its list of SARS-infected areas and lifted its travel advisory against this city. This decision took effect immediately.

### *3.3 Post-processing and learning after the crisis*

Beijing achieved the victory of controlling SARS, which did not mean the end of crisis management process. Quite the contrary, it unveiled a new stage—the stage of post-processing and learning. Beijing started the work of crisis post-processing and learning on June 24 when WHO announced it was removing Beijing from its list of SARS-infected areas and lifting the travel advisory against the city.

#### 3.3.1 Preventing another SARS outbreak

Obviously, Beijing had learned an important lesson from this unexpected event. Prevention, surveillance and disease control mechanisms gained new value in the fight against infectious diseases. Each disease prevention and control center in Beijing had implemented a SARS reporting system utilizing the internet and had healthcare workers on duty 24 hours a day. A SARS surveillance system was established at all levels consisting of healthcare administrative units, disease prevention and control centers, various medical institutions, and entry-exit inspection and quarantine departments.

Another significant crisis management lesson was the importance of early warning and precautionary measures. To prevent the reoccurrence of another SARS epidemic, the Beijing government issued the Preparing Project for Emergencies of SARS Prevention and Treatment in Beijing on September 11, 2004.

Besides, the government also learned that making information public and having good communications with the public were extremely important during a crisis. On September 19, the Ministry of Health announced the conditions of SARS surveillance on the mainland. On October 15, the Information Office of Beijing Municipal Government held its first press conference and provided public health information on how to prevent the reappearance of SARS that winter and the next spring. It also declared that it would publish public health information periodically.

3.3.2 Reinforce the public health system

Having suffered greatly from the SARS crisis, Beijing went deep into reflections upon the problems of the public health system. In accordance with these reflections, Beijing wanted to reinforce the establishment of the public health system, including "one mechanism, four systems." "One mechanism" meant the mechanism of meeting public health emergency. The government planned to establish a uniform, highly efficient and authoritative command system of meeting a public health emergency by 2005 and set up a command center in the Municipal Bureau of Health, which would be in charge of integrated command and coordination of first aid, medical treatment, pre-warning report, emergency response and on-the-spot management. The "four systems" were disease prevention and control system, public health emergency treatment system, public health information system and public health supervision system (Beijing's Public Health Work, November 2003).

3.3.3 Establish urban crisis management system

The SARS crisis heightened awareness and highlighted the importance of crisis management. The Beijing municipal government began to realize the importance of managing emergencies and crises. Consequently, efforts were made to establish an urban crisis management system. The Beijing municipal government started to consider setting up an all-round urban emergency response system and a consultative group of thirteen experts was created. This system would cover all social, civil and economic aspects of people's lives, including the subsystem of meeting emergencies such as serious transportation accidents, fires, severe animal epidemics, public health emergencies, safety of urban infrastructure, anti-terrorism, violent criminal activities, food production safety, earthquakes, floods, and drought.

## *4. Combating SARS in Beijing: Urban Crisis Management Challenges*

### *4.1 Crisis awareness*

Crisis awareness is a prerequisite for good crisis management: being in tune with the unraveling events, how they interact with other events, and sensing their potential impact. The crisis awareness of a government has a direct impact on its understanding, definition and formation of the crisis problem. Therefore, it is the foundation upon which a crisis pre-warning system is effectively established and crisis potency is recognized. It will influence a government's ability to make policies for crises and affect the management of crises.

The Beijing government's lack of crisis awareness was the main factor that resulted in the upheaval of the crisis and constantly worsened the SARS epidemic. When SARS was ravaging Guangdong, the government officials in Beijing lacked an understanding of the severity of the outbreak and were generally over-optimistic about it. As a result, Beijing lost its best opportunity for taking precautionary measures against SARS. Even when the first SARS cases appeared in Beijing, the government did not make an accurate definition of the crisis nor did it understand the magnitude of the crisis. Active crisis measures were not taken until the middle of April, after mounting pressure from abroad. The government's lack of crisis awareness was a contributing factor to the SARS epidemic in Beijing.

### *4.2 Mechanisms for initiating crisis management*

An authoritative, highly efficient and unitary core command and coordination system is often a critical factor for effective crisis response. For a long time China has lacked a complete and mature crisis command mechanism. In the early stage of the SARS crisis, the absence of a core command mechanism was the key reason for poor crisis management such as tardiness in crisis decision-making and obstacles in communication and coordination among departments. The Beijing authorities did not react to SARS with the necessary measures until April 13 when the Joint Working Team for SARS Prevention and Treatment was established under the leadership of the Secretary of Municipal Committee of CCP and the mayor. The team established a standing headquarter and worked around the clock to monitor the situation and to coordinate related work. However, the SARS epidemic was no longer a crisis just in Beijing, but a crisis that spread throughout the nation. The team's capability was limited in preventing SARS from scattering to other areas; coordinating the army in Beijing, the central government and international organizations; responding to international criticism; and managing domestic social disorder.

This crisis situation needed a core commanding institution at a higher level. On April 23, the State Council lead by Premier Wen Jiabao decided to set up the SARS Control and Prevention Headquarters of the State Council with the Vice-Premier Wu Yi as its Commander-in-Chief. The headquarters was in charge of the integrated command and coordination of the SARS prevention and treatment all around China. This high-level system of command and decision-making was the center of the anti-SARS campaign, virtually embodying the strategic resolution of the central government and its ability of handling a crisis. But what has to be emphasized is that, it was still more the command of high leaders of the nation than an effective core command system of crisis management that played the key role. A mature and complete crisis command system should be a system of automation; that is, when a crisis appears, it will automatically be put into motion and the various departments and units will immediately take appropriate action.

*4.3 Crisis communications*

In the age of globalization and information, an important aspect of crisis management is to foster good relations with the government, the media and the public. An effective crisis response network should include the government, social organizations, enterprises, individuals, and the international community; this network should provide the public and media with information and, if needed, mobilize the public.

The SARS crisis taught the government a hard lesson that it should be open with the public about the hard facts and communicate openly and promptly with the media. Even if a government cannot provide any information for the public, it should monitor informal information sources. Information transmitted by informal sources is often distorted and exaggerated and can easily intensify panic, causing an unimaginable psychological impact on society. Once rumors prevail, it becomes very difficult to keep a crisis under control. In Beijing, the government tried to conceal the news reported by the media but the public found news fragments, which aroused a number of rumors, by accessing information from the internet and other modern information channels. Consequently, the public became so disconcerted that they started to get suspicious of the government. Undoubtedly it would have been much better if the government had from the very beginning provided the public with information about SARS through the mainstream channels rather than waiting until the public started asking questions based on the rumors they had heard.

In the state of an emergency, governments often worry that negative news will create unnecessary social panic and cause social instability. But in reality, people become more rational in their thinking after an initial state of panic. For example, when the SARS epidemic was made public on April 20, the public did initially panic (rushing out to purchase masks and medicine) but soon the state of panic was pacified. The public started to trust the government again and the government's image was recovered.

On May 1 and 2, the Horizon Investigation Company telephoned 321 Beijing residents for a survey and the result showed that over 80 percent of the people felt the epidemic situation in Beijing were "very serious" or "quite serious," nearly half remained optimistic, and only 8 percent were pessimistic. Nonetheless, over 95 percent reported that they had confidence in the government and its ability to successfully defeat SARS (SPPM, 2003d: No. 13). As information was publicized, the public grew more conscious of self-protection and gradually understood and cooperated with the government. This was very helpful for the government since it needed to implement precautionary measures with the public's compliance (such as putting patients into isolation and cutting off transmission chains)in order to control the epidemic.

### *4.4 The government's credibility and international image during the crisis*

A crisis is usually characterized by high uncertainty and a lack of information. Once a crisis occurs, it easily creates speculations and rumors, which result in the public's intensive desire to find reliable information. Therefore, if the government does not provide reliable information, it will easily lose the trust of the people and the government's credibility will be severely challenged. A government's credibility is closely connected with how well it communicates with the public and if it provides trustworthy information.

On April 20, the central Chinese government adopted extraordinary measures to show its firm resolution against SARS and started to demonstrate a sense of responsibility by publicly confirming the SARS epidemic in Beijing. This actually helped restore the public's faith in the government. Surveys confirm that the government was able to gradually restore its credibility after its announcement on April 20.

On April 25 and 26, 2003, CCTV Market Research conducted a poll by telephone interviewing about three hundred people in Beijing. The results revealed that 96 percent of the respondents were confident that SARS would be successfully terminated (SPPM, 2003d: No. 13). The Department of Sociology at Nanjing University and the Center for Public Opinion Investigations and Analysis in Nanjing made two surveys in five major cities (Beijing, Shanghai, Guangzhou, Chongqing and Nanjing) from April 1 to 24, 2003. Their results confirmed the previous findings that the government evidently regained its credibility: 72 percent of the people considered that the government had a very strong or quite strong ability to deal with the crisis (Nanjing Daily, 26 May 2003).

During the SARS crisis, the Chinese government struggled to maintain its domestic credibility. Also, in the early stage of the crisis, the international community heavily criticized the Chinese government for not taking the necessary measures and for not properly informing the public of the newly found virus. The Chinese government was severely condemned, and even rejected, by the world community (SPPM, 2003c: No. 4).[4] After much international criticism, the Chinese government's attitude changed and it eagerly cooperated with the international community in an attempt to convince them that the Chinese government was sparing no resources in the fight against SARS and that it was fully capable of tackling the SARS epidemic.

Even the local authorities in Beijing were also condemned for being too sluggish in responding to the crisis and for concealing the truth. The foreign media expressed their deep concerns for the Olympic Games scheduled to be held in Beijing, questioning the city's ability to handle crises (SPPM, 2003f: No. 16).

### *4.5 Learning from the Past: Fighting SARS*

Beijing emphasized coordination and communication in its crisis response to SARS, and it proved to be effective. The Beijing government adopted the policy of publishing information in a timely manner and communicating with the public. Hotlines were established in Beijing in order to deal with the public's concerns and questions.

Beijing emphasized cooperating with international organizations and, in return, received significant support from several international organizations (e.g., WHO and the Red Cross). For example, MHO in Beijing and Beijing CDC held a conference in order to discuss matters concerning SARS prevention and control with WHO experts.

Definitely, some problems surfaced during the SARS outbreak, concerning prevention and control: lab management, hospital hygiene and quarantine routines, and reporting medical information. These problems also highlight the problem of disjoint between crisis management and daily management.

## *5. Conclusion*

Symbolically the SARS outbreak in Beijing was a significant test for China as a great world leader, since the city is the political and cultural capital of the nation. In addition, the central Chinese government is physically located here as well as many international organizations. The entire world had their eyes on Beijing. Despite the initial delay from the local and central Chinese authorities in dealing with SARS, Beijing became the turning point for China's management of the SARS outbreak.

## *Notes*

1. The case study draws mainly from the research made by the School of Public Policy and Management (SPPM) at Tsinghua University. The fruits of the research include over twenty "Studies on Emergency Management: SARS Special Publication" and more than thirty "Study Reports on China's Situation: SARS Special Publication."

2. This article cites the speech given for the colloquia of experts on "Strengthening the establishment of public health system and accelerating coordinated development of the economy and society" held by the State Council on June 17, 2003, with Premier Wen Jiabao as chairman.

3. On April 4, Vice Premier Wu Yi inspected the Center of Disease Control and said that "highest priority" should be given to SARS precautionary measures. On April 13 at a nationwide working conference for SARS prevention, Premier Wen Jiabao said that the SARS situation was still "extremely serious." On April 17, the Secretary General of Central Committee of CCP presided over the standing meeting of the Politics Bureau and presented a special report on SARS prevention and control measures.

4. Of the 202 reports about SARS in China published from March 31 to April 12, 2003, in four Western mainstream media sources (Washington Post, New York Times, CNN, and BBC), 132 reports were negative, 69 reports were neutral, and only one report was positive.

## *References*

Beijing's Public Health Work Conference (November 2003) Discussions carried out during the conference.

Beijing's Statistics Annual (2003).

Chi, Fulin (2003) "*The SARS crisis presses the birth of media reform in China.*" www.china.org.cn, 2003-6-16.

China Medical Association and China Association of Chinese Medicine (30 September 2003) *The Scheme for Diagnosis and Treatment of SARS.*

China News (14 May 2003) "The international community send understanding, compassion and aids to China for anti-SARS." www.chinanews.com.cn

Guo, Yong (2003) "The impact of the SARS crisis on China's governance framework." In *A Perspective View of SARS: Health and Development*, edited by Hu Angang, p. 271. Beijing: Tsinghua University Press.

Hu, Angang, Ed. (2003a) *Health and Development*. Beijing: Tsinghua University Press.

Hu, Angang (2003b) *China: A New Concept for Development.* Hangzhou: Zhejiang People's Press.

Liu, Ying (2003) "The international cooperation during China's response to the SARS crisis." In *A Perspective View of SARS: Health and Development*, edited by Hu Angang, pp 308-320. Beijing: Tsinghua University Press.

*Nanjing Daily* (26 May 2003) "Public opinion survey of residents in five major cities."

Sina (2003) "Vice Mayor of Beijing Confesses Five Defects in Beijing's Public Health System." Available at: http://www.sina.com.cn (Accessed on 20 November 2003).

SPPM (School of Public Policy and Management), Tsinghua University (2003a) *Studies on Emergency Management: SARS Special Publication.*

SPPM (2003b) *Study Reports on China's Situation: SARS Special Publication.*

SPPM (2003c) Why the Chinese government was struck by passivity - Comments on the concentration of negative reports on China by the western media." *Reports on China: Special SARS Issue.* No 4.

SPPM (2003d) "More rational, more optimistic and more confident - Beijing citizens' general opinions regarding the SARS Epidemic." *Reports on China: Special SARS Issue.* No 13.

SPPM (2003e) "Walking out of the shadow of SARS: Main Problems and Suggestions for Recovering from a Crisis." *Communications of Crisis Management Research. Special SARS Issue.* No. 14.

SPPM (2003f) "International media reports on SARS and their impact on China's international image." *Communications of Crisis Management Research. Special SARS Issue.* No 16.

Wang, Chenguang (2003) "The nomocracy under the impact of emergencies." In *Thoughts When Confronting SARS*, published by the Beijing Planning Office of Philosophy and Social Science. Beijing: Tongxin Press.

Xue, Lan and Qin Zhu (2003a) *Define Clearly the Position of the Government, Strengthen the Market System, and Promote Actively the Deep Reform of Public Health System.* Beijing: Tsinghua University Press.

Xue, Lan and Qin Zhu (2003b) *Crisis Management in China: the Challenge of the Transition.* Beijing: Tsinghua University Press.

Zhang Xiaoqun (2003) "The Role of Chinese media in the SARS crisis and their transform tendency." In *A Perspective View of SARS: Health and Development*, edited by Hu Angang. Beijing: Tsinghua University Press.

# Chapter 4
# The SARS Crisis and Crisis Management in Hong Kong

Simon Shen[1]

For many Hong Kong citizens, the outbreak of severe acute respiratory syndrome (SARS) in 2003 was to be an unforgettable experience. Between February and June 2003, more than 1,700 people were infected with the SARS virus and nearly three hundred died. The epidemic can be regarded as the most serious crisis that the Hong Kong Special Administrative Region Government (HKSARG) had ever faced. The aim of this paper is to evaluate the crisis management of the HKSARG in dealing with the SARS outbreak. The status of Hong Kong and its administration are described and the chronology of the outbreak mapped out. The most important decision-making occasions that occurred during the epidemic are highlighted and analyzed. The Disease Ordinances of Hong Kong and Sweden are then compared. Last but not least, the impact of SARS on civil society and Hong Kong's accountability system is discussed. However in order to understand the entire story, a general description is provided of Hong Kong's administrative system, in particular its connection with the mainland's after the handover.

## *1. Hong Kong and Its Administration*

Hong Kong is a Special Administrative Region of the People's Republic of China and is composed of three parts: Hong Kong Island, the Kowloon Peninsula and the New Territories. Formally it is called the Hong Kong Special Administrative Region (HKSAR). Hong Kong is very small and much of its huge population lives in densely populated areas. In 2004, Hong Kong had a population of approximately 6.8 million, with a population density of about 6,300 people per square kilometer (Hong Kong in Brief, 2004). Located at the southern tip of the Pearl River Delta, Hong Kong is one of the biggest cities in Asia. Geographically, Hong Kong and mainland China are close. Following the reopening of the mainland's borders and, more recently, Hong Kong's handover to China, there has been a growing trend of economic cooperation between Hong Kong and the mainland. Cross-border trade and investment have increased compared to previous decades. The manufacturing sector of Hong Kong has gradually moved its production facilities northwards into China, attracted by lower rents and salaries. In return, growing enterprises in China have relied to a certain extent on the service sector of Hong Kong for financial, banking, accounting, and transportation support. It can be said that to some extent the economies of Hong Kong and China have grown hand in hand.

Hong Kong was returned to China on July 1, 1997, becoming then a Special Administrative Region. The Principle of "One Country, Two Systems" was adopted in Hong Kong and the HKSARG exercises a high degree of autonomy and enjoys executive, legislative and independent judicial power, including that of final adjudication, in accordance with the provisions of the Basic Law (Basic Law of HKSAR of the People's Republic of China: Article 2). As stipulated by the Basic Law, the socialist system and policies shall not be practiced in Hong Kong and the capitalist system and the way of life shall remain unchanged for fifty years (Basic Law of HKSAR of the People's Republic of China: Article 5). Government contacts and cooperation as well as the population flow have been growing rapidly. The social and economic ties between Hong Kong and the Pearl River Delta region are especially close and encouraged by their geographical proximity. Cross-border traffic and consumption also have increased.

### *1.1 Hierarchy of Hong Kong's Health Care System*

The current structure of the public health system comprises three institutions: the Health, Welfare and Food Bureau, the Department of Health, and the Hospital Authority. Set out below is a brief description of the role of each of the three institutions in safeguarding the health of the community.

*The Health, Welfare and Food Bureau (HWFB)* is one of the eleven policy bureaus of the HKSAR and assumes responsibility for all matters relating to health, social welfare, food and environmental hygiene, and women's interests. The Department of Health, the Hospital Authority, the Food and Environmental Hygiene Department, the Social Welfare Department, and the Government Laboratory are all under the HWFB. The HWFB is responsible for the management and allocation of nearly one-third of the government's entire annual recurrent expenditure (SARS Expert Committee Report, 2003: p.8). The Secretary for Health, Welfare and Food (SHWF) is the head of the HWFB and is a Principal Official (PO) under the accountability system. POs are nominated by the Chief Executive and appointed by the Central People's Government (SARS Expert Committee Report, 2003: p.9). The SHWF is further supported by the Permanent Secretary for Health, Welfare and Food, a number of Deputy Secretaries and some two hundred other civil servants.

*The Department of Health (DH)* acts as a health adviser to the Government of the HKSAR, a health advocate in the community, and an executive arm in health legislation and policy. It also assumes responsibility in safeguarding the health of the community through various services. The DH is responsible for conducting disease surveillance and control of communicable diseases, preventive health programs, public health education and promotion, development of traditional Chinese medicine, public health regulation and licensing, port health measures, tobacco control, and family health and social hygiene services. The Director of Health is the head of the DH and reports to the SHWF, so preferably he/she should be a medical professional. The department is accountable to the HWFB.

In addition to the HWFB and the DH, a further health institution assumes responsibility for the provision of public hospital services within Hong Kong. This is the *Hospital Authority (HA)*, which is a statutory and independent body. The HA is responsible for the establishment and management of public hospitals. It advises the government on issues concerning public needs for hospital services and resources in running them, as well as assisting and providing the necessary training and education for persons engaged in providing hospital services. Unlike the HWFB and the DH, the HA is not a governmental department, but serves as an independent body and is governed by an HA Board appointed by the Chief Executive of the HKSAR, which includes three ex-officio members: the Director of Health; the Deputy Secretary for Health, Welfare and Food; and the Deputy Secretary for Financial Services and the Treasury. The HA is accountable to the government for its provision of public hospital services in an effective and efficient manner. During the SARS crisis, the three healthcare institutions worked together to fight the epidemic.

## 2. Epidemic in Hong Kong: A Chronology

### 2.1 Prelude (Mid-February to Mid-March 2003)

On February 10, 2003, the local media in Hong Kong began to report an outbreak of atypical pneumonia in Guangdong Province. When the details of this unusual epidemic, which produced a fatal pneumonia-like illness, came to light, they induced panic in the community (SingTao Daily, 10 February 2003: A01). In response to the news, the DH conducted a media briefing on February 11, 2003 and reassured the community that there were no signs to indicate that this influenza-like illness and respiratory tract infection had reached Hong Kong. However, the situation was being closely monitored because of the proximity of the cases of pneumonia in Guangdong. A Working Group on Severe Community-acquired Pneumonia (CAP)[2] was formed by the HA head office to give advice on the monitoring and approaches to be adopted should cases of SARS occur. Comprised of experts from microbiology, medicine, and intensive care medicine, the group agreed upon a set of procedures for the notification of SARS cases for epidemiological investigation and action. The group later further refined the reporting mechanism for SARS cases from hospitals to the HA's Secretariat of Infection Control Taskforce and prepared an information package on the management of SARS, which included the reporting mechanism and case definition. On February 13, 2003, the HA commenced notification to the DH of suspected and confirmed SARS cases, and private hospitals were also required to report any SARS cases upon admission. As a new disease, it was not previously statutorily reportable.

On February 22, 2003, Kwong Wah hospital admitted Liu Janlun, who was a professor from Guangzhou and was suspected of having SARS. He died on March 4, 2003, but confirmation of the diagnosis was not obtained until mid-April after a definitive diagnostic test became available. Professor Liu Janlun infected members of his family (including his wife, daughter and brother-in-law), a registered nurse in Kwong Wah Hospital, and a number of hotel guests and visitors at the Metropole Hotel in Hong Kong. He was one of the first SARS cases in Hong Kong and was later identified as the index case in the outbreak in the Metropole Hotel where he had stayed for only one night. The Metropole Hotel was later identified as the source of international spread. Infected hotel guests and visitors unwittingly had carried the SARS virus to other countries including Singapore, Canada and Vietnam.

On the same day as Professor Liu Janlun from Guangzhou was admitted to hospital, a woman was transferred from the Union Hospital to the Prince of Wales Hospital. She had been to Guangzhou in late January and was found to have symptoms of SARS. Ten days after her admission, on March 4, 2003, she checked out of the hospital against medical advice and was diagnosed with SARS in April 2003. Only one of four contacts of this woman was eventually found to have developed SARS and a nurse in the Union Hospital developed symptoms of SARS. The nurse was admitted to the Princess Margaret Hospital in late-February 2003. She made a full recovery and was discharged but was later, in April 2003, diagnosed to have had SARS.

On March 5, 2003, the World Health Organization (WHO) informed the DH that a Chinese American, Johnny Chen, would be transferred from Hanoi to Hong Kong for treatment. Accompanying this was a message that seven healthcare workers who had rendered care or assistance to him had reported symptoms of an unknown infection. Johnny Chen was admitted to the intensive care unit of the Princess Margaret Hospital and received care in isolation. The DH conducted contact tracing and surveillance, and epidemiological and intensive laboratory investigations were made on the Johnny Chen case. In addition, strict infection control measures were implemented so that no healthcare staff was infected during his period of treatment. Nevertheless, Johnny Chen was later linked to the outbreak in the Metropole Hotel and confirmed as the source of the SARS outbreak in Hanoi, Vietnam.

### *2.2 The Outbreak of the SARS Epidemic at the Prince of Wales Hospital*

On March 4, 2003, a local resident of Hong Kong was admitted to Ward 8A of the Prince of Wales Hospital with the provisional diagnosis of SARS. However, as his condition gradually improved after admission, he was never categorized as a SARS case. He was put on a nebulizer in the hospital between March 6 and 12, 2003. He was later confirmed to be a SARS case linked to the outbreak in the Metropole Hotel and the index patient in the Prince of Wales Hospital outbreak.

On March 10, 2003, the outbreak of an epidemic was apparent. The hospital management was notified that a group of eleven healthcare staff (seven doctors and four nurses), all of whom had worked in Ward 8A, had gone on sick leave simultaneously. A possible communicable disease outbreak was suspected and Ward 8A was immediately closed to admission and visitors. This was later modified to just visitor restrictions. A special meeting was convened by the hospital that morning, with the participation of clinicians, the infection control team, hospital management, and the community physician of the DH's New Territories East Regional Office. At the meeting, the hospital was advised to isolate the SARS cases, screen other wards, and monitor sick-leave records. Furthermore, an epidemiological survey would be conducted. Disease surveillance was also initiated. All staff members on sick leave were called back for physical check-ups and screening.

On March 12, 2003, the DH informed the WHO of the outbreak in the Prince of Wales Hospital and a press conference was called to inform the public of the contraction of SARS by healthcare staff at the hospital. A Disease Control Centre was set up to handle and manage the outbreak. Measures were adopted to prevent cross-contamination among staff members and cross-infection between patients. On the same day, the WHO issued a global alert about cases of an acute respiratory syndrome in Vietnam, Hong Kong, and the Guangdong Province in China of unknown etiology that appeared to place health workers at high risk.

On March 13, 2003, the SHWF reviewed the outbreak situation in the Prince of Wales Hospital with officers from the DH, the HA and a WHO representative. The DH's team confirmed as the index case, and the source of the outbreak in the hospital, a local resident who had been admitted to Ward 8A on March 4, 2003. Discharged patients, visitors, staff members, medical students, and in-patients who had been exposed to this patient were then examined. However, the number of SARS cases began to grow and subsequent investigations revealed that this Ward 8A patient had infected a total number of 143 persons: 50 healthcare workers, 17 medical students, four relatives, 30 Ward 8A patients, and 42 visitors to Ward 8A (SARS Expert Committee Report, 2003: p.2006).

On March 15, 2003, in the light of the spread of infection, the WHO issued an emergency travel advisory naming the illness Severe Acute Respiratory Syndrome (SARS) and listing the main symptoms and signs. No recommendations were given to restrict travel to any destination.

On March 19, 2003, the DH announced that at least seven SARS cases were related to the Metropole Hotel. The index case of this cluster was identified as Liu Janlun. On March 22, 2003, the University of Hong Kong announced the identification of a novel variant *coronavirus* as the causative agent in SARS.

Meanwhile, other healthcare establishments also experienced SARS outbreaks, but the extent and scale were much smaller.

*2.3 Community Outbreak: Outbreak in Amoy Gardens*

On March 26, 2003, the United Christian Hospital admitted fifteen suspected SARS cases from seven households. All of them resided in Amoy Gardens. The DH made a field visit to the housing estate on the same day to interview those in twenty accessible units on the seven floors with suspected cases, all in Block E. The affected households did not know each other and were not involved in any common activities. The DH then placed family members of suspected SARS cases under medical surveillance and initiated contact tracing. The building management was instructed to disinfect the common areas in all blocks.

Between March 27 and 29, 2003, the DH made further visits to Amoy Gardens and an inter-departmental work force was set up to monitor the whole situation. On March 27, 2003, the government announced new measures in handling and managing the SARS epidemic, including adding SARS to the list of infectious diseases specified in the First Schedule to the Quarantine and Prevention of Disease Ordinance (Chapter 141 of the Laws of Hong Kong) with immediate effect and introducing a health declaration for incoming visitors to Hong Kong, effective from March 29, 2003. As the outbreak in Amoy Gardens represented a community outbreak in Hong Kong, the government decided to suspend classes in all schools effective from March 29, 2003 to April 6, 2003, when the Easter holiday began.

On March 30, 2003, the number of cases in Amoy Gardens totaled 190, of which almost 50 percent were in Block E. (SARS Expert Committee Report, 2003: p.48). The severe outbreak of infection in Block E was followed by an order of the DH to isolate all of Block E for ten days from March 31, 2003. However, the DH later announced that the residents in Block E were to be transferred to three government holiday camps for isolation, while an investigation and disinfection of the estate took place. Then from April 12, 2003, the government started to release the names of other buildings with confirmed SARS cases, which was later extended to naming buildings with suspected SARS cases.

*2.4 The Decline of the Epidemic*

The SARS epidemic in Hong Kong can be said to have started from the outbreak in the Prince of Wales Hospital, with the peak of infection occurring at the Amoy Gardens outbreak. After that, there was a gradual decline in the epidemic, and a drop in the number of newly infected cases began in late April. At that time, there were some reported cases of SARS in different buildings, hospitals and estates, but they were of a smaller scale and extent.

On May 4, 2003, the daily number of new cases fell for first time to below ten, and from May 16, 2003, the daily number fell to below five. Soon afterwards, on May 23, 2003, the WHO lifted the travel advisory against Hong Kong and Hong Kong was finally removed from the SARS list on June 23, 2003. There had been 1,755 cases reported during the entire SARS epidemic, of which nearly three hundred had been fatal. Among the dead were eight healthcare workers; six of these were from public hospitals and two were private doctors (SARS Expert Committee Report, 2003: p.65). Following the end of the SARS epidemic, a period of evaluation was conducted by the HA, the government, and the Legislative Council.

## *3. The Most Important Decision-Making Occasions during SARS*

The outbreak of SARS in Hong Kong started in February 2003 and ended on June 23, 2003, when the WHO removed Hong Kong from the SARS list. During this period, the HKSARG implemented many policies and measures in order to control and prevent the epidemic from spreading further. Of all the government decisions, the handling of the SARS outbreaks at the Prince of Wales Hospital and Amoy Gardens was far more important than any other event. The outbreak in the Prince of Wales Hospital marked the beginning of the SARS epidemic in Hong Kong. Many patients were either infected at the hospital or by SARS carriers who had visited the hospital. In total, 114 healthcare workers, 17 medical students, 39 patients, and 42 visitors were infected. Therefore, the effectiveness of the HKSARG in handling the outbreak in the Prince of Wales Hospital had a great impact on the outcome of the epidemic. On the other hand, the Amoy Gardens case represented the outbreak of the SARS epidemic in the community. With more than five thousand families and around seventeen thousand residents living in Amoy Gardens, the government had to handle the outbreak there very carefully to prevent a dreadful disaster from occurring (SARS Expert Committee Report, 2003: p.35).

### *3.1 Handling the SARS outbreak at the Prince of Wales Hospital*

The government's response to the SARS outbreak at the Prince of Wales Hospital received the most criticism from the public. On March 10, 2003, when the hospital found that eleven healthcare staff from ward 8A had that day gone on sick leave, it was realized that there was an outbreak of an unnamed infectious disease. A decision was finally made to close Ward 8A and to prohibit admissions and visitors. At the cluster meetings on atypical pneumonia, the members of the hospital cluster management and medical experts refused to accept the proposed closure of the hospital but argued to continue its operation. The next day, the no-visiting policy to Ward 8A was modified. Visitors were allowed to enter the ward if they were wearing surgical masks, and disposable gowns and gloves. In order to prevent the epidemic from spreading further, various measures were instituted in the Prince of Wales Hospital (SARS Expert Committee Report, 2003: p.204). Non-emergency surgical operations were suspended, while non-atypical pneumonia emergency medical patients and those attending the emergency department at the Prince of Wales Hospital were diverted to the nearby Alice Ho Miu Ling Nethersole Hospital and the North District Hospital. Moreover, infection control guidelines and upgraded measures for droplet infection were issued, and staff members were also given twice-a-week training sessions on infection control. In addition, a "cluster meeting on atypical pneumonia" forum was established to meet twice a day to provide guidelines and make decisions on disease and infection control.

On the evening of March 13, 2003, Ward 8A was reopened as a cohort ward for patients with atypical pneumonia while Ward 8B was used for patients with confirmed or suspected atypical pneumonia. Ward 8D was opened as a screening ward and used to admit all patients with fever and respiratory symptoms for initial diagnostic screening. Patients were transferred to Ward 8A (male) or Ward 8B (female) for further treatment if they had symptoms of fever and lymphopaenia together with chest X-ray changes and a contact history. The next day, all clinical admissions to the medical department of the Prince of Wales Hospital were stopped. On March 17, 2003, medical emergencies in the hospital were diverted to other hospitals outside the New Territories East Cluster and later the accident and emergency services were suspended until March 30, 2003.

### *3.2 Handling the Community Outbreak in Amoy Gardens*

Amoy Gardens was the residential area which was most affected by the outbreak of SARS. Hundreds of residents from Amoy Gardens were infected with the disease during that period. The DH was first notified about the outbreak in Amoy Gardens on March 26, 2003, as the United Christian Hospital had admitted fifteen suspected SARS cases from seven households, all of which were in Block E of Amoy Gardens. Besides placing family members of all those with suspected SARS under medical surveillance and initiating contract tracing, the DH also sent a medical team to the estate to collect information. On March 27, 2003, a multidisciplinary team led by the DH went to Amoy Gardens to make a detailed site inspection and two medical stations manned by the Auxiliary Medical Service were set up at Block E to take the body temperatures of residents and to provide SARS-related information.

When by March 30, 2003, the total number of suspected and confirmed cases in Amoy Gardens had risen to 190, of whom half were from Block E, the government decided to issue that evening an isolation order for Block E of Amoy Gardens (SARS Expert Committee Report, 2003: p.48). Starting from March 31, 2003, residents from Block E were not allowed to leave the block or received visitors for ten days. The government later found evidence suggesting that the sewage and drainage system might have been involved in the vertical spread of SARS in Block E. In order to prevent the disease from spreading further in Amoy Gardens, the government decided to evacuate all Block E residents to three government holiday camps and this operation was carried out on April 1, 2004. In total, 247 residents were moved to these camps for medical surveillance (SARS Expert Committee Report, 2003: p.50).

After the evacuation, the Food and Environmental Hygiene Department launched a disinfection and pest control exercise in Amoy Gardens and its surrounding areas, concentrating especially on Block E. At the same time, a team was sent to carry out in-depth investigations in Amoy Gardens. Urged by the Owners' Committee, the government also released the names of other buildings where there were SARS cases. The isolation order for Block E expired on April 9, 2003 and residents then started to return to the building. The evacuation was claimed to have been successful in preventing a further outbreak of SARS in Amoy Gardens as only five more cases occurred among residents of Block E after the isolation order (SARS Expert Committee Report, 2003: p.52). After April 15, 2003, there were no more newly suspected or confirmed SARS cases from Block E.

## *4. Crisis Management Operation during the SARS Outbreak*

Crisis management by the HKSARG during the SARS outbreak is discussed here. The entire crisis management process has been divided into three parts: pre-crisis management, operation during the crisis, and post-crisis management.

### *4.1 Pre-crisis Management*

Infectious diseases differ from other crises, such as traffic accidents or natural disasters, which are often unpredictable or occur suddenly without any prior warning. Outbreaks of diseases (like SARS or the avian flu) and their effects on society can be minimized with better government control and if they are identified and dealt with in an early stage.

#### 4.1.1 Surveillance and Warning Systems

First of all, effective surveillance and warning systems play a significant role in managing crises involving infectious diseases. The outbreak of SARS in Hong Kong has shown that the HKSARG acquired insufficient information in the early stages from its surveillance and warning system. As a consequence, the HKSARG underestimated the effects of the disease.

Due to its geographical proximity to Guangdong Province and the fact that it is one of the most densely populated provinces in China, Hong Kong is at great risk if there is an outbreak of a disease in Guangdong. Before the SARS epidemic, there had been an agreement between the cities in the Pearl River Delta Region of Guangdong (e.g., Guangzhou, Zhuhai, Shenzhen, and Hong Kong) on cross-border notification of diseases. These cities had agreed to monthly exchanges of statistics and information on specific infectious diseases. However, shortcomings in this notification system had weakened the HKSARG's capacity to collect sufficient information on the outbreak of SARS in Guangdong. The government was thus not warned about the seriousness of the disease until its outbreak in March. For a start, only diseases such as cholera, malaria, and viral hepatitis were included in this notification system; the system did not allow for the exchange of statistics on other infectious diseases or emerging infections. Although the first investigative report on SARS was finished by the health authority of Guangdong Province as early as January 23, 2003, the HKSARG had not been notified about the epidemic until it was reported by the Hong Kong media on February 10, 2003. Secondly, as the agreement had been signed only by a number of cities in the Pearl River Delta Region in the Guangdong Province, it was difficult for Hong Kong to get information relating to outbreaks of infectious diseases in other parts of Guangdong or its surrounding provinces.

Moreover, the HKSARG lack of awareness of the SARS epidemic in Guangdong Province also reflected the poor collaboration that existed between health authorities in Mainland China and Hong Kong. After the media coverage on SARS in mainland China, the DH in Hong Kong tried on February 10, 2003 to gain information about the disease from the health authorities in Guangzhou by phone and by fax. However, Guangzhou did not reply. Finally, the DH was obliged to seek help from the Director General of the Department of International Cooperation of the Ministry of Health in Beijing. This event has shown that there is a need for better collaboration between the health authorities of the HKSARG and the authorities in Mainland China. One interesting point is that the fax sent by the DH to Guangzhou was written in English, which is an official language in Hong Kong, but not in Mainland China. This also reminds us that when organizations are dealing with each other, the culture of the other party should not be ignored.

Apart from showing the inability of the HKSARG to collect statistics on infectious diseases occurring outside Hong Kong, the outbreak of SARS also exposed the weaknesses of the local surveillance and warning systems for new diseases. The challenge was that under the existing protocol, it was difficult for the government to detect the occurrence of a new disease outbreak of unknown etiology and request its timely report by healthcare providers to the government without a clear case definition in the first place. Due to the sudden escalation of the crisis, the DH had to rely on healthcare providers to report cases on infectious diseases by letter or fax (SARS Expert Committee Report, 2003: p.106). An ad hoc passive surveillance system was set up by the HA in mid-February only after the notification of SARS cases in Guangdong. Although the system was extended to private hospitals with the assistance of the DH, it was not a comprehensive disease surveillance system as the government was unable to get adequate information from the private sector and laboratories (SARS Expert Committee Report, 2003: p.105).

4.1.2 Preparedness

Apart from having surveillance and warning systems, governments can also help cope with crises in advance by having emergency response plans. With these plans in place, it is possible for governments to manage crises or emergency situations more effectively and thus minimize their effects. In Hong Kong, although it was found that the HKSARG has made an effort towards crisis management by preparing its own emergency response system, outbreaks of infectious disease were not considered a major crisis management concern and thus the emergency response system did not work in dealing with the outbreak of SARS.

The emergency response system of the HKSARG had been largely prepared by the Emergency Support Unit of the Security Bureau. According to the government, an emergency is defined as "any event, natural or man-made, that demands a rapid response in order to protect life, property and public security" (The Government of HKSAR Emergency Response System, 2003: Chapter 2). For situations that lead to "a serious disruption of life, probably arising with little or no warning, that cause or threaten death or injury on a scale exceeding the normal responses required of the public emergency services," they are even defined by the government as "extreme emergencies or disasters" (The Government of HKSAR Emergency Response System, 2003: Chapter 2). By these definitions, the outbreaks of SARS in Hong Kong should have been regarded by the government as an "emergency" or even an "extreme disaster" as the effects of the epidemic were potentially tremendous. However, it seems that the HKSARG has never considered the outbreak of infectious disease as something emergent. At that time, the government had only prepared contingency plans for situations like an aircraft crash, natural disasters, terrorism, and an accident at the Daya Bay Nuclear Station. The government would also implement the emergency response system in the event of a serious traffic accident which resulted in heavy casualties, such as happened in the Tuen Mun Highway bus crash on July 10, 2003. Although departments like the HA and DH were included in the emergency response system and provided support in emergencies, the HKSARG had not prepared any contingency plans for dealing with infectious diseases before the outbreak of SARS in February 2003.

Although the outbreak of the avian flu in 1997 had already shown that infectious disease could be a threat to Hong Kong, the fairly successful measures taken by the government then without any advanced planning may have given government officials the impression that a further outbreak of infectious disease could also be handled without prior preparation.

When a crisis or disaster is looming, pre-planned systems can often be insufficient and additional ad hoc measures may be needed. In the case of SARS, the authorities in Hong Kong could have been more aware of the severity of the epidemic if early information had been obtained directly from Guangdong. However, the pre-established notification system meant that Guangdong was not obliged to report the outbreak of the epidemic to Hong Kong. After media reports of the epidemic, the DH could still have done more to get relevant information directly from Guangdong. Unfortunately, the DH seemed to be unwilling or ill prepared to communicate with officials from an unfamiliar organization. This is a factor likely to affect information flow between organizations when there is a crisis (Quarantelli, 1998:373-385). As a result, no one was dispatched to Guangdong from the DH and bizarrely the fax sent to Guangdong was written in English.

Moreover, experience from the earlier avian flu crisis could have encouraged the government not to employ the emergency response system. The relative success of their dealing with avian flu might have persuaded the government that ad hoc measures would be sufficient in the event of the outbreak of another epidemic. Contrary to research findings which conclude that previous disaster experience leads to higher levels of preparedness and a more effective response, it seems that experience can also provide false security that similar measures would be sufficient to deal with another comparable crisis, even if it was more serious (Mileti, 1999:228).

### *4.2 Operation during the Crisis*

Public healthcare services in Hong Kong are jointly provided by various government departments and organizations including the HWFB, the HA, as well as the DH, and each of them has it own tasks and responsibilities. However, the outbreak of SARS has highlighted the poor communication between these departments and organizations. The following discusses the decision-making, coordinating and communicating processes of the HKSARG in dealing with the SARS epidemic.

#### 4.2.1 Decision-making

The HWFB is a policy bureau responsible for all issues related to healthcare and hygiene in Hong Kong and the DH is one of the government departments within this bureau. However, laws in Hong Kong provide the Director of Health with more power than the SHWF in controlling and preventing infectious diseases. On the other hand, the HA is an independent organization which administers all public hospitals in Hong Kong, but policies made by the HWFB will also affect public hospitals. Therefore, the SHWF, the Director of Health, as well as the Chief Executive of the HA could all make decisions affecting public healthcare services at the time of the SARS epidemic.

At the time of the outbreak of SARS in mid-March, there was no centralized decision-making body responsible for the control of the disease. On March

14, 2003, soon after the outbreak at the Prince of Wales Hospital, the SHWF set up the HWFB Taskforce, which supervised the measures taken by both the DH and the HA when dealing with the epidemic and collected and organized experts' opinions to assist both the DH and HA. The taskforce was chaired by the SHWF and members included medical experts from the DH, the HA and local universities, as well as officials from the DH and HA. Decisions made by the taskforce were to be implemented by the HWFB, DH and the HA.

Despite the presence of the taskforce, not all decision-making power was centralized. For instance, the HA decided to suspend accident and emergency medical services in the Prince of Wales Hospital on March 18, 2003 without consulting the DH. But as the outbreak continued, the taskforce had to play a more active role in coordinating the work of the DH and the HA. When the Director of Health suggested during a taskforce meeting that selected medical centers should be established to identify patients infected with SARS, it was decided at the meeting that, with the consent from the HA, the Princess Margaret Hospital would become a SARS hospital.

While the taskforce was made up of the bodies responsible for public health, an Inter-departmental Action Coordinating Committee (IACC) was set up on March 24, 2003, and chaired by the Permanent Secretary for Health, Welfare and Food. Its members included representatives from more than twenty five policy bureaus, departments and public bodies (SARS Expert Committee Report, 2003: p.104). The aim of the IACC was to coordinate the implementation of decisions made by the would-be-established CESC and the SHWF (Ibid).

One day later, the Chief Executive created another decision-making body. The Chief Executive's Steering Committee (CESC), chaired by the Chief Executive himself, was the highest decision-making body and it replaced the HWFB Taskforce. Members of the CESC included various Principal Officials of the policy bureau and the objectives of this committee were to "ensure better coordination of the Government's response and to ensure that the necessary manpower and financial resources were made available" (SARS Expert Committee Report, 2003: p.96).

As there were now three main ad hoc bodies within the government dealing with the outbreak of SARS, the decision-making was not straightforward, as it was heavily influenced by bureaucratic politics. On March 30, 2003, the SHWF requested the Director of Health to isolate residents living in Block E of Amoy Gardens during a taskforce meeting. As the only person who held such power, the Director of Health discussed this issue with other officials from the DH. Although the DH was just a department under the supervision of the SHWF, the DH did not accept the proposal immediately. The concerns raised by the DH included the criteria for triggering an isolation order to restrict movements of residents of other blocks in Amoy Gardens and other housing estates, and the additional heavy workload on the law enforcement agencies and other departments to provide meals and other support services. Officials from the DH also questioned whether better options existed, such as compulsory attendance at designated medical centers or immediate removal of residents to camps. The signal that such action would send to local and international communities was also a matter of concern. The response of the SHWF was to claim that officials from the DH simply feared that Hong Kong would become a "laughing stock" in the public health sector. The decision was finally made after further discussion involving other top officials, including the Chief Secretary and the Secretary of Justice.

The potential conflict between the SHWF and the DH probably also influenced the decision to make SARS a statutory notifiable disease. While the WHO gave the name "severe acute respiratory syndrome (SARS)" to the epidemic on March 15, 2003, the disease was not made a statutory notifiable disease until March 26. Again, the Director of Health was the official who had the power to amend this ordinance. But as she subsequently revealed to the Legislative Council, the process of amending the ordinance was slowed up because of the controversy about the name and the definition of the disease. The SHWF was particularly concerned about the name, because "SARS" was similar to the short form for the Special Administrative Region, "SAR." The HWFB even sent an email to the DH, telling the DH to use the term "SRS" when announcing news to the public. Though the Legislative Council report concluded that the controversy regarding the name and definition of the disease did not affect the process of amending the ordinance, the signal received from the HWFB by the HA could have affected the decision made by the Director of Health. As the ordinance was not amended until March 27, measures like asking relatives of SARS patients to report to designated medical centers could not be imposed earlier.

After the outbreak of the SARS epidemic, a number of ad hoc organizations were set up within the government. As suggested by E.L. Quarantelli (1998:373-385), organizational authority conflicts can often be a problem with organizational decision-making when there are disasters. In Hong Kong's case, we can also see that it was unclear where the power lay for decision-making after the setting up of these organizations. According to Roland Warren (1967:369-419), organizational units may make decisions under four different contexts, namely unitary, federative, coalitional and social choice. While the HWFB Taskforce and then the CESC did play a commanding role during the crisis, which might suggest the context was unitary, both the DH and the HA clearly retained their authorities. However, they had to listen to the "orders" given by higher officials such as the isolation of the residents in Block E of Amoy Gardens, so the context was not federative either. In fact, this unclear distribution of decision-making power means that decision-making may have to be understood by employing the bureaucratic politics model developed by Graham Allison and Morton Halperin (1972:40-79). For instance, we saw how the

DH, who clearly held a different attitude than the SWHF regarding the isolation of residents, needed another meeting with higher officials from the CESC to agree upon issuing the isolation order. Although we do not know exactly what was discussed among the officials, units with different roles and stances finally reached a consensus, probably after some bargaining.

4.2.2 Communication

In dealing with the epidemic, the government's communication methods can be divided into two: internal and external. Internal communication refers to the information process between government bureaus, departments and organizations. Before the outbreak of SARS, there was not a formal system in place for handling information on an epidemic. At the early stage of the outbreak, both the HA and the DH established their own SARS database, but neither of them could directly access the other's. This hindered the government in controlling the disease and preventing further outbreaks of SARS. Later, in late-March and early-April, various databases were set up by the government to improve its efficiency.

First of all, in order to collect information about the newly admitted SARS patients and to facilitate tracing of contacts, the HA and the DH jointly developed a comprehensive electronic web-based system (the e-SARS system) under the supervision of the SHWF. This ensured both the HA and the DH shared information about SARS patients in the hospitals. Second, the SARS Case Contact Information System (SARS-CCIS) was also developed by the DH. It was a "data management system with a cluster analysis function which helped the field epidemiologists to construct cluster trees and extract cases of identified clusters for analysis" (SARS Expert Committee Report, 2003: p.106). Besides this database in the healthcare sector, there was also the Major Incident Investigation and Disaster Support System (MIIDSS). This was a crime investigation program used by the Hong Kong Police Force that had been adopted to "help quickly identify linkage between cases and contacts and high-risk locations of SARS occurrence to enable rapid implementation of public health measures" (Ibid.).

In addition to having the above databases, the government enhanced its internal communication by the setting up of various decision-making and coordinating bodies like the CESC and the IACC. Since members of these committee included officials from different government bureaus, departments and organizations, processing information within the government could be done more directly.

External communication refers to the information process between the HKSARG and the public. The government provided information about the epidemic to the public mainly through speeches made by senior officials, press conferences held by various government departments, and government websites. However, the public criticized the government during the SARS epidemic for its unsatisfactory mechanisms for press releases. Officials from various departments sometimes provided different information on the same day, causing the public confusion. Therefore, starting from April 19, 2003, daily press conferences with information about SARS were jointly held by the HA and the DH. This ensured that the public received information from the government through a more centralized channel.

Information flow is crucial to successful disaster management (Quarantelli, 1998:373-385). The HKSARG was criticized by the public for its poor collaboration between its different departments in the early stage of the SARS outbreak. Through the establishment of various inter-departmental taskforces and committees, government efficiency in decision-making, in coordination and in communicating processes was enhanced because officials could regularly exchange information during meetings. At the same time, the role played by the SHWF prompted the DH and the HA to share information with one another. This case may suggest that a superior body is needed to play an active role to enhance information flow among lower-level organizations.

### *4.3 Post-crisis Management*

After managing a crisis, there are two important post-crisis stage tasks that a government should carry out: evaluation and accountability of officials. After solving crises or dealing with emergencies, the HKSARG tends to set up committees or request specific departments to evaluate the incidents and complete reports on related issues. It can be shown that the HKSARG had considered the recommendations in the reports but reverted to its old practices or systems. On the other hand, these reports also evaluated the performances of senior government officials in managing the crises. However, not even one senior government official directly resigned due to his/her performance in dealing with a crisis or emergency.

#### 4.3.1 Evaluation

In May 2003, the Chief Executive of the HKSAR set up a SARS Expert Committee and appointed various experts, both local and overseas, to the committee to conduct a review of the SARS outbreak in Hong Kong. There were three main tasks of the committee (SARS Expert Committee Report, 2003: p.2). The first task was to review the work of the government, including the HA, in the management and the control of the outbreak. The second main task was to examine and review the capabilities and structure of the healthcare system in Hong Kong and the organization and operation of the DH and the HA in the prevention and management of infectious diseases such as SARS. This committee was also to identify lessons to be learned, and to make recommendations for areas of improvement in order to better prepare the Hong Kong system for any future outbreaks.

The SARS Expert Committee released a report in October 2003 making various recommendations to enhance the efficiency of the healthcare system and to prevent the outbreak of infectious diseases. Later, the Chief Executive set up the Monitoring Committee on the Implementation of the SARS Expert Committee's Report Recommendations to ensure the adoption of the recommendations. Besides the SARS Expert Committee report, there was also the Report of the Review Panel on the SARS Outbreak commissioned by the HA. So far, the HA has prepared an emergency response plan, called "the Hospital Authority's Response Plan for Infectious Disease Outbreaks." A Centre for Health Protection has also been established, which aims at "achieving effective prevention and control of diseases in Hong Kong in collaboration with major local and international stakeholders" (Centre for Health Protection, 2004).

#### 4.3.2 Accountability of Officials

In comparison with their implementation of recommendations suggested by the experts, identifying and making officials accountable seems to have been the weakest part of the HKSARG's post-crisis management. Although the SARS Expert Committee's report indicated that no official was responsible for the outbreak of SARS in Hong Kong or for the government's response in dealing with the crisis, the public criticized the report. As all members of the committee had been appointed by the Chief Executive, the public was reluctant to accept the conclusions of the committee on accountability.

Besides the SARS Expert Committee and the HA reports, the Legislative Council in Hong Kong also looked into the accountability of the officials by publishing its own report. After the HKSARG refused to set up an independent committee of inquiry, the Legislative Council set up the "Select Committee to Inquire into the Handling of the Severe Acute Respiratory Syndrome Outbreak by the Government and the Hospital Authority" and undertook investigations and hearings. A report was published by the committee on July 5, 2004, and it concluded that various officials from the HWFB, the HA and the DH were responsible for the SARS outbreak in 2003. However, these officials were not required to resign from their positions as they were not responsible or accountable to the Legislative Council under the existing system.

## *5. Impact of the SARS Crisis on Crisis Management in Hong Kong*

Apart from government action, support from the local community was also influential during the SARS epidemic. The concept "civil society" is commonly used by scholars to evaluate community responses to crises. Different schools have their own definitions of civil society but in the definitional sense, as summarized from various scholars' descriptions in The Civil Society Reader, civil society—the seedbed of interest groups—must have two prerequisites: a pluralistic democracy and a capitalist economy, and is widely referred to as the set of institutions, organizations and behaviors situated between the state, the business world, and the family (Hodgkinson and Foley, 2003). Although government retains its dominant role in planning and organizing various activities to tackle challenges in times of crisis, the local community also provides support to its citizens in different ways.

*5.1 SARS and Civil Society*

During the early stage of the SARS epidemic, citizens in Hong Kong knew little about the disease. The fear associated with an unknown epidemic can seriously affect the daily lives of citizens. For example, people may avoid meeting others in order to minimize the risk of becoming infected. The situation was especially worsened in late March after the closure of schools and the isolation of Amoy Gardens and its residents. Later, when the government and researchers released more information about the disease, people had a better understanding of the epidemic. They then began to join together and organize activities through various channels in response to the crisis.

The SARS epidemic had put the Hong Kong healthcare system under great pressure. The public healthcare sector in Hong Kong had faced the problem of insufficient resources for a long time. The epidemic resulted in a large increase in the number of patients who needed special treatment and medical care. Hospitals suffered from insufficient manpower and resources. Despite the fact that they were putting themselves in danger, many doctors, nurses and medical staff (from both the public and private medical sectors) saw the needs of their colleagues and voluntarily took part in providing medical care to SARS patients. Their contribution during the outbreak was recognized by both local and international media. *Time Magazine* went as far as naming them, together with the other medical staff members from the SARS-infected regions, as the "2003 Asian Heroes" (TIMEasia.com, 2003). Apart from frontline medical staff, researchers from local universities also took part in the fight against the terrible disease. Professors in the University of Hong Kong and the Chinese University of Hong Kong formed various research teams to study the SARS virus and reports were published in many international scientific journals.

In order to help citizens to protect themselves from SARS, talks and seminars aimed at providing information to the general public were held by social welfare organizations and schools. Telephone hotlines were set up by the Tung Wah Group of Hospitals, the YMCA of Hong Kong, the Hong Kong Playground Association, and other organizations to provide SARS-related information and counseling services to patients, their relatives, and those in need (SARS Atypical Pneumonia Special, 2003).

During the climax of the SARS epidemic, schools in Hong Kong were closed for more than one month to avoid the spread of the disease. To help students continue their learning at home, several organizations had developed a number of online learning platforms and provided free educational services to the students. The Faculty of Education of the Chinese University of Hong Kong Resources provided learning materials to both primary and secondary school students from 150 schools. In addition, the Hong Kong School Net cooperated with the Faculty of Engineering of the Chinese University of Hong Kong and on April 15, 2003, launched a homework assigning and submitting system. Students from more than 340 schools submitted 200,000 homework assignments during the epidemic (Fighting SARS: We Care We Serve, 2003).

Besides providing help to SARS patients, their relatives and medical professionals, citizens set up funds and projects to provide financial assistance to those in need. Examples of these funds and projects included "Operation UNITE", "Hong Kong is our home—support frontline healthcare workers," "Business Community Relief Fund for Victims of SARS," "Project Blossom and 1:99 Charity Concert" and "We Care Education Fund." Promoted by the famous talk-show host, Albert Cheng, funds were also raised to purchase masks to be given to people working in hospitals (Cheng, 2004). A total of HK$150 million was raised from the assorted funds and projects (Hong Kong Government Press Release, 2003).

Compared with non-governmental organizations (NGOs) in Mainland China, NGOs in Hong Kong performed better during the epidemic. The little participation undertaken by Chinese NGOs during the epidemic can be explained by the strict control of the Chinese government over them. In China, there are three administrative regulations concerning the management of NGOs: Regulations on the Registration and Management of Social Organizations, Regulations on the Registration and Management of Foundations, and Interim Provisions for the Administration of Foreign Chambers of Commerce in China. The regulations "demand a two-tiered management system" (Zhang, 2003). In order to be registered at the Ministry of Civil Affairs, NGOs have to find a governmental agency as their sponsoring agency and these sponsoring agencies supervised the work of the NGOs. Therefore, it is clear that NGOs in China are under strict supervision and control from the government. In the early stage of the SARS epidemic, the Chinese government denied that a large-scale outbreak in Guangdong had occurred and told the media that all patients were being effectively treated and that their conditions were under control (SARS Expert Committee Report, 2003: p.8). So it was difficult for the NGOs in China to play an active role in providing support to the community at a time when the government was reluctant to draw people's attention to the epidemic.

Another possible explanation is that of all the cities with cases of SARS, Hong Kong was the worst hit. This had obviously encouraged local citizens to unite together in the cause of getting rid of the epidemic. This confirms the findings that community solidarity is enhanced when it suffers a disaster (Mileti, 1999: 228).

### *5.2 Impact on the Accountability System of Hong Kong*

During the SARS epidemic, nearly three hundred citizens died and more than 1,700 were infected by the disease. Both the Secretary for Health, Welfare and Food (Yeoh Eng Kiong) and the Chairman of the HA (Leong Che Hung) were criticized for their poor leadership in handling the crisis. On July 7, 2004, two days after the Legislative Council published its investigation report on the SARS outbreak, Yeoh resigned under public pressure. Two days later, Leong also resigned from his position. Yeoh made his decision in order to "demonstrate [his] political accountability and to bring closure to this painful episode" (South China Morning Post, 8 July 2004: p.1).

In fact, Yeoh was the third principal official who resigned after Chief Executive, Tung Chee Hwa, introduced the accountability system for principal officials into the HKSARG in 2002. Tung hoped that the new system would strengthen the accountability of Principal Officials and the cooperation between the Executive and the Legislature. The introduction of the new system, from Tung's point of view, would also ensure a better response to the needs of the community, as well as effective implementation of policies and the provision of quality services to the public. Moreover, Tung also hoped that coordination in policy formulation would improve after the setting up of the accountability system (Hong Kong Government Press Release, 17 April 2003).

Although Yeoh's resignation helped to maintain the accountability system and lessen the pressure faced by the HKSARG, people still criticized him for his late resignation (Ibid.).

On the other hand, Leong was not a Principal Official under the accountability system. As the chairman of the HA, a public organization governed by ordinance, he was appointed by the Chief Executive and thus he was responsible to Tung not to the legislative branch. Despite criticizing Leong in the investigation report, the Legislative Council had no authority to dismiss Leong or other staff members of the HA. In fact, two senior officials in Mainland China were also forced to leave their positions due to their poor performances in handling the SARS epidemic. Zhang Wen Kang was removed from his position as Minister of Health by the Standing Committee of the National People's Congress (NPC). Meng Xuenong was dismissed as Deputy Secretary of the Communist Party of China (CPC) Beijing Municipal Committee and later he resigned from his position as Mayor of Beijing. Zhang was blamed for not being adequately prepared for a public health crisis, while Meng was blamed for failing to provide timely and accurate reports on the progress of the disease (UN Foundation, 21 April 2003).

Although these officials left their offices in Hong Kong and Mainland China due to the SARS epidemic, the timing and approaches used were different and thus people's reactions varied in the two places. In China, the two senior officials were removed in April 2004, at a time when SARS was still a crisis in the country. This showed that the Chinese government was determined to manage the crisis and reduce public discontent. However, Yeoh and Leong resigned one year after the end of the SARS epidemic. Many SARS patients felt their resignations came too late and could not help pacify people's anger. The removal of the two officials by the Chinese government conveyed the message that the central government was capable of managing the crisis and that officials would be punished if they performed badly. In Hong Kong, the resignations of Yeoh and Leong from office were voluntary; they were not dismissed. This gave the public the impression that the HKSARG would not punish officials who had made mistakes. This lowered people's confidence in the ability of the government to handle the crisis.

Another official who played an important role during the SARS epidemic was Margaret Chan, Director of Health in Hong Kong. In July 2003, she was offered an appointment as the Director of the Department of Protection for Human Environment of the WHO after a panel of experts examined Hong Kong's response to SARS (Asian Wall Street Journal, 21 July 2003: p. A4). She then resigned from the HKSARG in August to work for the WHO. Although the Select Committee of the Legislative Council considered that the performance of Margaret Chan was not satisfactory in the handling of the SARS outbreak (Report of Select Committee to Inquiry into the Handling of the SARS Outbreak by the Government and the Hospital Authority, Legislative Council, p.253), and legislators voted to condemn her for her handling of the SARS crisis and for missing opportunities that could have spared the city the worst of the outbreak (South China Morning Post—Hong Kong, 10 July 2004: p. 1), she was not penalized for her performance after resigning from the HKSARG.

## *6. Conclusion: Comparison of Disease Ordinances in Hong Kong and Sweden*

The outbreak of SARS was the most serious crisis the government had faced since the handover in 1997. Although the HKSARG had considered the importance of crisis management, had prepared its own emergency response system, and had put in to place various contingency plans, none of these measures focused on crisis management during an outbreak of an infectious disease. This shows that the government underestimated the potential effects of a disease outbreak on society despite the outbreak of the avian flu in 1997. Of the three crisis management stages, the pre-crisis and post-crisis stages were the government's weakest areas and were in the greatest need for improvement. Before the outbreak of SARS, there was no emergency response plan for infectious disease. This lessened the government's ability to make a quick response while dealing with the outbreak. Moreover, the government's surveillance system provided insufficient information and warning about the outbreak of an epidemic outside Hong Kong. In the post-crisis stage, the government adopted the recommendations suggested by the SARS Expert Committee. However, the question of accountability is still an issue with the public, as no government officials have been held responsible for the outbreak of the disease. Conclusions regarding the handling of the crisis can be drawn by comparing the disease ordinances of Hong Kong and Sweden, a nation with much systematic crisis management research.

In Hong Kong, the Quarantine and Prevention of Disease Ordinance (i.e., Chapter 141 of the Laws of Hong Kong) and its subsidiary legislation provide the government with a legislative framework, which is an essential element in ensuring public health, minimizing the spread of any possible epidemic, and preventing its importation from other infected regions. The ordinance was first issued in 1936 and has since been revised several times by the government. The law mainly focuses on the prevention of diseases like cholera, plague and yellow fever. The confinement and prevention of the spread of infectious disease is further ensured by subsidiary legislation of the above ordinance: the Prevention of the Spread of Infectious Diseases Regulations (Cap. 141B). The regulations provide the public health care system a regulatory framework in dealing with any possible outbreak. Under the law, a health officer (mainly the Director of Health) is given the power to decide issues relating to the treatment of sick persons, contacts and carriers, disposal of infected dead bodies, and ordering the isolation of specific areas. During the SARS epidemic, both the Quarantine and Prevention of Disease Ordinance and the Prevention of the Spread of Infectious Diseases Regulations were revised by the government to deal with the challenge.

The Communicable Diseases Act in Sweden was first published in 1988 and promulgated for many years. In January 2003, the Swedish Government conducted a review of the need for communicable disease control measures in extraordinary situations and proposed a bill named "A New Communicable Diseases Act" in Parliament in April 2003. The objective of the bill is to "create a better balance between the population's need for protection against communicable diseases and the integrity and statutory rights of the infected individual" (Government of Sweden, 2003).

*6.1 Exercise of Power*

Under Section 8 of the Quarantine and Prevention of Disease Ordinance, the Chief Executive is responsible for making regulations in order to prevent the introduction into, the spread in and the transmission from Hong Kong of any disease (Hong Kong Law: Chapter 141), while the Director of Health is the health officer appointed by the Chief Executive for carrying out the measures. In Sweden, the structure is similar to that in Hong Kong as county medical officers are responsible for planning and organizing activities to prevent and control the spread of infectious diseases. But there is a National Board of Health and Welfare at the national level to regulate and supervise all the policies. Moreover, the

Communicable Disease Act provides the Swedish Institute for Infectious Disease Control (SMI) with an active role in monitoring and analyzing the distribution of communicable diseases nationally and internationally and proposing measures to ensure that national disease control functions efficiently (Government of Sweden, 2003).

### 6.1.1 Classification of infectious disease

In Hong Kong, the Quarantine and Prevention of Disease Ordinance and its subsidiary legislations only apply to those infectious diseases that have been listed in Schedule 1 of the ordinance. According to this ordinance, the government has not granted the power to control and prevent all infectious diseases. However, government power can also be extended as the Director of Health is the only official who has the right to amend Schedule 1 and include other diseases in the list. According to the Swedish Communicable Diseases Act, control measures that may violate the integrity of the individual are only applied to diseases that are dangerous to public health. However, it also provides the government with the power to apply the law to other diseases in emergency situations.

### 6.1.2 Reporting of infectious disease

One of the fundamental objectives of a disease act is to ensure that the government is able to collect information about the outbreak of infectious disease rapidly. Therefore, the reporting of an infectious disease to the government is an important part of the disease act. Both the Hong Kong and Swedish disease acts require doctors and individuals to report cases of infectious diseases. According to the Prevention of the Spread of Infectious Diseases Regulations, any medical practitioner or medical officer who "has reason to suspect the existence of a case of an infectious disease or, that an infectious disease existed in a death, s/he shall immediately notify the Director of Health" (Hong Kong Law: Chapter 141). The responsibility to report an infectious disease to the health authorities also applies to inmates, hotel-keepers, care-takers, and anyone having knowledge of a sick person. In Sweden, medical practitioners as well as physicians at microbiological laboratories have to report cases to the county medical officer and to the Swedish Institute for Infectious Disease Control.

### 6.1.3 Issuing isolation orders

In order to prevent the spread of infectious diseases, isolation of areas is sometimes essential. Although both the Hong Kong and Swedish disease acts have given their governments the power to issue isolation orders, the methods and approaches used by them are different. Under the ordinance, the Director of Health in Hong Kong can order the isolation of specific areas or premises and no person may enter or leave the isolated areas or premises, nor may they bring in or take out anything from these places. However, the issue of an isolation order in Sweden is rather different. It is the county administrative court, not the county medical officer, which makes decisions on issuing isolation orders. These orders apply only to the isolation of an individual and not to a certain area or premise. The county medical officer can submit an application to the court and each isolation order is valid for a maximum period of three months. After that, the court can decide on extending the isolation order for periods of up to a maximum of six months. People can also send applications to the court for the termination of isolation. Apart from this, the county medical officer can decide on the temporary isolation of a hospital. But this decision has to be tried by a county administrative court within four days and such temporary isolation can only last for a maximum of two weeks.

### *6.2 Rights and Obligations*

Comparing the two disease acts, it is obvious that Sweden's provides more clear definitions of individuals' rights and obligations than Hong Kong's. It states that all individuals "have an interest in, and responsibility for preventing the transmission of infections" (Government of Sweden, 2003). A person who knows or suspects that s/he is infected with a communicable disease should be under an obligation to take the necessary measures to protect others from the risk of infection. It is his/her obligation to seek medical attention, undergo examination and submit information to the physician to facilitate contact tracing. An individual has to undergo a compulsory examination if s/he is suspected of being infected with a communicable disease dangerous to public health and refuses to undergo the necessary examination. However, this is decided by the county administrative court and not the medical officer. Comparing Hong Kong with Sweden, the Hong Kong ordinance mainly focuses on granting powers to the Director of Health in order to control the disease but places no emphasis on the individual's responsibility.

In Sweden, medical practitioners have to provide patients with medical and practical advice on how to avoid exposing others to the risk of an infection. Behavioral guidelines are drawn up by them for patients and should be included in the patient's medical record. Another difference from the Hong Kong disease act is that the Swedish act also emphasizes the responsibility of the government. When a disease that is dangerous to public health affects an individual, the government is obliged to provide psychosocial support, care and the treatment necessary to prevent transmission of the disease. Moreover, county councils must ensure that the residents have access to the information and advice necessary to protect themselves from infection. They also have to notify people who have close contact with people at risk of infection even if the infected person has not been informed of the disease. Obviously, in terms of systems and procedures, Hong Kong still has much to learn of crisis management from overseas.

## *Notes*

1. Special acknowledgement should be given to research assistants Wilson Chong and Lee Chun Wing, both from the Department of Government and Public Administration at Chinese University in Hong Kong, for their assistance in drafting this report. The author is also indebted to Dr. Isaac Fung for the comments he provided for improving this study.

2. It was officially named the Severe Acute Respiratory Syndrome (SARS) by the World Health Organization on March 15, 2003.

## *References*

Allison, G.T. and Halperin, M.H. (1972) "Bureaucratic Politics: A Paradigm and Some Policy Implications." *World Politics 24.*

Asian Wall Street Journal (21 July 2003) p. A4.

Basic Law of Hong Kong Special Administrative Region (HKSAR) of the People's Republic of China.

Centre for Health Protection (2004) Available at: http://www.chp.gov.hk/vision.asp?lang=enandid=22andpid=8.

Cheng, K.H. (2004) *SARS in the Storm*. Tom (Cup Magazine) Publishing Limited.

Fighting SARS: We Care We Serve—Education (2003) Available at: http://www.cuhk.edu.hk/health_promote_protect/sars_care/index.html.

Government of Hong Kong Special Administrative Region (HKSAR) (2003) Emergency Response System, Chap. 2. Available at: http://www.info.gov.hk/sb/eng/emergency/index.html.

Government Office of Sweden (2003) "A new Communicable Diseases Act." Available at: http://www.sweden.gov.se/sb/d/2946/a/17068;jsessionid=anqCiTQ2vms_.

Hodgkinson, Virginia and Foley, M., Eds. (2003) The Civil Society Reader. Hanover: University Press of New England for Tufts University.

"Hong Kong in Brief" in the homepage of Hong Kong Special Administrative Region Government. Available at: http://www.info.gov.hk/info/hkbrief/eng/ahk.htm.

Hong Kong Government Press Release (19 July 2003) Available at: www.info.gov.hk/gia/general/200307/19/0719079.htm.

Hong Kong Government Press Release (17 April 2003) Available at: http://www.info.gov.hk/gia/general/200204/17/0417251.htm.

Hong Kong Law, Chapter 141 Quarantine and Prevention of Disease Ordinance Available at: http://www.legislation.gov.hk/chi/index.htm.

Mileti, D.S. (1999) Disasters by Design: A Reassessment of Natural Hazards in the United States. Washington, D.C.: Joseph Henry Press.

Quarantelli, E.L. (1998) "Disaster Crisis Management: A Summary of Research Findings," *Disaster Management Studies* 25(4). p. 373-85.

Report of Select Committee to Inquire into the Handling of the Severe Acute Respiratory Syndrome (SARS) Outbreak by the Government and the Hospital Authority, Legislative Council, HKSAR.

SARS Atypical Pneumonia Special (2003) Available at: http://yukz.com/ap/hotline.html.

SARS Expert Committee Report (2003) Hong Kong Special Administrative Region.

SingTao Daily (10 February 2003) A01.

South China Morning Post( 10 July 2004) p. 1.

South China Morning Post (8 July 2004) p.1.

TIMEasia.com, Asian Heroes (2003) Available at: http://time.com/time/asia/2003/heroes.

United Nation Foundation (2003) "Two Top Chinese Officials Fired As Death Toll Rises." Available at: http://www.unwire.org/unwire/20030421/33301_story.asp.

Warren, R.L. (1967) "The Interorganizational Field as a Focus for Investigation," *Administrative Science Quarterly* 12(3). Pp. 369-419.

Zhang Ye (2003) China's Emerging Civil Society. Available at: http://www.brookings .edu/dybdocroot/fp/cnaps/papers/ye2003.pdf.

## *Chapter 4 - Appendix*
## *Chronology of the SARS Epidemic in Hong Kong*

This chronology of the SARS epidemic in Hong Kong is based on information obtained from the SARS Expert Committee Report (2003).

23 January 2003
-Health authorities in Guangdong Province finished an investigation report on the SARS cases which occurred in November 2002.

10 February 2003
-Local media reported the SARS outbreak in Guangdong Province.
-Department of Health (DH) tried to contact Director General of the Department of Health in Guangdong Province to inquire about the outbreak.

11 February 2003
-DH contacted Ministry of Health in Beijing
-Guangzhou Bureau of Health held a press conference informing the public that the situation was under control.
-Media briefing by Director of Health, who issued press release on the Guangdong Province outbreak.
-WHO received reports from the Ministry of Health in Beijing of a SARS outbreak with three hundred cases and five deaths in Guangdong Province.
-HA head office set up a Working Group on Severe Community-Acquired Pneumonia (CAP)

13 February 2003
-HA began notifying DH of suspected and confirmed SARS cases.
-DH asked private hospitals to report severe CAP cases upon admission.

17 February 2003
-A woman was admitted to the private Union Hospital after arriving in Hong Kong from a trip to Guangzhou.

18 February 2003
-Chinese Centre for Disease Control and Prevention in Beijing reported that they had identified Chlamydia Pneumonia as the probable cause of the outbreak in Guangdong Province.

20 February 2003
-DH alerted WHO and Ministry of Health in Beijing and had a media briefing. A press release was issued to all parties, and a letter was issued to all doctors informing them of the two cases of H5N1 infection.

21 February 2003
-Professor Liu Janlun from Guangzhou, China, arrived in Hong Kong with his wife and checked into room 911 of Metropole Hotel, where they stayed for one night.

22 February 2003
-Professor Liu Janlun was admitted to Kwong Wah Hospital (KWH).

4 March 2003
-Professor Liu Janlun died in KWH. His brother-in-law in the same hospital was transferred to intensive care unit.
-A local resident, JJ, was admitted to Ward 8A of the PWH with a diagnosis of CAP.

5 March 2003
-DH was informed by WHO that Johnny Chen (the Chinese American who was referred to as DD in the original medical report) would be transferred from Hanoi to Hong Kong for treatment. Presumptive diagnosis in Hanoi was Influenza B. WHO also indicated that seven healthcare workers who had rendered care or assistance to Johnny Chen had reported having high fevers, malaise and headaches.

7 March 2003
-The Director of the Ministry of Health in Beijing said that no definite cause had been identified to account for the outbreak in Guangdong Province, nor was there any evidence to suggest it was H5N1. However, WHO experts were of the view that H5N1 could not be excluded.

10 March 2003
-PWH management was notified of a possible infectious disease outbreak with eleven healthcare workers on sick leave from Ward 8A of the Medical Department. The hospital issued a press statement.
-PWH management closed Ward 8A to new admissions, discharges, and visitors.

11 March 2003
-Media reported that a group of medical workers from Ward 8A in PWH had reported having respiratory infection symptoms over the past three to four days.

12 March 2003
-DH alerted WHO on the outbreak in PWH, and conducted a media briefing to alert the community of the outbreak of the atypical pneumonia among healthcare workers in PWH as well as to explain the actions being taken.
-WHO issued a global alert about the acute respiratory syndrome cases in Vietnam, Hong Kong, and Guangdong Province in China with unknown etiology that appeared to place health workers at high risk.

14 March 2003
-At the weekly Senior Officials Meeting chaired by the Chief Executive of the Hong Kong Special Administrative Region, the Government made three strategic decisions:

- information on the outbreak should be disseminated to the public on a daily basis,
- advice should be given to the public on precautionary measures, and
- Hong Kong should work closely with international organizations and seek expert help if necessary.

-PWH management also decided to stop all clinical admissions to the medical department.
-HA head office set up the Outbreak Coordination Centre, later named the HA head office SARS Coordination Centre.

15 March 2003
-WHO issued an emergency travel advisory naming the illness Severe Acute Respiratory Syndrome (SARS) and listing out the main symptoms. No recommendation to restrict travel to any destination was given.

17 March 2003
-HA commenced diversion of medical emergencies from PWH to other hospitals outside New Territories East Cluster.

18 March 2003
-CUHK, working with PWH, identified the *paramyxovirus* as the possible causative organism of the outbreak.

19 March 2003
-PWH temporarily suspended accident and emergency services, but would be a subject for review on March 21.

23 March 2003
-HA's Chief Executive admitted to hospital with SARS infection.

24 March 2003
-The Government announced that SHWF would coordinate implementation efforts to control SARS involving twenty Government departments and four bureaus.
-HA made a public announcement urging members of the public to avoid visiting public hospitals unless necessary.

25 March 2003
-A high-level SARS Steering Committee, chaired by Chief Executive of the Hong Kong Special Administrative Region and involving the relevant Principal Officials, was established to steer the Government's response to the SARS epidemic.

27 March 2003
-The Government announced measures to combat SARS, including:

- Adding the disease to the list of infectious diseases specified in the First Schedule to the Quarantine and Prevention of Disease Ordinance,
- Health declaration for incoming visitors to Hong Kong effective from March 29.
- Designated medical centers for medical surveillance of contacts from March 31, and
- Suspension of classes in all schools from March 29 to April 6, 2003.

-Orders were given with immediate effect to add SARS to the list of infectious diseases on the above-mentioned schedule. The HA Board held a meeting and announced the suspension of non-urgent services in all hospitals and the suspension of visitors to suspected and confirmed SARS patients. HA Board also decided to defer the implementation of new remuneration arrangement for new recruits and serving employees.

28 March 2003
-SHWF made a visit to PMH, and initiated the establishment of an electronic

database to capture on-line in real time clinical and administrative details of all SARS patients admitted to HA hospitals. This on-line information would be accessible by DH for immediate contact tracing and follow up. The database was subsequently named e-SARS.

-Following the announcement of the PMH as a designated SARS hospital effective from March 29, DH's New Territories West Regional Office liaised with the hospital on establishing a control room and other logistics for data flow and case follow up.

29 March 2003

-Government required all arriving passengers to fill out Health Declaration forms at all immigration border control points at air, sea and land. Even departing air passengers had to answer questions relating to SARS. PMH's accident and emergency department closed at 00:00 on March 29, and started at 09:00am admitting SARS patients referred from all other hospitals. PMH informed DH that a control and coordinating centre would start functioning at the hospital on March 31. Schools and childcare centers are temporarily closed.

30 March 2003

-Government launched a territory-wide Household Cleansing Day. PWH's accident and emergency department reopened for walk-in cases.

31 March 2003

-A total of 213 Amoy Gardens' residents had been admitted with suspected infection, with 107 coming from Block E. DH served an order to isolate the whole of Block E for ten days starting at 06:00am (and due to expire at midnight on April 9). DH also appealed to residents, who have moved out prior to the isolation order, to report to the Department.

-DH mandated all close contacts of SARS patients under the Quarantine and Prevention of Disease Ordinance to report daily to one of the four designated medical centers for check-up for a period of up to ten days. All contacts were further required to remain at home and encouraged not go to work or school.

1 April 2003

-Government experts found preliminary evidence suggesting that sewerage and drainage system might have been involved in the vertical spread of SARS cases in Block E. The Government announced evacuation of its residents to holiday camps under the removal order to continue the ten day quarantine. The camps were declared as appointed places under the Quarantine and Prevention of Disease Ordinance. Investigation of the outbreak by different government departments continued in Amoy Gardens.

2 April 2003
-WHO revised its advice to international travelers and recommended postponing all but essential travel to Hong Kong and Guangdong Province.

3 April 2003
-Education and Manpower Bureau announced that class suspension period would be extended to April 21. Also it issued revised guidelines to schools in light of the ten-day surveillance period at designated medical centers required of close contacts.

4 April 2003
-With assistance from the Police, virtually all households that moved out of Amoy Gardens Block E before imposition of the isolation order had contacted DH for medical surveillance. All households required disinfection under Regulation 19 of the Prevention of the Spread of Infectious Diseases Regulations.

5 April 2003
-HA commenced hotline services in staff clinics. The IT team also linked e-SARS to HA's clinical management system to collate clinical information.

6 April 2003
-The Police commenced assisting DH in epidemiological investigations using its sophisticated computer system called the Major Incident Investigation and Disaster Support System (MIIDSS). The MIIDSS allowed SARS investigators to validate addresses, map out the geographical distribution, reveal potential sources or routes of spreading, and show the connectivity between cases and contacts.
-PWH resumed full accident and emergency service at 09:00. In view of SARS infections among healthcare workers and high SARS caseload, United Christian Hospital stopped all medical admissions through its accident and emergency department.

7 April 2003
-PMH started transferring convalescent SARS patients to Wong Tai Sin Hospital. HA decided to stop admitting referrals from other hospitals to PMH and to confine its admission to referrals from DH's designated medical centers

8 April 2003
-An on-line e-SARS database was launched. Through e-SARS, HA could provide real-time information of confirmed or suspected SARS patients to DH to facilitate prompt case investigation and rapid contact tracing. The Food and

Environmental Hygiene Department undertook disinfection of individual flats in Amoy Gardens Block E.

9 April 2003
-The isolation order on Amoy Garden Block E (activated on March 31) expired at midnight. Residents were discharged on the morning of April 10. Special arrangements were made for residents who wished to leave the camp at midnight.

10 April 2003
-The Government announced that all household contacts of confirmed SARS patients would be confined (quarantined) at home, with no visitors allowed, for a period of up to ten days with immediate effect.

11 April 2003
-The Government reached a consensus with the Guangdong Government on SARS-related matters regarding exchange of information, medical cooperation, notification mechanisms, and border quarantine arrangements. They agreed to establish an expert group to deal with these measures.
-The Government announced that individuals having close contact with a SARS patient would be barred from leaving Hong Kong during the quarantine period with effect from April 14. DH also implemented home confinement (Regulation 11 of the Prevention of the Spread of Infectious Disease Regulations) on household contacts.

12 April 2003
-Canadian scientists sequenced the genome of the SARS coronavirus. DH started to release on a daily basis the names of the buildings with SARS patients admitted to hospitals within the past ten days. List uploaded onto DH website.

15 April 2003
-The Government amended the existing Quarantine and Prevention of Disease Ordinance (Cap 141) to empower persons authorized by DH to take body temperature of persons arriving in or leaving Hong Kong, and to prohibit persons who have been exposed to the risk of SARS from leaving Hong Kong. The amendment is enshrined in the Prevention of the Spread of Infectious Diseases Regulation 2003.

17 April 2003
-The Prevention of the Spread of Infectious Diseases (Amendment) Regulation 2003 was gazetted, which:

- prohibited contact with a SARS patient or a carrier of,
- empowered an authorized person to take body temperature of persons arriving or leaving Hong Kong, and
- empowered a health officer or authorized medical practitioner to carry out a medical examination for the purpose of ascertaining whether a person was likely to be infected with SARS.

-The Government put in effect body temperature checks on departing passengers at the airport. Those with a fever were not allowed to board unless they received clearance from an authorized medical practitioner.
-The Government also made public the investigation findings of the Amoy Gardens outbreak. The vertical spread of SARS in Block E was attributed to a combination of dried-up U-traps, contaminated sewage, and updraft in light wells that facilitated the spread of droplets.
-The first issue of the SARS Bulletin published on HWFB's and DH's webpages to provide updated information, statistics, epidemiology of SARS cases, ongoing development, and health advice to the public.
-The first meeting of the Guangdong-Hong Kong Expert Group on Prevention and Treatment of SARS (April 17-18, 2003, in Guangzhou) met and agreed to:

- further improve notification mechanisms and exchange of information regularly,
- set up a point-to-point exchange mechanism between counterpart organizations to enhance communications and to draw on each other's experiences in disease control, and
- expand the existing scope of information exchange on infectious diseases.

19 April 2003
-Government implemented a territory-wide cleansing day.

21 April 2003
-Between April 21 and May 2, DH developed a dedicated computer program called SARS centralized case and contact information system (CCIS). It was used for keeping and updating a centralized database on SARS cases and contacts. The system could also generate lists of cases and contacts for other departments assisting in home confinement and mass mailings for generating permits for home confinement.

22 April 2003
-Classes resumed for students, in form/level 3 or above, in secondary schools.
24 April 2003
-Government put in effect body temperature checks on transit and arriving passengers at Airport Lo Wu, Hung Hom railway station, and land borders.

25 April 2003
-The home confinement scheme was extended to household contacts of suspected SARS patients. Listing of buildings on DH webpage extended to those with suspected SARS cases.

26 April 2003
-A six year old girl of a Hong Kong tour group visiting Taipei developed a fever while there and was admitted to hospital as a suspected SARS case. The tour group was placed under isolation by the Taipei health authorities.

28 April 2003
-Classes for secondary school students in form/level 1 and 2 were resumed. Any schools with a suspected or confirmed SARS case were still required to suspend classes for ten days.

29 April 2003
-Following further communication with the Taipei authorities, the Government arranged a chartered flight to take members of the tour group, including the girl and her relatives, back to Hong Kong. The girl was sent to Yan Chai Hospital for observation upon return, and all tour group members were put under home confinement. The girl was subsequently confirmed to be a non-SARS case. The home confinement order on the tour group members was thus lifted accordingly.

30 April 2003
-The HA's Chief Executive returned to duty

5 May 2003
-Government announced that Chief Secretary for Administration would lead a cross-bureau, inter-departmental task force "Team Clean" to improve environmental hygiene in Hong Kong.
-Government announced that Financial Secretary would head an economic relaunch strategy group. HK$1 billion earmarked to promote Hong Kong as soon as WHO announced lifting of the travel advisory against Hong Kong.
-Government announced that SHWF would look into establishing a CDC-type organization to improve preparedness for future outbreaks of communicable

diseases. It further announced the establishment of a research fund, totaling HK$500 million, to encourage, facilitate and support research work on SARS and other communicable diseases.
-Hong Kong Jockey Club Charities Trust pledged HK$500 million to support Government's efforts to establish a CDC-type organization and to support professional training and public education.

7 May 2003
-Multi-disciplinary Response Team led an investigation of Wing Shui House of the public Lek Yuen Estate in Shatin District upon identification of three cases from two units in the housing block.
-A total of twelve cases were eventually identified. However, the Team found no evidence of environmental factors being involved in the spread of the outbreak.

12 May 2003
-Classes resumed for students in grade 4 and above in primary and special schools.

16 May 2003
-WHO released investigation findings on the SARS outbreak at Amoy Gardens, which corroborated with the report findings of Hong Kong Government: a unique sequence of environmental and health events that happened simultaneously contributed to the SARS outbreak in Amoy Gardens.
-Government extended body temperature checks to departing passengers at China Ferry Terminal and Macao Ferry Terminal.

19 May 2003
-Classes resumed for students from grade 3 and below as well as students with mental handicaps.

21 May 2003
-The Government put in effect body temperature checks for departing passengers at the railway station in Hong Kong.

23 May 2003
-WHO lifted the travel advisory against Hong Kong.

24 May 2003
-Media reported that a joint study by HKU and Shenzhen Centre of Disease Control found coronavirus in civet cats. DH requested details of the study from

the Ministry of Health in Beijing. The importation of game meat derived from civet cats was suspended in Hong Kong as a precautionary measure.

25 May 2003
-New Territories East Cluster announced the resumption of limited accident and emergency services at Alice Ho Miu Ling Nethersole Hospital.

11 June 2003
-The last SARS case was confirmed and reported. The patient had been at the hospital in isolation since June 2.

16 June 2003
-HA's Kowloon West Cluster announced the resumption of all its clinical services in phases: Wong Tai Sin Hospital's TB and chest services and all PMH's clinical services including accident and emergency services were resumed.

23 June 2003
-WHO removed Hong Kong from the list of areas with local transmission of SARS, declaring Hong Kong SARS-free.

# Chapter 5
# An Analytical Memoir of the WHO Operation in China[1]

Edward Deverell

## *Introduction*

The outbreak of severe acute respiratory syndrome (SARS) in China in 2002-2003 made it clear that in a world of globalization, with rapid movement of people and air travel, a single lapse in the chain of security can transform a critical regional situation into a fully-fledged global crisis. In the case of SARS in China, a single carrier of the virus led to several national and international outbreaks of the previously unknown and deadly disease. The epidemic of 2003 was a harsh reminder of the importance of rapid response, openness, cooperation and information sharing on all levels of governance when dealing with potentially trans-boundary threats and crises.

This chapter presents a view from the ground of the World Health Organization's (WHO) management of the SARS epidemic in China in the spring of 2003. Based to a large extent on first hand impressions from the field it gives a personal account of the WHO's work in China in May and June 2003. In the midst of the SARS epidemic, Peet J. Tüll, who at the time was Medical Director at the Swedish National Board of Health and Welfare, was appointed by the WHO to spend five weeks in China to assist WHO's Beijing office. As a WHO temporary advisor and leader of the Epidemiology team at the Beijing office, his mission was to assess the activities of the Chinese government and agencies on central, provincial and local levels regarding epidemiological results and practice, and to advise on what future measures should be taken for the world at large to be content with China's actions. By assisting the team leader of WHO's Communicable Disease Control in China, Alan Schnur, with epidemiological evaluations, assessments and judgments, Tüll was also assigned to relieve some of Schnur's workload. The informal terms of reference then included analyzing epidemiological data, monitoring daily events, gathering more knowledge about the disease and participating in meetings with ministries, provincial leaders, Health Bureaus, and China Centers for Disease Control and Prevention (China CDC). Another important task was to help the Chinese provinces present their campaigns in a way that was understandable and acceptable to the international community.

## *The WHO and the Disease Control and Prevention Regime*

When Tüll arrived in China the outbreak had been going on for some time and China and WHO were busy launching efforts to contain th SARS outbreak.

The WHO, which is the United Nations' specialized agency for health, played a central coordinating role in the response against the SARS outbreak in the spring of 2003 (WHO, 2003d). As a Specialized Agency of the UN, the WHO is part of the UN structure but it also has its own Constitution. This implies that the WHO has a considerable amount of autonomy (Vanderburg, 2004). The WHO is organized geographically in six regional offices (WHO Presentation, 2004).[2] The regions have a fair amount of autonomy (Vanderburg, 2004). Since the WHO is a membership organization by country, its employees work for each of the countries in which the WHO is present. While employees' tasks are given from the Regional Office, most often the WHO works directly through and with the Ministry of Health of each country. The head of each WHO country program, i.e., the representative of the WHO office, is a member of the diplomatic corps with a legal standing equal to that of an Ambassador. This arrangement assures WHO direct access to the highest levels of government. It also formally acknowledges that employees of WHO are answerable to the WHO, not to specific governments (ibid.).

The WHO's work within the field of disease control and prevention is carried out at the Department of Communicable Disease Surveillance and Response (CDS). The CDS produces guidelines and manuals on the surveillance and control of epidemic-prone diseases and guidance on how to assess surveillance systems (WHO, 2004c). The work of the CDS for global health security via epidemic surveillance, alert and response can be divided into three major parts:

- Containing known risks
- Responding to the unexpected
- Improving preparedness.

A great deal of the disease control and prevention regime's operational clout, however, was a result of work by partners within the Global Outbreak Alert and Response Network (GOARN) (WHO, 2003d). GOARN was set up in 1997 and formalized in 2000 (Heymann and Rodier, 2004). It is a network of collaboration for rapid identification, confirmation and response to serious and internationally threatening outbreaks. It sustains intelligence work on call twenty four hours a day, seven days a week (WHO Presentation, 2004) and has over 120 partners throughout the world.[3]

GOARN's objective is to contribute to global health security by combating international spread of outbreaks, rapidly ensuring appropriate technical assistance to affected states and contributing to long-term epidemic preparedness and capacity building (WHO, 2004b). Although GOARN identifies and responds to some fifty outbreaks in developing countries each year, the SARS outbreak was the first time that GOARN responded to a very rapid global outbreak (Heymann and Rodier, 2004).

## *Efforts to Contain the SARS Outbreak in China*

The following section provides a chronology of some of the main events that took place from November 16, 2002, to May 9, 2003. The delimitations of the timeline signify when SARS, via back-tracking was first discovered and when WHO consultant Peet J. Tüll arrived in China.

### *Outbreaks in Guangdong*

Although it was not noticed at the time, the first case of a previously unknown atypical pneumonia that later on became dubbed as SARS showed up in Foshan City, Guangdong Province in China on November 16, 2002 (WHO, 2004a). In late November, GOARN received several reports about influenza outbreaks in China. WHO then requested more information on the subject from Chinese authorities on December 5 and 11 (Heymann and Rodier, 2004). The unknown disease drew the attention of Chinese health personnel in mid-December (Huang, 2003). Between November 16, 2002, and January 19, 2003, seven cities in Guangdong identified index cases of SARS (WHO, 2003b).

On January 20, 2003, the first team of experts sent by the Ministry of Health (MOH) arrived at Guangzhou and the provincial government in Guangdong ordered an investigation of the disease almost at the same time. The report, which was kept top secret, was only sent to the provincial health bureau and, presumably, to the MOH in Beijing on January 27 (Huang, 2003). On February 10, the WHO asked China to verify reports of pneumonia in Guangdong (WHO, 2003a). The following day WHO received reports from the MOH of an outbreak of acute respiratory syndrome with 300 cases and 5 deaths in the province (WHO, 2004a). On February 14, the MOH informed WHO that the outbreak in Guangdong was coming under control (WHO, 2003a).[4]

### *The Disease Spreads Over China and Abroad*

On February 20 the Regional Director of the WHO Western Pacific Regional Office (WPRO) proposed an official visit to Guangdong and three days later a WHO team arrived in Beijing (WHO, 2003a). Now the disease also started turning up in other countries. The Vietnam based WHO official Carlo Urbani was alarmed by the unusual disease and notified the WPRO office in Manila on February 28 and WHO headquarters moved into a heightened state of alert (WHO, 2004a). The practical implications of the Vietnam outbreak were that the WPRO in Manila had the WHO's formal responsibility to respond to the SARS outbreak. The Regional Director, Shigeru Omi, appointed Hitoshi Oshitani to head the SARS effort and response team in WPRO (Vanderburg, 2004).

In early March it was evident that the disease was a serious health threat. Medical staff members in Beijing's military hospitals were briefed about the dangers of SARS, but they were told not to publicize what they had learned since it could interfere with the National People's Congress meeting to be held in Beijing (Huang, 2003). On March 10, the Chinese MOH asked WHO to provide technical and laboratory support to clarify the cause of the outbreak. On March 12, WHO issued a global alert about cases of severe atypical pneumonia (WHO, 2004a). The next day WHO sent emergency alerts to its partners in GOARN. On March 15, WHO named the illness Severe Acute Respiratory Syndrome (SARS) and declared it a worldwide health threat. WHO also issued a travel advisory as evidence mounted that SARS was spreading by air travel. The following day over 150 suspect and probable cases of SARS were reported from around the world (WHO, 2004a). Nevertheless, in China the outbreak was still managed as Guangdong's problem.

*The Dragon Awakens From Its Slumber*

On April 2, WHO recommended that persons traveling to Hong Kong and Guangdong should consider postponing all but essential travel until further notice. At the same time the cumulative world total of SARS cases passed the two thousand mark (WHO, 2004a). Now actions were taken at the central level in China. The State Council held its first meeting to discuss the problem. The government established a small group led by the health minister and an interministerial committee led by a vice secretary general to address prevention and treatment. The government also gave a WHO expert team permission to travel immediately to Guangdong.[5] After arriving in Guangdong on April 3, the team was given access to sites and health staff (WHO, 2004a). Nevertheless, a comprehensive Chinese response was still lacking since all provinces and involved institutions were not acting in accordance with new guidelines (cf. Enserink, 2003). A lot of the information that made its way to the central level then was flawed. For instance, Minister of Health Zhang Wenkang announced that Beijing had seen only twelve cases of SARS, despite the fact that the city's No. 309 PLA hospital alone had some sixty SARS patients (Huang, 2003).

In April China began daily electronic reporting of cases and deaths, nationwide, by province and on April 9 the interim report of the WHO investigative team in China was presented to the MOH. The team expressed serious concerns about the situation in Beijing. At the time only a minority of hospitals in the capital reported daily to the MOH. Moreover, contact tracing was not carried out systematically, and health authorities failed to investigate rumors of SARS cases (WHO, 2004a). After the meeting Bekedam, nonetheless, was optimistic and told the press: "We now have very high-level commitment and with this high level of commitment, very soon we'll get some real answers" (OLNH, 2003).

*Beijing Falls into Line*

Rumors about underreporting in Beijing's military hospitals had been floating around the capital for some time. Of Beijing's 175 hospitals, 16 were under the control of the army, which maintained a relatively independent health system (Huang, 2003). When the senior military physician, Jiang Yanyong, released a written statement to news organizations and in a subsequent interview on April 9 (Rosenthal, 2003) told the world about the number of probable SARS cases at Beijing's No. 309 PLA hospital, it was no sense in keeping up the policy of secrecy and denial. However, military hospitals in Beijing still refused to hand in SARS statistics to the Ministry, although they had admitted a large number of SARS patients (Huang, 2003).

On April 14, the cumulative number of worldwide cases passed the three thousand mark and the total number of reported SARS cases in China was 1,418 (CU, 14 April 2003). Now the mood began to change also for SARS researchers in China. Safety regulations that had banned transfers of the virus were lifted, which facilitated epidemiological research cooperation. Suddenly it was easier to report research results that differed from official policy (Enserink, 2003). On April 15 the WHO Beijing Assessment team was also granted permission to visit military hospitals (CU, 15 April 2003). The following afternoon the expert team held a press briefing. According to the team's rough estimation there were some one to two hundred SARS cases in Beijing, i.e., considerably more than the thirty seven cases officially reported two days previously (CU, 16 April 2003; WHO, 2004a).

*The Politburo Means Business*

At an urgent meeting of the Standing Committee of the Politburo on April 17, explicit warnings against covering up SARS cases were declared (Huang, 2003). In the meantime the spread of SARS in China continued and eleven of China's thirty one provinces, autonomous regions and municipalities reporting to MOH had reported at least one case. The WHO team in Beijing, however, told media that it still noticed serious under-reporting, especially in military hospitals. In addition, Bekedam stressed that the Beijing municipality was still not doing a good job in surveillance and contact tracing (Bekedam, 2003).

On April 20, Vice-Minister of Health Wang Longde presented the number of probable cases of SARS to Bekedam. Progress had been made in reporting SARS cases by including cases from all hospitals (CU, 20 April 2003). The government now inaugurated a nationwide campaign to begin truthful reporting about SARS (Huang, 2003). The increased government efforts also resulted in an evident increase in reported cases (CU, 21 April 2003). The increased efforts touched upon various fields of SARS combat: The week-long May Day holiday was shortened and the mayor of Beijing Meng Xuenong and the Minister of Health Zhang Wenkan were removed from their Communist Party posts (WHO, 2004a).

On April 23, WHO expanded its travel recommendations. In addition to travelers to Hong Kong SAR and Guangdong, travelers to, e.g., Beijing and Shanxi were advised to consider postponing all but essential travel. The advisory would be reviewed after twenty one days. Moreover, due partly to improved surveillance and reporting, there was a steep increase in the number of reported cases to the WHO. The MOH reported 306 new probable SARS cases to WHO/China, including the first cases from Tianjin, Hebei, Hubei and Shandong and the cumulative number of the reported probable cases was 2,305 (CU, 23 April 2003). Bekedam commented the numbers by saying: "At this moment appropriate actions are being taken and the numbers are going up" (Bekedam, 2003).

In the meantime authorities continued to impose measures to contain the disease. The inter-ministerial group under the health minister was replaced by a task force known as the SARS Control and Prevention Headquarters of the State Council, to coordinate national efforts to combat the disease. Vice Premier Wu Yi was appointed as head of the task force (Huang, 2003). Drastic measures were also taken in Beijing. Officials in the capital suspended all primary and secondary schools for a two-week period (WHO, 2004a). But the number of reported cases in Beijing was still on the increase.

On April 28 the WHO assessment team that had traveled around Shanghai for four days, met with MOH officials. The WHO had expected Shanghai to have a higher number of SARS cases than the numbers reported (two probable cases and twelve suspect cases). However, based on examination of the city's case data and random visits, experts did not find evidence of systematic under-reporting. Bekedam responded by telling the press that "the focus of attention is now Beijing and western China" (ibid.). The cumulative total number of cases worldwide exceeded five thousand (WHO, 2004a). On May 8, travel recommendations were extended to Inner Mongolia and Tianjin (WHO, 2004a).

## *China's Crisis Organization for the Outbreak*

The chronological paragraphs above make it possible to pinpoint where the Chinese authorities and WHO were in the process when Tüll was recruited to join the WHO's Beijing office. The collaboration between WHO and the Chinese government and agencies was improving after the rocky start, but uncertainty about the SARS virus and epidemiology still prevailed.

Initially, Chinese authorities did not pay sufficient attention to the fact that the disease was highly infectious and deadly. In addition, the Chinese government did not take the outbreak seriously, be it for lack of information or lack of political will. It took a long time to comprehend the gravity of the situation and a clear commitment from the political authority was lacking in the beginning of the outbreak. Until the Politburo decided what it wanted to do, very little happened. Meanwhile, the business community took a great interest in the SARS outbreak (Tüll, 2004). International and regional meetings and conferences, consultants' visits along with planned activities for various agencies and organizations were postponed or cancelled. Tourism businesses and international business people had concerns about staying in SARS affected countries (Vanderburg, 2004). Although the level of sincerity is ambiguous, some companies even considered closing up operations and moving to other countries.[6] Possibly, the Chinese government sensed the gravity of the situation, and after a sluggish start it switched to a more active response in mid April.

It soon became evident that the central government had understood that they faced a national threat of great proportions. Massive campaigns were launched, officials were fired, radical measures were taken and articles and new legislation about SARS were being written. China had an advantage in being a communist state organized by party cadres which reach all the way to the smallest villages. The response rested on the administrative organization on the one hand and on the cadres on the other. Many people were involved and information was rapidly spread in cities and in the countryside. But in early May 2003, it was still a widespread impression among the public, media and expert organizations such as the WHO, that China had not taken sufficient measures to eradicate SARS (Tüll, 2004).[7]

Notwithstanding the advantage of the cadre system and that the government was seemingly committed, combating SARS in China did not become flawless overnight. Chinese authorities still lacked a system to manage a disease of such great proportions. Neither legislation nor bureaucracy was sufficiently adjusted for this kind of disease. For example the reporting system was inadequate and the data were not collected in one place. There was a lack of a cohesive central authority over health issues. Several central-level agencies, besides the Ministry of Health, had significant health authority.[8] Hence, no single authority had an overview of the situation and there was no place where authorities and involved actors could get the full picture. So, even if great measures had been taken on the provincial level, political infighting and uncertainty concerning mandates on the governmental level were problematic. Another shortcoming was the analysis, which was ad hoc and relatively primitive (Tüll, 2004).

## *The WHO's Crisis Organization for China*

The WHO worked with several teams in China during the SARS outbreak. All in all WHO sent seventy seven consultants and staff to China from February to August 2003 (WHO, 2003a). Teams were assigned to assess the SARS situation and control and prevention efforts in Chinese provinces and cities. They were instructed to conduct site visits at all levels of government, public health offices and clinics and hospitals. In addition, they reviewed surveillance and case reporting systems and evaluated hospital management and infection control. Team members also held meetings with officials from government, regional, municipal and local levels, health workers and experts (Tüll, 2004).

The first team traveled around Guangdong in the beginning of April 2003. The Guangdong team reviewed case-based data that they assumed was useful for articles for publication that could help disseminate information on the Guangdong lessons. Another WHO expert team worked mostly in Beijing. In addition, joint teams visited Shanghai, Anhui, Guangxi, Hebei and Henan provinces in May. Poor provinces with weak infrastructure and limited health facilities and considerable movement of people in and out of bordering big cities were seen as especially vulnerable (e.g., Guangxi) (CU, 12 May 2003).

The teams consisted of different specialists. Special teams were assigned for particular issues such as care, hygiene, the laboratory system, air conditioning (Tüll, 2004) and health controls at urban international and domestic airports, train stations and bus terminals (CU, 25 May 2003). At the end of each provincial tour, the teams delivered their reports to the provincial governors. Upon the return of the assessment teams to Beijing, they also briefed the Chinese ministries and the WHO (Tüll, 2004).

## *A Memoir of the WHO Operation*

In the following sections Tüll's impressions from working on the field in China are portrayed. It is a chronological description that starts out with a description of what happened when Tüll took on the WHO temporary assignment, continuing with a depiction of his arrival to China and his first WHO-China meeting on Chinese soil on May 9. At this meeting trust between WHO and the representatives of the Beijing authority was limited and WHO staff had to figure out ways to get the parties to trust each other. The description ends with a final meeting on June 12, when a team of senior WHO officials, headed by David L. Heymann, WHO's Executive Director of Communicable Diseases, arrived in Beijing to assess the situation of SARS control in China.

### *Requests for Epidemiological Expertise*

Things were getting increasingly hectic at the WHO office in Beijing in the midst of fighting the SARS outbreak. The WHO used all available resources to assist in combating the disease. A crisis organization was being established. Meanwhile, new divisions dealing with, for instance, infection control and managing the laboratories were being established. In addition, a new division for overarching epidemiology and holistic management of the epidemic by the name of the Epidemiology team was set up. The Epidemiology team was established to construct an overview of the national epidemiological situation of SARS in China. The WHO needed someone to head the new team. Many consultants that came to China to assist in containing SARS, stayed for a week or two. The ongoing turnover of staff was not a problem for the provincial assessment teams, but it was problematic for the people that had to make an overview of the national situation. Hence, in order to staff the new division in an appropriate way, the WHO required professional expertise that could stay in China for a longer time than two weeks (Tüll, 2004).

In April GOARN requests for expertise made their way to Swedish institutions. Meanwhile, Henk Bekedam held meetings on a regular basis with several country ambassadors to Beijing. The Swedish ambassador to Beijing, Börje Ljunggren, had good relations with Bekedam. Moreover, he was an old friend of the director of the Swedish Institute for Infectious Disease Control (SMI), Ragnar Norrby. The Ambassador had heard that WHO was in dire need of epidemiological expertise in Beijing. On the behalf of GOARN, the Ambassador then began sending e-mails to Norrby and other Swedes in central positions regarding requests for international expertise. But after several e-mails, no one in Sweden had shown interest in going to China. Apparently, no one wanted to take on the assignment. On April 24, Ambassador Ljunggren sent what was formulated as a final plea for a Swedish expert to Norrby, who in turn forwarded it to a broader circle of epidemiological experts including Peet Tüll. The assignment was vaguely described but it seemed to entail traveling to several provinces and making epidemiological assessments (Tüll, 2004).

Tüll thought that the situation was a bit ridiculous. Since he had experience within the field as well as fieldwork experience,[9] he e-mailed the ambassador and asked what, more specifically, the WHO in China needed help with. The Ambassador answered that the WHO requested someone that could assess for instance the quality of reporting, contact tracing and health care in a province or big city. At the same time, the Ambassador understood that Tüll was interested in the assignment, so he asked about his experience and requested a copy of his CV. The response came within a few hours and Tüll was asked to travel to China as soon as possible (Tüll, 2004).

*The Assignment*

It all happened very quickly and there was not much chance to talk with WHO representatives before traveling to China. There was, however, time to speak to Pat Drury, who was in charge of GOARN and to correspond with Alan Schnur at the WHO field office in Beijing concerning practical issues. It was also unclear what the WHO would expect from their newly recruited expert. Before arriving in China, Tüll was under the impression that he would end up in an assessment team that traveled the provinces. But the WHO probably thought that since the Swedish expert was a senior epidemiologist there might be better ways to make use of this expertise. Partly they were probably worried that he could be infected by SARS as older people were infected easier than younger. The work and the issues at hand also played a role (Tüll, 2004).

When Tüll arrived in China on May 9, he was assigned to work directly under Schnur. In the beginning it was somewhat unclear what the assignment would entail:

> No one really knew what I was supposed to do when I got there. My task evolved into creating an overview [of the outbreak] understanding what had been done in China, and estimating whether it was sufficient (Tüll, 2004).

The appointment entailed being in charge of the Epidemiology team. More specifically it involved analyzing epidemiological data, monitoring events, gathering more knowledge about the disease and participating in meetings with ministries, provincial leaders and China CDC (Tüll, 2004).

*The First Meeting*

Arriving in the Chinese capital of Beijing was an almost eerie experience. The vast and usually lively city resembled a ghost town. All hotels were empty and so were the streets. As soon as stepping into the WHO office in Beijing, however, it was a different story. There the pace was hectic and everyone seemed to be in a great hurry. On Tüll's first morning in China a meeting was scheduled with the team responsible for disease control in Beijing and when he came to the office, after some two hours on Chinese soil, it was decided that he should attend the meeting to get to know the ropes: "I came to the office, put down my bags, they were on their way to a meeting and thought that I should join" (Tüll, 2004).

At an earlier meeting Beijing's acting Mayor Wang Qishan expressed that a breakthrough in negotiations had occurred. After discussions with the new mayor, Bekedam told the international media: "We have agreed to work more closely together to improve the analysis and develop policy options on handling the outbreak" (CU, 10 May 2003). At the meeting on May 9, the way ahead was discussed. But trust between WHO and the representatives of the Beijing authority was still limited and now the WHO staff had to figure out ways to get the parties to trust each other. The meeting concerned the outbreak of SARS in Beijing. The WHO team for Beijing, consisting of staff from CDC Atlanta, did the talking. In what can be interpreted as a sign of new priorities, the Chinese counterparts had called in the former chief of Public Health in Beijing. He reported directly to the Mayor. The WHO team had attended many meetings earlier. It was evident that they were very frustrated because they thought that they did not receive accurate information about what was going on in Beijing (Tüll,

2004). While Tüll's impression was that the Chinese were willing to start discussing, the Beijing team, possibly due to many prior disappointments, did not believe what the Chinese told them. When Tüll expressed a more optimistic attitude the team assumed he was just being naïve and that he had not understood the Chinese system and mentality (Tüll, 2004).

Tüll also had objections to the methods used by the WHO team at the meeting. In the beginning of the meeting the WHO representatives requested Chinese databases. They wanted their counterparts to hand over all their numbers regarding the disease on a CD. The Chinese refused to simply hand over the data to the WHO and let it do the analysis and work alone, but instead offered cooperation together. As it turned out the databases were not provided. The WHO then publicly stated that China was not cooperating. Tüll was surprised and disappointed by the WHO team's response:

> It's foolish to approach someone with that question, to distrust them to such an extent that you demand basic data. That attitude is completely wrong! You can't do that! You don't have that position or role to do such things (Tüll, 2004).

Most countries would meet such a demand with a refusal, as did China. The attitude was surprising because it was not in compliance with how such issues should be managed. The issue, then, was solved in accordance with the Chinese offer. The Beijing team was allowed to go to their counterparts' offices and sit down with their people and work with the numbers (Tüll, 2004).

*Planning the Work of the Epidemiology Team*

The Epidemiology team consisted of four persons of different nationalities. Cooperation within the team was satisfactory but since everyone had very different tasks it never really turned into a team in the strictest sense of the word. As the senior member of the team, Tüll's thoughts became highly influential. He did most of the pondering and reading by himself. In order to establish some structure regarding the assignment Tüll drew up a work plan for the team, which listed the goals, objectives, activities and long and short term desired outcomes for the mission (Tüll, 2004).

The principal mission was to eliminate SARS from China. To that end the WHO needed a sustainable strategy that had to be approved by the Chinese government. The Epidemiology team also pledged to assist the MOH and China CDC to work out an elimination plan that would include an analysis of basic data. The desired outcome was to get access to sustainable criteria and, in the long term, being able to control future development (ETW, 2003).

A central concern for the team was that the collected data were not being analyzed, interpreted or disseminated in a timely and systematic fashion. The second task, then, referred to the WHO data output, namely to follow SARS epidemiology in China. To that end, the Epidemiology team had to disseminate credible China SARS data (regarding primarily magnitude and geography) to the international community by obtaining information from the MOH website and transferring the data to translated Excel sheets. The work aimed to improve timeliness of data transfer and control appearance of new cases as well as enhance credibility and the profile of China's scientific community. Another issue was to follow up and evaluate all rumors. By exchanging data between provinces, China CDC, MOH and WHO, the team also went through WHO lists on all new probable and suspected cases containing relevant epidemiological data (e.g., number of cases under medical observation and other types of observations and quarantined) (ibid.).

Thirdly the Epidemiology team aimed to improve data analysis and reporting. Therefore the team, in regular meetings with a joint MOH-China CDC-WHO group, analyzed incoming data by looking at key indicators and analyzing the need to improve surveillance and data design. The aim was to establish case count verification and real-time analysis in order to enhance SARS surveillance and foster trust and recognition of benefits in collaboration. The team also looked for geographical data of reported cases and tried to map the data. In addition, to construct a system for identifying data that needed further assessment, a daily analysis of incoming data was conducted and presented to the MOH and China CDC (ibid.).

Other tasks were to support and cooperate with the provincial assessment teams in their search for reliable data, to offer technical assistance to the MOH when updating guidelines and order, and to develop WHO intelligence on SARS. The latter task entailed getting access to recently published data and documents, observing the decisions made by the Chinese government, carrying out daily control of websites and articles of interest and transferring relevant material to shared maps. The objective was to make sure that WHO was kept up to date on SARS epidemiology and containment strategy and that the data were shared with the MOH and China CDC (ibid.).

The seventh and final task was to maximize the epidemiological knowledge base on SARS. The team tried to identify and prioritize key points and areas in which research was needed. This was supposed to be carried out in collaboration with MOH, China CDC and the Ministry of Science and Technology (ibid.). However, such activities did not come about (Tüll, 2004.).

### *Meetings Early On*

After mapping out the assignment and constructing an overview of the situation, the next step was to define the key issues at hand, i.e., to separate what was essential and had to be focused upon, from what could be handled at a later stage. Firstly it was important to establish an understanding of the Chinese administration's new legislation and implemented measures and decisions. In order to establish a trustful relation to the MOH, it was important to communicate that the WHO was not in China to weaken the country or the administration and to make it clear that the WHO was there to be of assistance. This was not always easy:

> At one of the early political meetings in the Ministry they thought we were ignorant. They had these 50 new rules and legislations and we were not aware of them. So of course we asked a lot of stupid questions that they had already thought of (Tüll, 2004).

Naturally, the WHO mission, to determine whether the Chinese administration was able to contain the outbreak, was extremely sensitive. Hence, some of the Chinese counterparts, people at the MOH that belonged to the old guard, were not interested in cooperating at all.

Second on the agenda was to contact China CDC to get an overall picture of what kind of professional and research based knowledge about SARS was available in China. It was important to convince the experts at China CDC that they were negotiating with competent people who understood epidemiology. To that end it was necessary to ask the right questions and get constructive dialogues going. Complications would easily arrive, as the story below illustrates:

> When I was at China CDC and criticized them for not telling the world about SARS they gave me the journal of the Chinese Medical Association with 30 articles about SARS. No one had read them! That wasn't very clever. It had been better to try to comprehend the situation before airing different views. In our defense, we could say that everything came pretty late and it took weeks to translate the documents. It meant that we were always behind schedule (Tüll, 2004).

The same problem emerged concerning legislation on SARS. It was part of Tüll's assignment to read the legislation and WHO received translated legislation continuously. In the beginning legislation was scant and it took time to receive translations (Tüll, 2004). Another example can be found at the online directory of the Chinese Medical Journal (www.cmj.org). There were nine articles on SARS in the journal's June 2003 issue. Of course, by writing articles in Chinese, they are not open for the international scientific and academic community or indexed in databases used by international researchers. Such articles then cannot aid international researchers in their quest. In the words of Rao Zihe, structural biologist at Tsinghua University in Beijing: "China had patient number one, death number one. . . . Publications? Zero" (cited in Enserink, 2003: 296).

Although Chinese data were sparse in the beginning, Tüll used the epidemiological data and the legal measures that were reported to WHO to make an epidemiological analysis and then compare that analysis with the Chinese impression of the data. When it was clear that the Chinese authorities actually knew what they were doing, it was time for the next step: to convince the authorities to present their compiled measures to the international community. Thus, it was important to listen to the Chinese assessments and find out what the problems were on their end. A serious problem regarded communication between different ministries, and between the provinces and the central level. The quote below offers accounts of discussions on the issue at meetings with the Ministries.

> I said, I think it would be a good idea if you present how many fever controls you have carried out at railway stations and trains and how many cases you have found. Then they started to squirm and they said that the Ministry of Transport had that information. Ok, so call them and ask them. Well, it's not that easy. Or, when we met with the Ministry of Science and Technology. We said, there are investigations in Guangdong about infected animals. What are the results? How many people are investigating? That's the Ministry of Agriculture. They don't reveal their information. What has the Military done? Defense, no way! (Tüll, 2004).

When shortcomings were commented upon, it was obvious that the Chinese counterparts were well aware of the problems. The job was made easier with knowledge of general bureaucratic and political shortcomings. Tüll explains: "If you know how governments work, how inter-ministerial relationships are, how the relations to the rural areas are, then it is easier to come to speaking terms." With an altruistic mission the WHO Epidemiology team and the Chinese authorities were working toward the same goal. Initially, the Chinese counterparts might not have been aware of that. But in time they became aware. As a result, the assignment became easier after a while (Tüll, 2004).

*The Chinese Counterparts*

Meetings and negotiations between the WHO and their Chinese counterparts were either formal or informal. Formal negotiations were mostly held with high-level civil servants, working directly under the health minister. These meetings, which were translated by interpreters, were tough and highly politicized. Naturally, it was destined that an outbreak such as SARS would become politicized. The massive losses in BNP growth were a disaster for the administration. So were plummeting numbers of international tourists and the business community's great concerns about the situation (cf. Einhorn, 2003; Clifford and Engardio, 2003). Political adjustments had to be made.

During formal meetings the WHO's counterparts were part of a group within the MOH that managed negotiations. It was possibly the most politicized group in the Ministry. Formal meetings were characterized by political correctness and strictness. The counterparts weighed all issues and questions politically. Neither the civil servants nor the experts that accompanied them would say anything that the Politburo had not approved. The overall question was why there were different demands on different countries. More specifically, the Chinese wanted to know why certain measures were imposed on China and not on other countries.

Formal negotiations were handled by between six and fifteen persons depending on the issue, while the WHO was represented mostly of three or four people. At an ordinary formal meeting the counterparts represented the information division at the MOH and thus the central government. The spokesperson set the political standard, although other participants could express their opinions. The representative of the MOH was a politically tough counterpart who upheld the attitude that the government wanted to present to the rest of the world (Tüll, 2004).

During informal meetings the Chinese were more obliging. While at the formal meetings WHO representatives spoke English with Chinese translation and the counterpart spoke Chinese with English translation, at the informal meetings it turned out that the language barrier was not a problem. Translators were not necessary at informal meetings as everyone spoke English. As Tüll claims, "They spoke better English than I do!" and Tüll did not feel the need to have a translator. Informal meetings dealt with problem solving and were held when the WHO needed specific information to go further. Moreover, informal meetings evolved from formal meetings. After the formal meetings, requests were made to meet a certain person or expert that accompanied the civil servants. When the Chinese counterpart had accepted the informal meeting, the issue at hand moved from being a political issue to an expert issue. Then it was easier to obtain information and the Chinese were more obliging and talkative. The cooperation between the WHO and the Chinese improved with time and it was especially good during informal meetings (Tüll, 2004).

### *Cooperation and Conflict within the WHO*

Communication with the higher WHO level at the office was informal. Meetings were held with Bekedam and Schnur and conversations took place on a daily basis, like at any office. But time was limited. When the Epidemiology team held discussions with, e.g., Schnur, it was evident that he was under stress, running from one meeting to another. Staff meetings were held in the beginning of every morning where staff members reported their tasks at hand. The internal WHO meetings were very informal. Then there were more organized meetings that were held when a specific issue had to be discussed (Tüll, 2004).

One of the Epidemiology team's chores was to support the provincial assessment teams in their search for reliable data. The Epidemiology team met members of provincial assessment teams at the office and they read their reports. This was not an easy task, however, as the reports lacked structure. They differed in style and content, which made it difficult to make comparisons. The Epidemiology team thus started to reflect over what kind of information the WHO really required and ways that assessment teams could improve the arrangement of their work. Team members then gave advice on methods and prepared questionnaires and checklists for the assessment teams. The Epidemiology team listed five areas that they wanted the assessment teams to pay special attention to, namely: discarded fever patients, no contact patients,[10] numbers in other forms of containment, degree of isolation of other containment forms and degree of follow up on discarded patients (ETW, 2003). However, more detailed checklists were not put to test. Since the epidemic passed so quickly, the new system was barely finished.

It was not part of the Epidemiology team's mandate to assess and coordinate the SARS response in Beijing. Given the peculiarities of Beijing in comparison to other Chinese regions, in terms of for instance the amount of cases and cooperation difficulties with the mayor, a special organization was set up for Beijing. The WHO team in charge of assessing the SARS situation in Beijing was made up of personnel solely from CDC Atlanta. The WHO Beijing team worked separately from other WHO staff, which was responsible for other provinces. Although the Epidemiology team had no part in assessing the SARS outbreak in Beijing, it was supposed to manage scientific research issues. This included making assessments of the research that had been undertaken on SARS, by for instance reading national and international scientific articles and identifying and prioritizing key issues for further research. An overview of the whole country would then be helpful. Creating that overview, however, was a bit difficult as there were some people at the office that felt more called upon to deal with the scientific issues. It seemed like some WHO consultants did not want to share the data. When Tüll approached the Beijing team concerning access to Beijing's figures, they were still not provided. Certain consultants seemed more interested in holding on to the figures that were given to them, possibly in order to write articles later. The Epidemiology team therefore had little grasp of Beijing's actions and measures. The Epidemiology team members were not satisfied with the situation. In Tüll's own words:

> I don't know if we would have had so much use of their data since they managed Beijing. Rather it was the working climate that annoyed me. I don't think it disturbed our work (Tüll, 2004).

Almost a year later articles about the management of SARS in Beijing were published in *Emerging Infectious Diseases*. If some WHO consultants had a hidden agenda and prioritized boosting their own careers by publishing articles rather than keeping China's best interests in mind by improving its public health, it could have affected the relations between China and WHO and the trust between the parties. When it comes down to science and publications, institutions and individuals within them tend to be driven by self-interest (Tüll, 2004). Organizational rewards such as funding is on the line, which invites individuals to take part in the struggle. Moreover, means of rewards for scientists are scarce and publication is one of but a few ways to reach such rewards. Herein lies a value conflict between institutional self-interest and altruism. According to the official WHO stance such pathogens, however, were not a factor when combating SARS:

> The urgency of SARS has further challenged WHO to set in motion high-level international scientific and medical collaboration in which natural competition for publication and prestige is set aside in the interest of solving the scientific mysteries of a shared threat (WHO, 2003d:5).

However, consultants now and then retreat from such altruistic paths. Regarding the SARS outbreak it was not only in China that WHO consultants at times worked with their home institutions' interest in mind. Institutional self-interest and loyalty to parent organization came to the fore also in Vietnam and Hong-Kong (Tüll, 2004).[11] One might then suspect that such problems arise now and then during WHO operations. According to the former WHO Representative for Brunei Darussalam, Malaysia, and Singapore, Joel A. Vanderburg, however, problems of institutional self-interest or loyalty are infrequent and concern issues of inadequately communicating with individuals of another culture and problems of adjusting to another culture and are expressions of weaknesses of some individuals rather than a demonstration of organizational routine or frequent behavior (Vanderburg, 2004).

### *Cooperation and Conflict between WHO and China*

Initially relations between WHO and China were marked by conflict over China's cover up policy early on in the outbreak. When China shifted to a more open and cooperative policy, the negotiators spoke about constructive and open attitudes during meetings. However, the politics of secrecy and denial left a mark on the negotiations that were difficult to erase. Even after the central government had committed to cooperating with the WHO, the situation was still characterized by suspicion and confrontation. But a new climate between the parties was developing and when Tüll joined the operation, in early May, cooperation between the WHO and the Chinese counterparts was already running along pretty smoothly. That said, formal negotiations could be really tough. At one such meeting on the national level, discussions concerned what kind of data the WHO received. The WHO received data about what day authorities had reported a case of SARS. But they wanted to know the day of onset, i.e. what day the subject fell ill. Hence, to get an overall assessment of the development, the WHO asked for statistics showing how many people fell ill each day and in what towns. The response was irritable to say the least. The Chinese counterparts called the demands an outrage. Moreover they claimed that since no one had raised demands on the United States to report such figures there was no reason for China to release such data until the United States had made their figures public. After the meeting the WHO team went back to the office. They contacted the headquarters in Geneva, which in turn had to put pressure on Washington. When the WHO had made sure that the United States was open about its figures, China showed its statistics (Tüll, 2004).

Getting access to the right data compilations was a serious problem. The Chinese did not want to admit that they lacked the requested data. Rather they would say that they did not want to hand the data over. The basic problem was that no one on the central level had access to all the data that the WHO requested. The WHO received data from two different directions: One set of data was reported to the epidemiological department at the MOH. The staff members there were statisticians with no training in infectious epidemiology so they did not fully understand what the numbers represented. Epidemiological data and other data were also reported to China CDC. Two separate routes of data then emerged and they were never coordinated (Tüll, 2004).

The latter data route also had certain flaws. Since China CDC is organized on the central, provincial, city and municipal levels, some of the epidemiological data did not make it all the way to the central level. On May 5, a new law was decreed, which stated that all SARS relevant data should be reported to the central level of the China CDC. However, it took a while for the system to run accordingly. Some provinces were still not keen on delivering the data. Possibly inertia in the information chain emerged due to the fact that China CDC was a very young organization that had only been operational for a few years (Tüll, 2004).[12]

### *WHO Center-Field Communication*

As Chinese authorities were implementing several far-reaching measures and launching immense campaigns to combat SARS, some disagreements arose between the WHO center and field. The impression in the field was that the Chinese authorities were indeed taking responsible and thorough action in fighting SARS and this was reported to the head office and the regional office. Despite the field's advantage in access to information, especially in the beginning of Tüll's stay, neither headquarters in Geneva nor the West Pacific Regional Office (WPRO) in Manila believed fully in the reports (Tüll, 2004). This became evident during telephone conferences between the Beijing office and Manila, and Geneva that took place two or three times a week. The conversations were held either by Schnur, Bekedam, or Tüll on speakerphones so several people could listen in. The conversations concerned national numbers and lasted for about two hours. For most of the time, WPRO and headquarters in Geneva were skeptical of the assessments from Beijing. Reports from the WHO's Beijing office stated that things were moving in the right direction. The Beijing staff forwarded information that the Chinese numbers probably were correct, and that many important measures were being taken. Although Tüll, Schnur, Bekedam and the rest of the staff at the Beijing office had access to much more data and first hand information than anyone in Manila or Geneva, reactions from the center were still skeptical (Tüll, 2004).

An article in the *International Herald Tribune*, published as late as June 3, can characterize such center/field skepticism. The article was based on an interview with WHO Regional Adviser for Communicable Disease Surveillance and Response at the WPRO in Manila, Hitoshi Oshitani. Oshitani criticized China's lack of information sharing on the disease and although he trusted that the Chinese numbers were going down, he stressed that the lack of critical epidemiological information made it hard to assess the real situation. According to the *International Herald Tribune*, Oshitani said that "Chinese health officials are still not cooperating adequately in the fight against SARS." He stressed that the WHO was "still in urgent need of information that [they] were just not getting from China" and that "[o]n a policy level things have changed in China, but that has not altered attitudes on an operational level." In addition he reportedly said that:

> China was still disclosing far too little information on the number and background of cases as well as findings about treatments and the possible sources of the disease. We have good cooperation from Singapore, Hong Kong, Canada and even Vietnam. . . . But we still don't get enough information about the outbreak in China. The lack of information makes it difficult to judge the accuracy of China's fast-falling tally of daily new cases (Hitoshi Oshitani quoted in Crampton, 2003d).

More such center/field skepticism was depicted for instance in interviews with David Heymann of the WHO head office in Geneva by the *New York Times* and the *International Herald Tribune*. The articles were published on June 9 and June 7 respectively (Altman, 2003; Crampton, 2003c). According to David Heymann the reason for Geneva and Manila being skeptical was because of the Chinese downplaying the disease in the beginning of the outbreak. From that rather low point, the WHO's confidence in China increased during the process, especially after the breaking point when the MOH was replaced and Wu Yi was inaugurated. However, it was a dual battle and WHO could still not be convinced that transparency would prevail (Heymann, 2004). Joel A. Vanderburg offers a more general explanation:

> Public Health professionals are trained to be skeptical as to completeness of information. This is not from a political perspective, but more so from a scientific one—a need to be assured that information about a health issue is as complete as possible to assure that assumptions and responses are as accurate and as appropriate as existing information allows. This need for assurance is evidenced by a steady and persistent questioning of the circumstances and the conditions (Vanderburg, 2004).

Although the above quotes are signs of variations in center and field assessments, they are also accounts of the major flaw that the field organization had to cope with while dealing with the SARS epidemic. To reach results in the management of extraordinary events or crises of this kind, support from the central political level is required. As long as a commitment from the central political level is lacking the response will be insufficient. In the case of SARS in China, as long as the disease was managed as a regional problem in Guangdong, the province could handle it. The real problems for China started when cross-provincial and governmental coordination and cooperation about political decisions was required. This problem is not specific for China. On the contrary, when complex crises occur there tends to be a "Beijing" in every country, i.e., a regional entity or organization that does not want to adapt, that goes its own way, or that has not quite understood what is required from it (Tüll, 2004). The main problem in China then was Beijing. While cooperation with the other provinces was working, Beijing was not as cooperative. It was obvious that Beijing could not solve the problem on the civil servant level and that, in order to overcome the problems, the issue of combating SARS had to be elevated to the highest political level by gathering different administrative levels together. As the fieldwork continued, Chinese decisions were examined and numbers and authorities' data about each specific case were presented, staff at the Beijing office became increasingly convinced that the Chinese authorities and government had taken considerable measures and that they had made serious efforts to contain the outbreak. Later, it also became obvious that that was the case (ibid.).

*The Last Week and the Final Meeting*

In the end of May, the Chinese authorities initiated a meeting with the WHO concerning regulating the national system of surveillance and reporting. The Chinese government required that their surveillance system for emerging diseases should be uniform for the whole country. A series of meetings were held on the issue, but in early June new issues were prioritized as it was told that David Heymann, Executive Director of Communicable Diseases at WHO Geneva (at the time), was coming to Beijing to assess the situation of SARS control in China.

The gist of the visit would be to assess the WHO travel recommendations that had been imposed on several Chinese regions. The travel recommendations were not popular in China. In fact, China had rejected them from the start (Crampton, 2003a). As a high representative of WHO, Heymann was seen as accountable for the travel recommendations (Tüll, 2004).

On May 23, WHO removed the recommendation that people should postpone all but essential travel to Guangdong and Hong Kong. At the same time WHO also reviewed its travel recommendations for other areas of China, including Beijing, Hebei, Inner Mongolia, Shanxi, Taiwan and Tianjin. Recommendations to consider postponing non-essential travel to these areas remained in place, although WHO had asserted that it would review those travel recommendations regularly (CU, 23 May 2003). The Secretary General in Geneva made decisions regarding the traveling recommendations but when asked about the criteria by the field office in Beijing, Geneva could not spell out what the criteria were for being on the list or not. This put WHO staff in the field in a rather awkward position when asked about the criteria by their Chinese counterparts:

> We couldn't answer because it was a decision from headquarters and the secretary general. We asked headquarters what the criteria were. And they couldn't explain it. It was not a good situation. . . . The Chinese were very frustrated and I understand them. It was foolish to not be able to explain what the criteria were. But I guess that the attitude at headquarters was that if we tell them, they'll adapt to what we're saying. It wasn't satisfactory to defend that position (Tüll, 2004).

The WHO head office did not agree with this view. Heymann has stressed that the travel advisory criteria were clear and readily accessible on the WHO web site (Heymann, 2004).[13] The problem began when the first travel advisory was issued and it became apparent that once a country or area was labeled as an

"Affected Area," there needed to be some criteria for being able to remove that label once all local transmission of the disease had ceased. As SARS was a new disease, very little was known about it. One specific area of uncertainty was the incubation period of the disease. Thus, it was uncertain how long a period must take place following a SARS infection before authorities could be reasonably assured that the public was safe from further occurrences of SARS (Vanderburg, 2004). Different labels possibly added to the confusion. From March 16 through May 1, 2003, the WHO website referred to "Affected Areas." But as of May 2, 2003, "Affected Areas" became refined to "Areas with recent local transmission" (WHO, 2004g).[14]

When it was decided that the WHO delegation headed by Heymann was about to visit Beijing, the WHO Epidemiology team and the Chinese counterparts became engaged in finding out what to do when Heymann came. The answer was to present credible SARS assessments from the different provinces. Prior to the meeting with Heymann another high-level meeting with the Chinese counterparts was held. They wanted the WHO to help them find out what kept them on the travel recommendation list. Since Tüll knew what data the Chinese authorities had and what the international community requested in order to believe in them, he wrote a memo with recommendations of what the Chinese should present. The memo was presented to the high-level public servants and China CDC at the MOH the following day. It included WHO recommendations of what data China should present and how the data should be produced, analyzed and presented. The task of the Epidemiology team, in this respect, was not to do their work but to help them present their efforts, activities and measures in regard to SARS control in a way that was understandable and acceptable to the world at large (Tüll, 2004).

When the WHO representatives declared how they wanted the data to be presented eventually the most senior civil servant from the ministry said that they would come together and present the required data. Nevertheless, Tüll had learned how the system worked during his visit in China. It was likely that the Chinese did not have all the data that the WHO required. Moreover, it was clear that the administration could not handle SARS management on the national level, until authorities across the board pulled together, gathered and reported the required data to the central level. Therefore, they had to call in the provincial (civil servant) leaders (Tüll, 2004).

While the meeting with Heymann was expected to take place on Thursday, June 12, the provincial leaders were summoned to a meeting on Sunday, June 8. Tüll then held a lecture for the provincial leaders with instructions of how the WHO wanted the provinces to present their data. The provincial leaders evidently listened to the WHO's recommendations:

> They must have had a certain amount of trust in me. Otherwise they wouldn't have accepted it. When they understood how they should do it, they did it exactly as I said. There was no questioning (Tüll, 2004).

Then a lot of hard work followed. They worked twenty four hours straight, three days in a row. Although, the amount of work done by each province differed. Guangdong for example, was pretty well prepared since it had more experience and had been dealing with the disease for a longer period (ibid.).

When the different provinces worked with their presentations, the WHO Epidemiology team was there to be of assistance. Credibility was a key aspect. If all provinces' presentations were to be streamlined in the same way, people would not believe in them. Therefore some differences in the various provinces' presentations, in terms of layout, but also in terms of certain aspects that were important in one province but maybe not in another, were required. So, although the basic contents were the same, different provinces gave somewhat different presentations. The message was that they had been thinking and investigating independently and that they understood what they were doing (Tüll, 2004).

When the data were compiled, the provinces presented their work for a small group of WHO staff. Some things had to be redone and changed. In the meantime, media reports stated that Heymann had told the press that he did not trust the Chinese numbers. One such example was an interview with Heymann in the *New York Times* on June 9:

> [The WHO] says it needs to learn much more about how China is reporting SARS cases for it to gain full confidence that the epidemic there is truly waning. It's not the quantity of cases, it's the quality of the data. . . . We depend on what is reported (Heymann, cited in Altman, 2003).

Another example was the interview with Heymann in the *International Herald Tribune* on June 7. There he reportedly said: "We have information only as good as the reports by China or other governments. . . . We cannot certify its accuracy" (Heymann quoted in Crampton, 2003c). In retrospect, however, Heymann emphasizes that the WHO leadership at the time had confidence in what they were hearing and that is why the high level delegation went to Beijing in the first place (Heymann, 2004). The team of senior WHO officials arrived in Beijing on June 11 and the provincial presentations were given the following day.[15]

The presentations were basically demonstrations of credibility. They included a map of the region, basic facts such as size, population and number of big cities and administrative levels. Then more detailed information followed about the disease. An epidemic curve was provided, i.e., the number of probable cases per day. It showed the date of onset and the rise and decline in the number of cases. The probable cases were then dissected into subcategories such as: geographical place of onset, residence (which referred to contact tracing, where the cases originated from) occupational profession, age and gender.

Cluster cases were broken down into some detail and probable connections between the cases were presented. In addition, a thorough presentation of the cases that had no known contact was provided. So was an evaluation and explanation of each case of "no contacts."[16] The presentations also gave an account of the results of community surveillance by listing the number of fever clinics, SARS designated hospitals and how many patients had been found by fever screening. Moreover, the presentations showed the decrease in broad quarantines for the public and the increase in isolation and medical observation for people that had been in contact with SARS victims. They also showed what had been done in terms of guidelines, principles and regulations by listing the number of regulations, established fever clinics and control stations by transportation hubs and how migrant workers were followed up by quarantines and isolation (Tüll, 2004).

Another important aspect, which Tüll specifically asked the provincial leaders to shed light on, was a presentation of the time lag from dates of onset to isolation care per two-week period. This showed the decrease in time between when a person fell ill and when that person's contact tracing was accomplished. While the time lag in some cases lasted up to five days in the beginning of the outbreak, the presentations showed that they had decreased to a day or in some cases to a couple of hours. The presentations fostered credibility. After the presentations there was a thorough time slot for questions and the audience was impressed by the presentations. They showed that on every level in this huge country there was a structured response to SARS and that the reports were based on a solid foundation (Tüll, 2004).

Although all presentations had not yet been made, Heymann was returning home after the first day of presentations. Before leaving Beijing he spoke to the international media in a considerably more positive tone regarding China's response to SARS than had been the case a few days earlier. Heymann said on CNN that the disease had finally been contained in China and he praised China's efforts in mobilizing the population as well as monitoring the situation, identifying new cases, and providing treatment (CNN, 2003b).

After hearing first-hand about what was being done in China to contain the disease the WHO leadership was more confident in China and the presentations had increased its conviction that China was acting appropriately (Heymann, 2004). However, Heymann also acknowledged that huge questions remained unanswered over how the disease originated and spread to humans (CNN, 2003b). Daniel Felkin of the WHO also participated in the meeting and like

Heymann he was predominantly satisfied when he spoke to the press after the meeting:

> We are confident that the numbers are being reported accurately. . . . It does seem like they have really made an effort to report fully that their surveillance systems are quite good now and they have learned from some of the mistakes made early on in the outbreak (Felkin, 2003).

On June 13, the same day that Heymann returned to Geneva, travel recommendations for the provinces of Hebei, Inner Mongolia, Shanxi and Tianjin, were removed. In addition Guangdong, Hebei, Hubei, Inner Mongolia, Jilin, Jiangsu, Shaanxi, Shanxi and Tianjin provinces were removed from the list of areas with recent local transmission (WHO, 2004a). Concurrently Tüll's assignment in China came to an end and he departed from China the same day (Tüll, 2004).

## *Conclusions*

The case of combating SARS in China sheds light on several issues that might have implications for international crisis management practice and theory. Some of these issues are discussed in this concluding section.

### *Bureau politics and organizational pathogens*

Although crises many times make stakeholders strive for consensus decision-making, while public action involves coming together in united efforts, organizational politics flourish in crisis. In crises agencies' decision-makers often try to safeguard institutional interests (Rosenthal and 't Hart, 1991: 358). Organizational or bureaucratic politics can be detrimental to problem solving, early warning and information sharing. But, interestingly enough, interagency tensions do not invariably lead to negative consequences. On the contrary, bureaucratic turf battles can also lead to various positive side effects; for example, they might counteract groupthink tendencies, promote openness or facilitate democratic control (Rosenthal, 't Hart and Kouzmin, 1991: 211). Notwithstanding the above arguments, there is also a risk that bureaucratic politics amount to segmentation and non-contact if the conflict becomes institutionalized (ibid: 217).

In the case of SARS combat in China, Chinese domestic bureaucratic politics initially provided a barrier against swiftly tracking and eradicating the disease. Lack of cooperation and information sharing between the government and agencies operating from other parts of the hierarchical institutional layers that at worst escalated into non-contacts does not necessarily imply that there was an outspoken will not to cooperate. An alternative explanation is that the bureau-politics was a result of agencies that lacked a history of cooperation and suddenly were compelled to work together. As 't Hart, Rosenthal and Kouzmin (1993: 23) stress pre-existing bureaucratic tensions hardly wither away during crisis. On the contrary, bureau-political tensions often intensify.

As any large-scale crisis, the case of SARS in China was a rare opportunity for many actors to bolster the public opinion of their agency and also a chance for individuals to climb a step or two in the career ladder. But it is essential for consultants, working for international organizations, to work against the same goal. Signs of organizational politics were evident among individual consultants working for the WHO. Some consultants apparently had difficulties in pushing institutional self interests aside and working for the greater good of the WHO and the member states that the international organization was assisting. Such behavior might not only hamper efficient problem solving and crisis management but also jeopardize relations between the WHO and their local counterparts as well damage the international organizations' credibility worldwide in the long run.

*Center-field relations*

Crisis management literature often refer to the centralization thesis as a tendency to centralize administrative decision-making during crisis by concentrating power to a limited number of decision-makers, to the central government or searching for strong leadership in crisis ('t Hart, Rosenthal and Kouzmin, 1993: 12-14). The reason behind such aspirations is to avoid formal and slow decision-making routines (Rosenthal, Boin and Comfort, 2001: 19). In the case of SARS combat in China all three kinds of centralization were seen, but for most times centralization in this case refers to consolidation of power to the central government. It was not until such centralization of decision-making to the Politburo came about that a coordinated, comprehensive and vigilant response to the outbreak was established. But even after SARS had scaled up the hierarchical chart, problems for decision makers were manifold. Learning about measures taken in various provinces and getting access to statistics from the provinces was essential for building a cohesive response to the outbreak. This was difficult as established channels of communication between the different actors at various levels in the hierarchy were missing. Such channels had to be constructed in the midst of the crisis. Naturally, then it took some time before they were working efficiently.

Center-field relations were also an issue for the WHO. Leadership and public administration literature often refer to variations in the appreciation of the problems at hand as the appreciative gap between center and field. When this gap is established it is likely to be prolonged by following misunderstandings (cf. Boin, 1998: 29ff). While leaders placed in the center might be physically and/or psychically distant from the crisis, leaders on the field may find themselves caught up in the middle of the suffering and hardship that follows in the wake of a crisis. In such situations strident appeals for more resources and appreciation from the center will most probably develop (cf. Deverell, 2003: 85). In the case of SARS in China, there was another form of appreciative gap between center and field. Variations in proximity to the crisis and access to accurate information influenced the interpretations of the crisis. Opinions about the daily events differed and the WHO's field office in Beijing had to work hard to persuade the WHO center (i.e., the WHO regional office in Manila and headquarters in Geneva) that they were making good progress.

*Credibility traps and credibility gaps*

It is naturally detrimental to credibility to build up expectations without fulfilling promises. Such gaps between words and actions lead to credibility traps. It is a common pit fall for crisis managers to resort to ill-advised statements early on in a crisis when the full scope of the situation at hand has not yet been fully realized. These statements tend to come back and haunt stakeholders as long as the crisis is not solved (cf. Newlove, Stern and Svedin, 2000: 126). The Chinese government along with several agencies found themselves caught up in a serious credibility trap after the initial dormant response to the SARS outbreak. When it was evident for the world at large that official statements declaring the disease under control were incorrect a more active response was launched. But then it was too late. The damage to Chinese credibility was already done and the international trust in agencies and decision-makers at the time was low. The Chinese government tried to speed up the struggle for retaining credibility by letting a couple of officials take responsibility for the initial failure to respond accurately to the new disease. But real results were required in order to regain international credibility. Despite massive efforts in SARS combat and control, the fact that China's starting position was tainted by the lack of credibility, meant that this was an uphill battle. It took some time for the parties to shake off the mutual feelings of suspicion. In addition, the international crisis politics setting is conducive to miscommunication and misunderstandings as the high pace and piercing noise level make accurate communication difficult (Allison and Zelikow, 1999: 310).

*Experts and decision-makers*

Like most organizations, the WHO is staffed and structured according to normalcy. When a contingency or crisis occurs within the field of the WHO's expertise, the organization has to adapt to the extraordinary conditions. Expertise from member states and global partners is then contracted on a relative short-term basis. Bringing in consultants on rather short-term contracts and some times ad hoc, can be problematic. There is a risk that different working ethics and variations in organizational styles might collide. In addition, there is no simple or clear-cut relationship between experts and decision-makers in crisis. Expert advice is only one of many sources of influence on decision-making. Many times stake-holders, deliberately or not, choose advice or interpret it in an unfavorable way (Rosenthal and 't Hart, 1991); it may also put strain on the experts as they suddenly, in a situation of stress, time pressure and values at stake, may find themselves in a strong position. In crises expert advice might have great importance and lead to comprehensive implications.

WHO consultants seemed careful not to overstep the lines between advisor and decision-maker for most of the times, although the lines may have been fuzzy at times. The mission was advisory and trust-building, and although advice was many times highly influential, the mission did not evolve into making real decisions.

Another problem related to experts is risk of dual institutional loyalties, loyalty to the WHO and loyalty to the parent institution. If consultants from other institutions find it difficult to meet their obligations to WHO because of their emotional or professional ties to their parent institution, it would indeed be a problem. The question is if it is an organizational problem or an individual one regarding individual employees. Whatever the answer, it affects the WHO and therefore it needs to be solved on the organizational level.

*Experiential learning*

Although individuals constantly make use of experience when solving problems, they tend to find it difficult to draw accurate lessons and refraining from over-generalizing from past experiences (Rose, 1993; Khong, 1992; Hacker, 2001). Drawing and making use of the crisis experience of oneself and of others is vital for creating reliable organizations and societies as well as for decreasing the risks of future crises. Many of the problems that emerged while working in China were hardly specific for the huge Eastern Asian state. On the contrary, many problems that the WHO faced were general problems that could just as well have turned up in any other country. Prior fieldwork experience (not least from other communist or post-communist countries) and understanding generic patterns of bureaucratic peculiarities were beneficial for experts dealing with SARS combat in China. It was an advantage to understand the ways of governments. There are often tensions over funds between ministries and authorities and there is often lack of communication between ministries and authorities. Furthermore, when new organizations are born, changes in the emergency or coordination planning are required. This might be a reason behind flawed communication practices (cf. Rosenthal, 't Hart and Kouzmin, 1991: 20-21). China CDC had been operational less than a year and never before faced such a challenge. Organizational experiences of a large scale crisis of this kind were thus lacking within the China CDC.

It was also favorable to have insights into the culture and the relations between provincial and central government. Many times and in many different settings it is difficult to get these levels to cooperate. In the case of SARS in China there were tensions between, e.g., Shanghai and Beijing and the central government. Finally, it was beneficial to grasp the position that the Armed Forces has in the bureaucracy. In China the military resembles "a state within the state" (Tüll, 2004). A long way into the struggle against SARS, the military hospitals refused to align with the Chinese civil authorities and the WHO. Eventually, the highest political leadership forced the military hospitals to release data.

*Operational and strategic agencies*

In the aftermath of the SARS crisis, the role of the WHO has been heavily emphasized. It is undisputed that the WHO plays an important role in general and that it played an important role in combating SARS. WHO has established a gamut of guidelines that support countries that are affected by outbreaks and diseases. Nevertheless, it is necessary to keep in mind that the WHO is not an operational agency. The operational role is taken on by the member states. If the member states do not show sufficient interest in dealing with emergent diseases, there is (so far) not much the WHO can do about it. In the case of SARS in China all the legislation, rules and guidelines that were made in China had most likely been decided and implemented even without assistance of the WHO. The WHO gave support by offering technical assistance to China, and other countries. Thus China and other countries received assistance from capable people. Clearly it was favorable to the affected countries to receive assistance from people with understanding of, for instance, scientific methodology. When the WHO staff and consultants looked at existing and new guidelines they could spot the flaws. But the WHO did not gather the data. Basically, all the data rested in the hands of Chinese authorities. The WHO could only assist authorities, stressing that in order to make sure that the international community would believe in the data, especially after the cover up, the data had to be presented in a reliable way. And by explaining what way, contents and analysis was required to make sure that the data would be regarded as credible, and the authorities could adapt to the recommendations (Tüll, 2004).

## Notes

1. This chapter is to a large extent based on interviews with Peet Tüll, and the author would like to thank him for his extensive participation. The views presented are not necessarily the views of the WHO.

2. The regional office for Africa, the Americas, South East Asia, Europe, the Eastern Mediterranean and the Western Pacific.

3. Partners include the Canadian Global Public Health Intelligence Network (GPHIN), which is a search engine for real time early warning that continuously scans Internet communications for rumors and reports of suspicious diseases (WHO, 2003c), the U.S. Global Emerging Infection Surveillance and Response System (GEIS) and the WHO Global Influenza Surveillance Network (GISN). The latter is a global alert system for emergent influenza viruses with pandemic potential.

4. In retrospect, James Maguire (2003) of WHO's Beijing Assessment Team and CDC Atlanta agrees that the epidemic in Guangdong in fact, at that time, was beginning to come under control.

5. The five-person team had been invited to China by the MOH and had arrived in Beijing on March 23. Upon arrival, the team members required permission to travel to Guangdong, but they had to wait eight days for access (Huang, 2003; WHO, 2004a; Crampton, 2003b).

6. According to discussions between Tüll (2004) and executives for companies such as, e.g., ABB, Ericsson, and SAS Radisson at the Swedish Embassy on June 6, 2003. See also Einhorn (2003) and Clifford & Engardio (2003).

7. Partly because Chinese legislation and articles were not being translated and thus were not well known to the international community (Tüll, 2004).

8. Health authority was divided amongst the State Food and Drug Administration, Ministry of Labor and Social Security, State Family Planning Council and the Administration for Quality, Supervision, Inspection and Quarantine. In addition the Ministry of Science and Technology is an important player in coordinating and supporting health research (WHO RC, 2003:6)

9. Before joining WHO's Field office in Beijing on a consultant basis, Tüll had extensive experience of WHO consultancy assignments. His field experience included assessment work for WHO's Polio Eradication program in Kazakhstan, Azerbaijan, Georgia, Bulgaria and Bangladesh as well as small pox eradication for WHO in Bangladesh and assessing HIV programs in India and Estonia.

10. The proportion of probable and suspected cases with unknown exposure was relatively high and that needed to be addressed and followed up on.

11. In Hanoi WHO consultants reportedly tried to obtain and smuggle samples (since they were not allowed to export samples). There was also a dispute regarding the outbreak in Hong Kong. Apparently the leader of the Hong Kong team did not distribute data to CDC Atlanta, which upset a few people there (Tüll, 2004).

12. China CDC is a huge network of organizations. There are over four thousand CDCs in China with more than two hundred thousand staff (WHO RC, 2003:5). A ceremony marking the establishment of China CDC was held on January 23, 2002 (Koplan, 2002). However, in the April 2002 issue of the *Bulletin of the World Health Organization* it is mentioned that China CDC is being set up and that the China CDC building is being built (Walgate, 2002). It then seems more likely that China CDC had not been operational for more than six months when the first outbreak of SARS began in Guangdong in November 2002.

13. Sources on the web are somewhat ambiguous regarding the criteria. On April 23, the criteria for why a region, country or city should be on the list or not was based on the magnitude of active cases, i.e., the number of prevalent cases and the daily number of new cases, the extent of local chains of transmission, and evidence of exported cases (WHO, 2004d). However in the province of Hebei, the given criteria were the magnitude of the outbreak "and evidence that local chains of transmission are occurring outside a confined setting, such as the health care environment" (WHO, 2004e). In the case of Taiwan the "adequacy of surveillance measures, including screening for new cases and tracing and follow-up of contacts" was also mentioned as a criteria (WHO, 2004f).

14. According to Vanderburg WHO recognized that the concerns were legitimate, but knowledge about the disease was so limited that accurate responses took some time to acquire. The issue was both raised and resolved within a period of no more than one month. This can be considered as a short time as the amount of knowledge that was gathered on SARS from the time it became recognized until its containment was quite remarkable (Vanderburg, 2004).

15. The following officials were present: Heymann, Henk Bekedam, Guénaël Rodier, director of WHO's Department of Communicable Disease Surveillance and Response (CDS), Denis Coulombier, CDS Epidemiology Team Coordinator, Thomas Grein, who coordinated global response operations for SARS, Roy Anderson, head of the Department of Infectious Disease Epidemiology at Imperial College in London and world authority on modeling, and Peet Tüll. The minister of health, and the highest provincial executives represented the Chinese (CU, 11 June 2003; Tüll, 2004)

16. "No contacts" might have appeared due to, e.g., the uncertainty of the disease and the diagnosis, flawed tracing, symptomatic patients, or other diseases (Tüll, 2004.)

## *References*


Allison, G. and P. Zelikow (1999) *Essence of Decision: Explaining the Cuban Missile Crisis*. 2nd edition. New York: Longman.

Altman, L.K. (9 June 2003) "SARS decline but doubts remain." *New York Times*.

Bekedam, H. (24 April 2003) Interview with Dr. Henk Bekedam, WHO representative in China, about the SARS situation in Beijing on *As It Happens*. Accessed on 4 March 2004. Available at: http://www.cbc.ca/news/background/sars/media.html.

Boin, A. (1998) *Contrasts in Leadership: An Institutional Study of Two Prison Systems*. Leiden: Eburon Publishers.

China Update/CU (20, 21, 23 and 28 April 2003; 6, 8, 10, 12 and 25 May 2003; 11 June 2003) Accessed on 9 March 2004. Available at: http://www.wpro.who.int/wr/chn/

Chinese Medical Journal (2003) Vol. 116, No. 6, June issue. Accessed on 8 July 2004. Available at: http://www.cmj.org/information/issuelist.asp?py=2003andpi=6.

Clifford, M. L. and P. Engardio (5 May 2003) "Standing Guard against SARS: How a big factory in Southern China is keeping the disease out." Accessed on 15 July 2004. Available at: http://www.businessweek.com/magazine/content/03_18/b3831065_mz014.htm

CNN.com (2003a) "SARS travel warning lifted for more of China". Published on 13 June 2003. Accessed on 6 May 2004. Available at: http://www.cnn.com/2003/HEALTH/06/13/sars/index.html

CNN.com (2003b) "SARS under control in China: WHO." Published on 12 June 2003. Accessed on 6 May 2004. Available at: http://www.cnn.com/2003/HEALTH/06/12/sars.wrap/index.html

Crampton, T. (2003a) "With SARS on rise, China disputes UN's travel warning." *The International Herald Tribune*, 5 April 2003.

Crampton, T. (2003b) "UN body warns travelers on SARS Southern China and Hong Kong are to be avoided." *The International Herald Tribune*, 3 April 2003.

Crampton, T. (2003c) "SARS wave could be peaking, UN says." *The International Herald Tribune*, 7 June 2003.

Crampton, T. (2003d) "WHO assails China for faltering on SARS." *The International Herald Tribune*, 3 June 2003.

Deverell, E. (2003) *The 2001 Kista blackout: Corporate Crisis and Urban Contingency*, Stockholm: CRISMART/ Swedish National Defence College.

Einhorn, B. (26 May 2003) "Taiwan's SARS Luck Runs Out." *Business Week Online*. Accessed on 15 July 2004. Available at: http://www.businessweek.com/magazine/content/03_21/b3834160_mz033.htm

Enserink, M. (18 July 2003) "China's Missed Chance." *Science*, vol. 301: pp. 294-296.

ETW (2003) "Epidemiology Team Workplan." Peet Tüll's private document.

Felkin, D. (13 June 2003) Interview with Dr. Daniel Felkin of the WHO if the SARS outbreak is near its end in China. Accessed on 4 March 2004. Available at: http://www.cbc.ca/news/background/sars/media.html.

Hacker, J. S. (2001) "Learning from Defeat? Political Analysis and the Failure of Health Care Reform in the United States." *British Journal of Political Science*, January: no. 31, pp. 61-94.

't Hart, P., U. Rosenthal, and A. Kouzmin (1993) "Crisis Decision Making: The Centralization Thesis Revisited." *Administration and Society*, Vol. 25, May: No. 1, pp. 12-45.

Heymann, D.L. (2004) Telephone interview with David Heymann, former WHO Executive Director of Communicable Diseases, on September 3, 2004.

Heymann, D.L. and Rodier, G. (2004) "Global Surveillance, National Surveillance, and SARS", *Emerging Infectious Diseases*, 10:2; February, pp. 173-175.

Huang, Y. (2003) "Implications of SARS Epidemic for China's Public Health Infrastructure and Political System" Prepared Statement dated May 12, 2003, pp. 33-41 in *Dangerous Secrets—SARS and China's Healthcare System*, Roundtable Before the Congressional Executive Commission on China, 108th Congress, 1st Session, May 12, 2003.

Khong, Y. F. (1992) *Analogies at War: Korea, Munich, Dien Bien Phu, and the Vietam Decision of 1965*. Princeton, N.J.: Princeton University Press.

Koplan, J. (23 January 2002) "Remarks of Dr. Jeffrey Koplan, Director of the U.S. Centers for Disease Control and Prevention (CDC), at a Ceremony Marking the Establishment of the China CDC." Accessed on 14 May 2004. Available at: http://www.usembassy-china.org.cn/sandt/KoplanSpeech-CH-CDC.htm

Maguire, J. (14 November 2003) "SARS in China: CDC Official Maguire Describes the Story of What Happened." *Harvard Public Health NOW*. Accessed on 11 May 2004. Available at: http://www.hsph.harvard.edu/now/nov14/

Newlove, L. M., E. K. Stern and L. Svedin (2000) *Auckland Unplugged.* Stockholm: ÖCB/CRISMART.

Online Newshour Update (9 April 2003) China accused of concealing extent of SARS spread. Accessed on 4 March 2004. Available at: www.pbs.org/newshour/updates/sars_04-09-03.html

Rose, R. (1993) *Lesson-drawing in Public Policy: A Guide to Learning across Time and Space*. Chatham, N.J.: Chatham House Publishers Inc.

Rosenthal, E. (12 April 2003) "Doctor says China lied about SARS in Beijing." *New York Times*.

Rosenthal, U., A. Boin and L. K. Comfort (2001)"The Changing World of Crises and Crisis Management." In *Managing Crises: Threats, Dilemmas, Opportunities*, edited by U. Rosenthal, A. Boin and L. K. Comfort, pp. 5-27. Springfield, Illinois: Charles C Thomas Publisher Ltd.

Rosenthal, U. and P. 't Hart (1991) "Experts and Decision Makers in Crisis Situations." *Knowledge: Creation, Diffusion, Utilization*, Vol. 12, June Issue: No. 4, pp. 350-372.

Rosenthal, U., P. 't Hart and A. Kouzmin (1991) "The Bureau-Politics of Crisis Management." *Public Administration*, Vol. 69, Summer issue: pp. 211-233.

Tüll, P. J. (2004) Interviews with Peet J. Tüll, Medical Director at the National Board of Health and Welfare and later WHO. Interviews took place on February 24 and April 1, 2004, at the National Board of Health and Welfare in Stockholm, Sweden and on July 7, 2004, at the WHO Regional Office for Europe in Copenhagen, Denmark.

Vanderburg, J. A. (2004) "Responses to Questions" received on September 29 and October 26, 2004. E-mail correspondence with Joel A. Vanderburg, Acting WHO Representative for Brunei Darussalam, Malaysia, and Singapore stationed in Kuala Lumpur, Malaysia from February through June 2003.

Walgate, R. (2002) "China sets up Centres for Disease Control and Prevention." *Bulletin of the World Health Organization*, 80 (4):335.

WHO (2002) "Revision of the International Health Regulations." Report by the Secretariat, Executive Board EB111/34, 111th Session on December 15, 2002.

WHO (2003a) "SARS - A Challenge for the Region." SARS Preparedness and Response Team, World Health Organization, Western Pacific Regional Office, 54th Session of the Regional Committee Meeting for the Western Pacific, on September 8-12, 2003. PPT presentation available at: http://www.wpro.who.int /sars/docs/presentation/challengefortheregion.pdf.

WHO (2003b) *Consensus document on the epidemiology of severe acute respiratory syndrome (SARS).* Department of Communicable Diseases Surveillance and Response.

WHO (2003c) "Severe acute respiratory syndrome (SARS): Status of the outbreak and lessons for the immediate future." WHO, CDSR. Geneva. 20 May 2003.

WHO (2004a) "Update 95, SARS: Chronology of a serial killer." Accessed on 23 February 2004. Available at: http://www.who.int/csr/don/2003_07_04/en/.

WHO (2004b) "Global Outbreak Alert and Response Network." Accessed on 22 March 2004. Available at: http://www.who.int/csr/outbreaknetwork/en/

WHO (2004c) "CSR information resources." Accessed on 14 April 2004. Available at: http://www.who.int/csr/resources/en/.

WHO (2004d) "Update 37 - WHO extends its SARS-related travel advice to Beijing and Shanxi Province in China and to Toronto Canada." Published on 23 April 2003. Accessed on 9 September 2004. Available at: http://www.who.int/csr/sars /archive/2003_04_23/en/.

WHO (2004e) "Update 58 - First global consultation on SARS epidemiology, travel recommendations for Hebei Province (China), situation in Singapore." Published on 17 May 2003. Accessed on 9 September 2004. Available at: http://www.who.int /csr/sars/archive/2003_05_17/en/.

WHO (2004f) "Update 82—Change in travel recommendations for Taiwan." Published on 17 June 2003. Accessed on 8 September 2004. Available at: http://www.who.int /csr/don/2003_06_17/en/.

WHO (2004g) "Areas with recent local transmission of SARS." Accessed on 27 October 2004. Available at: http://www.who.int/csr/sarsareas/en/.

WHO Presentation (2004) "Main directions of the communicable disease surveillance: International collaboration in the framework of the WHO and EC." Bulgaria, 30 April 2004, by Peet Tüll.

WHO RC (18 July 2003) [The Office of the World Health Organization Representative in China] "Public Health Options for China: Using the Lessons Learned from SARS." *Mail.*

# Chapter 6

# Lessons Learned from the Greater Toronto Outbreak

Dan Markel and Christopher Stoney

## *Introduction*

Outside of Asia, Canada was the country hardest hit by SARS. Nonetheless SARS–like illnesses, such as avian influenza, continue to fuel concern that Canada is vulnerable to serious infectious diseases. Severe Acute Respiratory Syndrome (SARS) arrived in Canada via airline passengers traveling from Hong Kong on February 26, 2003. Estimated by the World Health Organization (WHO) to kill fifteen percent of people who contract the virus (and more than fifty percent of elderly patients), it spread without detection for more than two weeks. By the time it was contained, some four months later, it had cost forty four lives, made countless others sick, led to thirty thousand Canadians being placed in quarantine and had paralyzed a major segment of Ontario's health care system (National Advisory Committee on SARS and Public Health/NACSPH, 2003; Crowe et al., 2003).

Furthermore, the Greater Toronto Area (GTA), Canada's major urban centre, was economically devastated by the SARS outbreak and its important tourist industry has yet to fully recover. With Toronto being at the heart of Canadian industry, tourism and finance, the economic impact of the SARS outbreak, reached far beyond the GTA. According to the TD Bank, for example, the estimated net cost of the GTA SARS outbreak to the national economy ranged from $1.5 to $2.1 billion Canadian (US$ 1.2 -1.7 billion) (NACSPH, 2003). Factored into this estimate is the direct impact that the GTA SARS outbreak had on tourism and travel, the immediate costs through public health and health care measures necessary to contain the outbreak and treat those affected, as well as a wide-range of indirect costs that were incurred as a result of:

> lost productivity from illness, quarantine, self-isolation, and related workflow disruption; payments to health care facilities and physicians in lieu of ordinary throughput-related revenues that were interrupted by SARS; salary and other compensation for those who were quarantined or otherwise unable to carry on their normal duties of employment as a result of SARS; and service backlogs in health care and public health [had to be] cleared (NACSPH, 2003: p.96).

Public and commercial concerns about the inadequate and apparently uncoordinated response of Canada's health and emergency services to the SARS outbreak have been reinforced by a number of critical inquiries and investigations. The SARS Commission Interim Report (Campbell, 2004), for example, was scathing in relation to the way the SARS crisis was handled. In terms of Canada's public health capacity and emergency management procedures, SARS exposed serious weaknesses that confirmed growing concerns about the relatively low priority afforded by politicians to developing and funding longer-term strategies.

In particular, a lack of resources, weak leadership, poor communication and inadequate coordination between agencies and the three tiers of Canadian government (municipal, provincial and federal) have been identified as some of the key factors which undermined the effectiveness of Canada's response to SARS. Fortunately, SARS was only moderately contagious and did not turn into a full-blown pandemic (Gandey, 2003). Nonetheless, it severely tested local, provincial, and federal capacity to deal with the outbreak, and consequently, illuminated many of the strengths and deficiencies of the existing public health and health care systems (NACSPH, 2003; Frank et al., 2003; Gandey, 2003; MacKay, 2003; Nature, 2003).

No one could argue that the Canadian authorities had not been given sufficient warning about the probability of such an outbreak, or had not been advised of Canada's widely predicted inability to cope effectively. A plethora of reports, inquiries and similar emergencies had pointed to many weaknesses and limitations, yet relatively little was done to act on these warnings and bring about the necessary reforms.

Consequently, in addition to chronicling the SARS crisis in Canada, this chapter will analyze the combination of underlying systemic factors that together undermined the health system's attempts to prevent and manage SARS. In so doing, it goes beyond the strictly medical or health issues raised by SARS and analyses the economic, political and social factors that have created the public policy context and infrastructure within which healthcare professionals operate and decisions are made.

However, in addition to analyzing the inherent limitations of Canada's response to SARS, this chapter also identifies the measures, decisions and efforts that eventually enabled the spread of SARS to be contained. In particular, the exceptional efforts of healthcare professionals and the informal systems and cooperation that emerged are examined. In order to examine these points in more depth, we focus on the GTA, as it proved to be the main epicenter of the SARS outbreak in Canada and was by far the most seriously affected urban centre.

This chapter will also review and assess the key reforms being made to Canada's public health, healthcare and emergency preparedness systems and infrastructure in the light of the SARS outbreak. In the process of examining these reforms, we assess the degree of political commitment and institutional learning that is taking place in the wake of the SARS crisis. These factors are particularly relevant at a time when growing international travel and greater trade between countries, combined with the threats of biological terrorism and avian based pandemics, make the ability to cope with infectious diseases one of the most pressing issues facing governments around the world:

> Many factors facilitate the spread of infectious diseases, including globalization of travel and trade, weakening of national and international public health infrastructure, deterioration of socio-economic conditions, and heightened political and civil strife in some developing nations. These conditions render populations more vulnerable to infections and provide an environment conducive to the transmission of infectious diseases (Kombe and Darrow, 2001: p. 113).

For example, figures from the 2001 census (2003) estimated that at the time of the SARS outbreak, there were over one million (1,094,700) Canadian residents of Chinese origin and that 436,000 of those lived in Toronto while 348,000 resided in Vancouver. Continued immigration from China to Canada during the last five years has continued to increase these numbers and, in addition to growing business travel, will obviously have increased travel and the potential for infection between the two countries.

Faced increasingly with global health threats, there is a pressing need for health authorities around the world to develop adaptive responses and, in this context, we draw out the key lessons to be learned from the SARS outbreak and consider the extent to which Canada's public health system is now in a stronger position to deal with outbreaks of new and anticipated infectious diseases. Finally, we consider what further steps could be taken.

*SARS Enters Canada*

In mid-November 2002, a mystery illness emerged in China and quickly spread throughout parts of the country. Soon, messages were scattered worldwide by the Chinese media, and the Internet warning of a potentially deadly virus (NACSPH, 2003; CBC News Online, 2003a and 2003b; Crowe et al., 2003). Even as far away as Canada, indications of its potential seriousness could be seen. For example, large quantities of surgical masks, had been disappearing from the shelves of Vancouver stores, Canadian friends and family had been getting concerned telephone calls from mainland Chinese, requests were being made to pharmacists for masks to be sent overseas, and the front pages of Toronto's Chinese newspapers were being saturated with stories regarding the Chinese outbreak (Crowe et al., 2003).

The failure to confine the SARS outbreak can be traced to a number of factors. First, the inability to identify the virus was compounded by the silence of the Chinese authorities and their apparent reluctance to take effective action (NACSPH, 2003; CBC News Online, 2003a and 2003b).

Second, SARS is a potentially fatal, droplet-spread viral condition, but its initial symptoms are non-specific (i.e., muscle aches and pains, severe fatigue, dry cough, shortness of breath, and fever) and thus resemble those of many other respiratory infections including the common cold. In addition, no physical examination or biochemical test existed to identify the disease and, together, these factors made SARS harder to detect, despite attempts by Canadian health officials to warn doctors, infection control specialists, hospitals, emergency room physicians, public health authorities, the provinces and other relevant individuals for influenza-like symptoms in travelers returning from China (CBC News Online, 2004; NACSPH, 2003). Consequently, it was only by late February 2003, that this mystery illness had acquired the name SARS and it took a further month for the illness to be traced to the corona-virus. The failure to identify and detect SARS quickly assisted the virus to spread once in Canada, as catching an infectious disease at its early stages of manifestation is obviously crucial to containing its spread (Crowe, 2003).

Third, standard public health measures such as infection control, isolation, and transmission precautions were virtually non-existent in Canada as well as in China (Talaga et al., 2003b; Bonnell, 2003). For example, the first (undiagnosed) SARS patient admitted, the son of an infected woman who returned from Hong Kong (Canadian index case), was kept in an open emergency room for 24 hours and only separated from other patients by a curtain (NACSPH, 2003). Neither his symptoms nor those of his mother, who had died a few days earlier, were afforded any special attention. Consequently, hospital patients unknowingly infected with SARS mixed with other patients and family members. Even in the emergency room, where patients were being treated by tracheal intubation, little was done to prevent cross-infection (NACSPH, 2003).

Together, these factors contributed significantly to SARS establishing a bridgehead in Canada and enabled it to spread quickly in the GTA (NACSPH, 2003). Nevertheless, on April 25, 2003, health officials in Toronto insisted that the SARS outbreak was under control and by mid-May, Ontario announced that the provincial emergency was over. However, on May 23, 2003, new SARS infections were traced to a Toronto hospital where investigators discovered that the disease has been spreading unchecked for weeks.

The number of cases in this second phase of the outbreak, initially thought to be in the twenties, eventually rose to over one hundred probable and suspected cases. At least five thousand people in Toronto were ordered into quarantine, including fifteen hundred students and one hundred teachers, while health officials were required to investigate dozens of suspected new cases across the GTA region. On July 2, 2005, the WHO finally removed Toronto's name from the list of SARS affected cities for the second time.

In finally eradicating SARS several key tools were used to try to control the epidemic, including: case detection; patient isolation; contact tracing; and the quarantining of contacts; strict infection control measures in hospitals (i.e., including contact and droplet precautions such as hand washing, wearing gowns, gloves, N95 masks, eye protection, and the use of single or negative pressure rooms for all SARS patients; the suspension of non-essential hospital services, the limitation of hospital visitors, the creation of isolation units for potential SARS patients); the closure of hospitals; the creation and eventual closure of outpatient clinics to lessen the burden on emergency departments, and help prevent further transmission; the suspension of all non-SARS activity in infectious diseases; a private health-care personnel agency was retained and international laboratory collaboration flourished (e.g., between the Canadian National Microbiology Laboratory, the Centre for Disease Prevention and Control, the WHO and several countries, including the United States) and this promoted a better understanding of SARS. There were also attempts to improve communication and detection via regular updates on websites; daily teleconferences; airline passenger screening and travel advisories (NACSPH, 2003).

Important as these measures may have been, it was the courageous efforts of health professionals that were crucial in helping contain the outbreak. Frontline public health officials and health-care workers in particular worked extraordinary hours and placed themselves at personal risk (many nurses, for example, contracted SARS and several died from it) in order to protect, promote, and restore people's health. Without such professionalism and the basic, but effective, public health measures listed above, it would not have been possible to manage and combat SARS (NACSPH, 2003; Gandey, 2003).

Notwithstanding the efforts of public health and healthcare professionals, the fact that the SARS virus claimed lives and took over four months to contain led to criticism of the public health authorities and the governments responsible for handling the crisis. Sheila Copps for example, the then Federal Minister of Heritage, criticized key actors in the Liberal government, and blamed then Health Minister Anne McClellan for the delayed federal response to the SARS outbreak. At the provincial level widespread criticism led then Ontario Premier, Ernie Eves to call the first of several inquiries into how SARS was handled. The following section reviews the findings of these inquiries and analyses some of the deep inadequacies and systemic factors that may have undermined Canada's ability to identify and manage SARS more effectively.

### *Factors Contributing to the Spread of SARS in the GTA*

#### Forewarned, but not forearmed

Long before the emergence of SARS, evidence of weaknesses in public health infrastructure, outbreak management and emergency preparedness had been mounting, but a well-coordinated multi-level response had not been fully developed or tested. The warning signs and pressures for change came from a number of sources. First of all, a number of serious infectious diseases and threats, internationally and at home, had raised concerns about the government's ability to respond (NACSPH, 2003; Crowe, 2003; Kennedy, 2005a and 2005b). For example, the global spread of HIV/AIDS, the transmission of Hepatitis B and C through contaminated Canadian blood supplies, two widely publicized tainted water triggered *E. coli* outbreaks in Walkerton (Ontario) and North Battleford (Saskatchewan), *9-11* and the rise of terrorist threats (i.e., anthrax and other biochemical scares) placed infectious disease control firmly in the public and political spotlight.

Second, a number of inquiries and investigations had warned of impending health threats and recommended widespread changes to the system, most of which were ignored. For example, as far back as 1993, the Lac Tremblant Expert Working Group on Emerging and Infectious Diseases called for:

> A national strategy for surveillance and control of emerging and resurgent infections, support and enhancement of the public health infrastructure necessary for surveillance, rapid laboratory diagnosis and timely interventions for emerging and resurgent infections, coordination and collaboration in setting a national research agenda for emerging and resurgent infections, a national vaccine strategy, a centralized electronic laboratory reporting system to monitor human and nonhuman infections, and strengthening the capacity and flexibility to investigate outbreaks of potential emerging and resurgent infections in Canada (NACSPH, 2003: p.3).

More recently, the Federal, Provincial, and Territorial report on Public Health Capacity, presented in June 2001, highlighted the weaknesses in public health infrastructure across Canada. Of particular concern were the disparities in capacity from one province to the next, the relatively low priority given to longer-term disease and injury prevention strategies, deficiencies in public health human resources and growing difficulties with recruitment and selection in this area (NACSPH, 2003). Serious concerns, regarding the federal, provincial and municipal collaborative framework, were also raised at this time by the Auditor General (*cf.* the 1999 and 2001 Auditor General Reports referred to in NACSPH, 2003: Chapter 5) and by the 2002 Romanow Commission that recommended a national immunization strategy and the improvement of prevention programs (Romanow, 2002). The Michael Kirby Senate Committee on Social Affairs, Science and Technology recommended an additional $200 million of annual funding to enhance public health infrastructure across Canada and summarized the inconsistent funding, poor coordination among jurisdictions, and an overall lack of accountability and leadership as ongoing problems (NACSPH, 2003).

More specifically, in respect to the GTA, in March 2002, the Toronto District Health Council produced a report on emergency response coordination. Following a systematic review of the state of emergency preparedness in Toronto's health sector, the report found that:

> Each healthcare agency is responsible for developing its own emergency plan, but this is often done independently, and without formal collaboration with other healthcare organizations. As a result, there is no coordinated emergency plan for Toronto's health sector and appropriate emergency response linkages do not exist (Toronto District Health Council, 2002: p.2).

These conclusions were based on the following set of assumptions about the current state of emergency preparedness in Toronto's health sector (Toronto District Health Council, 2002: p.2):

- There are limited resources in Toronto's emergency department and inpatient units to deal with large-scale emergencies/disasters.
- There is inconsistent knowledge in Toronto's health care organizations regarding externally available resources.
- There is no clear notion of "best practice," i.e., no minimum standard of emergency response for CBRN (chemical / biological / radiological/nuclear) incidents.
- Staff training and education in emergency response is *(sic)* limited and full-scale testing of emergency plans is infrequent.
- There is limited understanding of the "big picture" with respect to decision-making regarding resource allocation for emergency preparedness.
- There is a lack of inter-agency communication and information sharing.
- There is no formal inter-agency coordinating body.
- There is no central communication link for health care organizations in the event of a large-scale citywide emergency.
- There is limited political buy-in from organizational leadership.
- There is a variance between community expectations and the current capabilities of the service provider agencies.

In spite of these warnings and recommendations in the build up to SARS, the governments of the day appeared ready to gamble with public safety, as little action was taken to address the problems identified (Campbell, 2004). The primary reason for government inaction is contextual and can be traced back to the vociferous demands for more affordable forms of government during the 1990s.

Rather than focusing on building government capacity, for something that may never happen, all levels of government were preoccupied with policies aimed at cutting costs and expenditure and reducing Canada's mounting debt. As a result, the period leading up to SARS was characterized by downsizing, restructuring and reengineering, tax reductions, spending cuts and fiscal prudence.

During this period of fiscal restraint, public health had to compete intensely with personal health services for provincial health dollars while federal transfers for local, provincial and territorial public health activities remained, until recently, virtually non-existent (NACSPH, 2003). Furthermore, these policies had a damaging impact on investment in prevention measures such as hospital infection-control programs. Consequently, critics argue that the erosion of Canada's public health infrastructure, and public health capacity resulted from more than two decades of financial, administrative, and political neglect (Binder et al., 1999; Crowe, 2003; Lim et al., 2004; Naylor et al., 2004).

Given the broader political context, and the subsequent years of underinvestment in health capacity and emergency preparedness, it was hardly surprising that when SARS struck, the GTA and Ontario's public health and healthcare systems were caught by surprise. No infectious disease pandemic plan existed, and the Ontario Public Health Branch was devoid of the professional capacity and expertise one would expect in a province the size of Ontario (Campbell, 2004). The province lacked a functioning epidemiological unit and the scientific backup to provide prompt advice to those managing the outbreak (Campbell, 2004). It also lacked inter-jurisdictional agreements for sharing and compensating public health and clinical personnel appropriately during an emergency. Likewise, pre-existing protocols, accords, and the other machinery required to ensure a necessary flow of information and analysis were non-existent (Campbell, 2004; Naylor et al., 2004).

Moreover, hospital infection control programs in the GTA, failed to meet the US standard of one infection control practitioner per 250 active care beds, and 80 percent remain unable to fulfill the new Canadian standard of one infection control practitioner per 175 active care beds. Consequently, the GTA was short of infection control practitioners and infectious disease specialists, and deficient in physical infrastructure—only 3.8 percent of acute hospital beds were in single, negative-pressure rooms, and many emergency departments lacked infection-control areas (D'Cunha, 2004; Lim et al., 2004; Naylor et al., 2004). In addition, Ontario regional public health reference laboratories were short-staffed, due to layoffs two years earlier of its PhD level scientists who had been engaged in the diagnosis and surveillance of new and emerging infectious diseases (NE-ID), and its facilities, equipment, and communications systems were outdated (Campbell, 2004; Hearne et al., 2004).

Health system complexities and jurisdictional tensions

Numerous other complexities and systemic deficiencies severely taxed regional capacity for outbreak surveillance, containment, information management, and infection control, as demands of an unprecedented nature were placed on the public health and healthcare systems, further limiting their capacity (NACSPH, 2003; Palmer, 2003). In addition to the under-funding of public health and healthcare, and its far-reaching impact on all aspects of the health system (e.g., human and physical resources, technology and infrastructure), a further problem is that the responsibility for public health in Canada is multi-level and hence complex (Talaga et al., 2003a and 2003b; Branswell, 2003a).

Power is shared between federal, provincial, and municipal governments, but like the provision of healthcare, the provinces and territories possess front-line responsibility for responding to health threats that occur within their jurisdiction (Lim et al., 2004; PHAC, 2004a and 2004d; NACSPH, 2003; Rachlis, 2004). Municipalities in Ontario hold the bulk of financial and operational power for public health as the provincial system, like the healthcare system as a whole, has gradually been decentralized. In effect, this means that the four public health units, like the twenty-eight general hospitals in the GTA, function semi-autonomously, not only in relation to the province, but also in relation to each other (Lim et al., 2004; Naylor et al., 2004). This was significant since, at the time of the SARS outbreak, Ontario was the only province that did not have a regional health authority to help coordinate efforts to control SARS (Lim et al., 2004; Naylor et al., 2004).

Divisions in local and provincial powers have also resulted in dual roles and functions. For example, local public health units are responsible for collecting data, conducting epidemiological investigations, containing outbreaks, and enforcing effective public health measures, while the provinces and territories are supposed to plan and administer budgets, analyze data, provide advice on programs, and offer technical assistance to local public units as needed (NACSPH, 2003; PHAC, 2004a). The federal government, on the other hand, is responsible for communicating with foreign governments and multilateral health agencies (PHAC, 2004a), and maintains:

> authority to legislate aspects of public health owing to its powers over, variously, the criminal law, matters of national concern for the maintenance of 'peace, order and good government,' [disease surveillance], the quarantine provisions and national borders, and trade and commerce of an inter-provincial or international nature (NACSPH, 2003: p.2).

In theory, each level of government also works together to monitor and conduct surveillance activities in order to identify and respond to potential threats to the health and safety of Canadians, exercise regulatory duties, set and implement public health policies, develop programs and educate and inform the Canadian population for the purposes of protecting and promoting the health of the population (PHAC, 2004a and 2004d). However, limited as the federal role in public health and clinical care is constitutionally, challenges for national and international coordination efforts are likely to manifest at the federal level during a health emergency (Naylor et al., 2004).

Many of the health complexities and jurisdictional tensions did come to a head during the GTA SARS outbreak, necessitating extraordinary measures to control and prevent further transmission (Lim et al., 2004). The systemic deficiencies that surfaced in the response to SARS include many of those predicted during the previous decade. In particular, a lack of capacity, and leadership, poor coordination and jurisdictional confusion blighted the response of the major stakeholders when confronted with the SARS crisis:

> Lack of surge capacity in the clinical and public health systems; difficulties with timely access to laboratory testing and results; absence of protocols for data or information sharing among levels of government; uncertainties about data ownership; inadequate capacity for epidemiologic investigation of the outbreak; lack of coordinated business processes across institutions and jurisdictions for outbreak management and emergency response; inadequacies in institutional outbreak management protocols, infection control, and infectious disease surveillance; and weak links between public health and the personal health services system, including primary care, institutions, and home care (NACSPH, 2003: p.1).

Moreover, neither Health Canada, the Ontario Ministry of Health and Long Term Care, the Provincial Operations Centre, which was established to deal with SARS, or the regional public health units ever fully understood the division of roles, responsibilities, reporting structures and jurisdiction (Palmer, 2003; Talaga et al., 2003b; NACSPH, 2003). Ultimate responsibility for the management of the outbreak was never clarified. "No one knew who was in charge. . . . [There was] no leader, no general just lots of lieutenants" (Branswell, 2003a and 2003b). Consequently, questions remained unanswered regarding who had the responsibility for: the classification of a case; issuing directives to hospitals; determining the consequences of not following directives; deciding what specific information had to be transmitted, by whom, when and to whom; establishing the extent to which public officials and private experts could share data and for what purpose; notifying relatives that a family member was classified as a suspect or probable case and; determining whether privacy rights prevented the sharing of information necessary to control and prevent the further spread of SARS (Campbell, 2004).

As a result, confusion, conflict, duplication, and inconsistency in approach translated into poor coordination between the federal, provincial and municipal governments, as well as across the regions of the GTA (Palmer, 2003; Branswell, 2003a and 2003b). The issue of coordination, however, did not rest exclusively with the federal, provincial, and municipal governments; it also extended to a broad range of public health stakeholders who, together, could have played a more significant role in managing the SARS outbreak had they been involved earlier.

### Inadequate data and poor communication

The absence of an effective provincial or national surveillance system, shared database and reportable disease information system undermined attempts to handle data collection needs and facilitate rapid reporting of disease activity across and within multiple jurisdictions (Campbell, 2004; D'Cunha, 2004; NACSPH, 2003; Palmer, 2003; Parashar et al., 2004). In fact, each of the four GTA public health units developed their own data collection system and became married to unique and divergent methods of collecting and reporting data, despite the challenges this posed (Campbell, 2004). For example, the Toronto Public Health unit, which had the majority of the SARS cases, relied on an antediluvian paper-based system of case tracking which resulted in cardboard boxes overflowing with paper that had to be collated and analyzed by hand (Campbell, 2004). Obviously, this created difficulties for the provision of adequate and timely data to experts and officials.

A single, effective, information technology system, however, was not the only obstacle to information flow. According to Justice Campbell (2004):

> Confusion, duplication, and apparent competition prevailed in the work of those in the central apparatus who sought information from local public health units and hospitals. These unfocused demands consumed valuable time of public health and hospital staff, distracted them from urgent tasks at hand, and impaired their ability to get on with the work of fighting the disease (Campbell, 2004: p.121).

Furthermore, information flow issues such as divergent reporting structures, and multiple information systems, were compounded by the absence of a pre-existing epidemiological unit whose responsibility it ought to have been to coordinate the local health units. Coupled with the lack of clear public health leadership these communication problems facilitated the disconnection of crucial front-line forces responsible for fighting SARS (Campbell, 2004).

The situation was further compounded by the inability and apparent unwillingness of Toronto Public Health officials to release data to the Ontario Public Health Branch and other Ontario provincial bodies, and by the reluctance of provincial officials to share data with federal officials. The main reason given for this lack of cooperation was legitimate concern for the protection of patient confidentiality (Palmer, 2003; NACSPH, 2003). However, such concerns contradict the need to protect the health of the population at large. High quality, accurate data remained essential to the experts on the Science Committee who had to provide evidence- and science-based direction for the management of SARS (Campbell, 2004). The federal government also required the timely dissemination of SARS information to fulfill its national and international obligations (Campbell, 2004).

Due in part to the inability of the regional public health reference laboratories to provide optimal support during the SARS outbreak, information was disseminated in an inefficient, and at times incomprehensible manner to health care workers, health professionals, and government employees (Talaga et al., 2003a and 2003b; NACSPH, 2003). Laboratory capacity had simply been outstripped, by the previous testing volumes required in outbreaks of West Nile and Norwalk virus, in addition to everyday demands for routine testing (Hearne et al., 2004; NACSPH, 2003). Although local hospital laboratories stepped in to conduct SARS testing, many were not provided with sufficient epidemiological or clinical data and on occasion, even basic identifying data were incorrect or missing (NACSPH, 2003; Naylor et al., 2004). In the absence of a central database and epidemiological data, and considering the absence of effective links between laboratories and clinicians, the difficulty of trying to verify data and weed out errors was predictable, as was the inadequate dissemination of results (Naylor et al., 2004).

Because the lack of an effective system for communicating routine infectious disease alerts from Health Canada to the operational levels of the health system (i.e., to hospitals, long-term care facilities, Community Care Access Centers, ambulance services, family physicians), up-to-date and desperately needed data did not reach doctors, nurses, hospital employees, and public health officials in a timely manner, if at all. This meant it was impossible to accurately chart the spread of the disease and to assess the efficacy of policies such as the widespread quarantining of contacts of SARS cases.

In fact many people working on the frontlines and/or in high-risk environments such as educational institutions, community access centers, residential homes, religious organizations, and private sector organizations were never kept directly informed about important developments (Talaga et al., 2003a and 2003b; NACSPH, 2003). Even when information was made available, healthcare workers were initially not informed about directives devised to try to stop the spread of infection in hospitals (Branswell, 2003a; NACSPH, 2003). The rapid change in directives, without explanation of what had changed or why, forced health and safety committees to spend hours examining lengthy documents looking for new advice and information (North Bay Nugget, 2003). In most cases, insufficient information and instruction was provided on how to manage severe outbreaks and, in any case, the majority of protocols had not been recently revised and updated. Consequently, it was some time before a clear understanding of the risks, the means of contagion, the population at risk of infection, and the cause of SARS emerged amongst health care professionals and the general public (Nature, 2003; NACSPH, 2003).

The inability to communicate information accurately and effectively fuelled confusion and panic: Was SARS infectious or wasn't it? Could it be caught like a cold or not? Was SARS under control or wasn't it? As it turned out, too many opinions were being publicly expressed on what was happening through daily news conferences (Lim et al., 2004). Communications with no clearly identified source, and often with conflicting and/or out-of-date advice, filtered in from a wide range of organizations responsible for the health care system. The resulting confusion and misinformation was exacerbated by non-stop requests for information on a minute-by-minute, 24 hour basis and this seriously limited the efforts of a small number of overworked staff to forge on with their job of collecting, analyzing, interpreting and disseminating the epidemiologic information required to combat SARS (Branswell, 2003b; Talaga et al., 2003b).

Operational and human resource issues

Ultimately, Toronto's over-stretched hospitals and its health-care tracking system were unable to keep up with the ballooning number of SARS cases (Donovan, 2003). With no regional disaster plan or previously identified methods for cooperation between facilities in place, it proved very difficult to transfer non-SARS related patients to other facilities and thereby control and contain the outbreak of SARS (NACSPH, 2003). In fact, according to Richard Schabas, with no adequate tracking system hospitals didn't have time to figure out who got transferred to which hospitals. "By the time a sick SARS patient was identified, that patient had already spread the disease" (Quoted in Donovan, 2003: p. A01).

A more mundane, but equally serious problem with many of the hospitals in the GTA, was that standard infection control procedures (i.e., isolation, basic hand washing, the use of personal protective equipment) were virtually non-existent. This, in large part, was due to widespread ignorance about the basic principles of infection control on the part of health care workers, the lack of immediate access to personal protective equipment including the province-wide required submicron-filtering N95 mask and poor understanding of how to use personal protective and isolation equipment (D'Cunha, 2004; Lim et al., 2004; Naylor et al., 2004).

With regard to the N95 submicron filtering mask, this illustrated many of the planning and logistical problems that undermined the GTA response. Following the outbreak, demand for the mask was understandably high; however, with no pre-existing supply stockpile, Canadian suppliers quickly ran out of stock. Hospitals were forced to obtain supplies from foreign manufacturers but, due to the worldwide threat of SARS, great difficulty existed in acquiring masks from other countries (Lim et al., 2004). As a result, the question was raised as to whether staff should be allowed to see patients and to provide patient care, if they could not be provided the appropriate mask (Lim et al., 2004).

In addition, GTA hospitals severely lacked infectious disease specialists, infection control physicians, hospital epidemiologists, intensive care nursing professionals, and others with relevant expertise and experience to handle the outbreak. This was exacerbated by the fact that the senior medical students, upon which many hospitals often depend to fill staffing rosters, were prohibited from providing patient care during the outbreak out of concern for their safety. In addition, a significant proportion of the part time and casual nursing staff, who typically worked shifts at several hospitals, were made to choose one facility to work at in order to reduce the potential for transmission. Unfortunately, this confronted nurses with the dilemma of either obeying public-health orders or protecting their incomes.

Hospitals also found it extremely difficult to reassign non-salaried physicians to SARS units, given their ineligibility for government disability insurance should a work-related injury such as SARS transpire (Lim et al., 2004). The shortage of adequately trained staff meant that the risk of becoming ill or "burned out," with no one locally available to replace them, was great and efforts at controlling the disease outbreak could be further jeopardized (NACSPH, 2003). As a result of finite numbers of hospital staff, delays occurred in contacting potentially infected people and in some cases individuals were missed altogether (Talaga et al., 2003a; NACSPH, 2003). These elements not only contributed to the spread of SARS, but hospitals and nosocomial infections actually proved to be the primary sources of transmission for the majority of those infected with SARS (Naylor et al., 2004).

### *International context of SARS*

In focusing on the inadequacies of the Canadian response to the GTA SARS outbreak, it is important not to forget the international context within which SARS and other viral outbreaks emerge. Many of these contextual factors are beyond the direct influence of the Canadian authorities, but they had an important influence on its rapid spread into the GTA and, ultimately, the human and economic damage it was able to inflict. First, for example, the inability to acquire timely and accurate information early in the outbreak was in large part, political, but also due to inadequate infrastructure, low diagnostic capabilities and the use of extremely vague case definitions in diagnosing the illness. Second, the rapid spread of press reports globally that were often inaccurate, sensationalist, and lacking in sound advice, exaggerated the threats and multiplied the economic impacts of SARS, particularly in respect of tourism. Third, the failure of countries to adhere to international expectations relating to appropriate conduct in response to disease outbreaks, namely reporting the spread of potential infectious health threats, makes global transmission more likely. Fourth, the lack of substantive support for developing countries economically damaged by disease outbreaks often discourages openness about outbreaks and their potential seriousness and makes early containment less likely (Cash et al., 2000). Although these issues go beyond the scope of this chapter, they are clearly issues that played a part in the spread and devastation caused by SARS and will require international cooperation and action if they are not to undermine efforts to contain future outbreaks. The combination of contextual and specific factors outlined in this section played a major role in undermining the effectiveness of the GTA response to SARS and, together, they help to explain why so many errors occurred in an under-prepared, under-resourced and overstretched public health and healthcare system.

## *Lessons Learned*

### Direction and rationale of post-SARS reforms

Ultimately, the fact that SARS was eventually contained is testimony to the highly effective social and often informal relationships that operated to overcome political, bureaucratic and practical flaws in the emergency management system. Nevertheless the SARS outbreak, and the ad hoc way it was eventually controlled, has led many observers to conclude that the Canadian public "dodged a bullet" and that next time, a more systematic and better coordinated response will be required. In this respect, the GTA experience with SARS, and the subsequent investigations, has provided important information and led to significant changes in emergency preparedness and responsibilities across Canada.

Following SARS, the main recommendations that have been advanced pertain to: improving physical facilities in emergency departments and hospitals; renewing health human resources; clarifying the legislative and regulatory context; improving F/P/T relations; developing regional outbreak management strategies; creating integrated emergency planning; coordinating crisis communications; improving continuing education on infection control; building research capacity; renewing laboratory infrastructure; and enhancing linkages between public health and segments of the personal service system (hospitals, home care agencies, primary care) as well as with international advisories (NACSPH, 2003).

The case for a coordinated and collaborative approach to public health is without doubt a priority given Canada's still-fragmented personal health system (NACSPH, 2003). Since public health threats have generalized impacts (NACSPH, 2003), Canada cannot afford to have weak links in a countrywide chain of health protection and disease control. Hence, it appears that new structures and funding mechanisms are intended to strengthen the public health system and remove it from the jurisdictional "crossfire." For example, $700 million per annum has been recommended by 2007 to reinvigorate the public health system in all jurisdictions (NACSPH, 2003). In addition, the NACSPH, along with the federal government and many public health stakeholders, are supporting the idea of a new Canadian agency for public health that would be an arm's length legislated service agency, analogous to the Canadian Food Inspection Agency. The aim is to enhance the credibility and independence of federal activities in public health and offer greater flexibility in terms of developing partnerships with NGOs and other stakeholders (NACSPH, 2003).

### Federal-led measures to improve Canada's emergency response

In the two and a half years since SARS devastated the GTA, many commitments and changes continue to be made by both the federal government and the province of Ontario to strengthen public health capacity in an attempt to prevent another SARS-like situation from ever occurring again. At the federal level, for example, an initial $665 million in funding was committed in the February 2004 Budget to strengthen the country's public health system. In particular, $100 million Canadian (US$ 86 million) was allocated to increase and strengthen front-line public health capacity, $300 million Canadian (US$ 240) to support new vaccine programs including childhood immunization (e.g., to prevent meningitis, ear and blood infections, pneumonia, whooping cough, and chicken pox) $100 million Canadian ($US 86 million) to improve infectious disease surveillance systems and $165 million Canadian (US$ 137 million) to begin to address gaps in the public health system (e.g., preparedness for infectious diseases, emergency response capacity, the national emergency stockpile system inventory and federal public health laboratory capacity) and support the creation of the Public Health Agency of Canada[1] (Public Health Agency of Canada/PHAC, 2004a, 2004b, 2004c and 2004d; Bennett, 2005; Rachlis, 2004).

Symbolically, Prime Minister Paul Martin established the first-ever Minister of State for Public Health on his first day in office. He appointed Carolyn Bennett, in December 2003, to implement recommendations from the Naylor report, establish the Public Health Agency of Canada (PHAC), oversee the process for the selection of Canada's first Chief of Public Health and improve the health of Canadians (Bennett, 2005). Subsequently, in September 2004, PHAC was officially launched and the country's first Chief Public Health Officer (CPHO), appointed (PHAC, 2004a, 2004b, 2004c and 2004d; Rachlis, 2004).

Despite the fact that the CPHO reports directly to the Minister of Health and not to the Minister of State for Public Health, this reform can be seen as an attempt to depoliticize and simplify health issues. For example, as well as being accountable for leading the PHAC, the CPHO, a non-politician, now also acts as a federal government spokesperson on public health issues and emergencies (PHAC, 2004c).

The creation of the PHAC was the result of wide consultation with federal, provincial, and territorial public health officials, parliamentarians, and public health stakeholders from across the country. Following recommendations from prominent public health experts, including Dr. Naylor, the Agency has been established to provide federal public health leadership, and improve collaboration within and between jurisdictions (PHAC, 2004c). The mandate of the PHAC now includes: emergency preparedness and response, health promotion and chronic and infectious disease prevention and control. Working jointly with other departments, including Public Safety and Emergency Preparedness Canada (PSEPC), on emergency planning and preparedness, PHAC is also responsible for developing an effective response to national public health emergencies and enhancing public health capacity.

In addition to having more resources and operating at arm's length from Health Canada, PHAC has evolved a different strategy than its predecessor, the now defunct Population and Public Health branch. In particular, it aims to establish a pan-Canadian[2] public health network by better connecting federal, provincial, and territorial operations. Currently, much needed inter-jurisdictional agreements are being worked on to: (a) clarify roles and responsibilities for preventing and responding to public health threats; (b) create a national network of public health science centers; (c) ensure there are sufficient human resources in health with the capacity to respond to regional and national public health emergencies (e.g., through greater inter-provincial and territorial collaboration during public health emergencies, so that temporary licensing for instance can be provided to doctors in one province to enable them to respond to a disease outbreak in another); (d) enhance national surveillance capacity and expand the infrastructure for information; and (e) guarantee a consistent methodology for the collection of data on infectious disease outbreaks so that information can be shared and compared in a more efficient, effective and timely manner with all those involved in helping to manage situations of public health import (Branswell, 2005a and 2005b; PHAC, 2004a; Rachlis, 2004).

The impetus for these changes in strategy stems from a greater understanding of the linkages between disease prevention, health promotion and the sustainability of Canada's healthcare system. This has been reinforced by agreement, at the First Ministers' meetings in September 2003, to "make public health a top priority," and, in 2004, to better co-ordinate inter-governmental efforts to improve health and safety (Bennett, 2005; PHAC, 2005k).

In an attempt to facilitate knowledge exchange and evidence-based public health decision-making, six National Collaborating Centers (NCCs) for Public Health have been created by PHAC to specialize in different priority areas. The NCC for infectious diseases aims to address present and future risks of new and emerging infectious diseases by complementing and building on ongoing research into diseases such as SARS, West Nile Virus and BSE, training the next generation of new and emerging infectious disease specialists, and through closer collaboration with universities to facilitate the commercialization of discoveries (PHAC, 2004b and 2005b).

However, the translation and exchange of knowledge, is only one area in which PHAC is focusing its efforts. Steps have also been taken to strengthen and expand public health infrastructure by opening a second Emergency Operations Centre in Winnipeg. Through ongoing development and provision of tools and applications to support the management of infectious disease, major outbreaks, and immunization programs, steps have also been taken to enhance capacity for alerting communities, domestically and internationally of public health events, and to ensure that accurate and timely data can be acquired and reports produced (Canada Newswire, 2005b; PHAC, 2005i and 2005k). In particular, PHAC has initiated the Canadian Integrated Public Health Surveillance (CIPHS) program that develops integrated computer and database applications to facilitate the systematic collection, analysis, and dissemination of public health surveillance data.

Its principal product is the integrated Public Health Information System (i-PHIS), a web-based software suite comprising customized health information management modules that together, support the full range of public health programming including case management, surveillance, screening, tracking and shortly, outbreak and quarantine management (Canada Newswire, 2005b; PHAC, 2005k). Efforts are also being made to merge i-PHIS with the electronic health record so that access to laboratory results and demographic information can be provided in order to assist in tracking outbreaks and assessing the optimal response (Canada Newswire, 2005b; PHAC, 2005k).

Much effort has also gone into developing a comprehensive, multi-pronged public health human resource strategy. The aim is to fill a wide number of gaps in epidemiology, surveillance, and health information management, and create a more robust, adequately trained, and responsive public health workforce. In part, this has involved working with provinces, territories, professional associations, and Canadian universities to develop Master of Public Health programs across the country, oriented to both classroom and on-line learning, as well as the PHAC Skills Enhancement Program, which is geared to current public health professionals for the purpose of updating public health knowledge, skills, and capacity (PHAC, 2005k).

At the same time, additional funding has been made available for federal public health laboratories (i.e., the National Microbiology Laboratory and the Laboratory for Food borne Zoonoses) with a view to building overall research capacity. The enhancement of human and physical infra-structural resources is intended to increase the provision of expert microbiological reference testing and assist with innovative research to improve Canada's capacity to identify dangerous viruses and bacteria.

Measures are also being put in place to arrest hospital acquired (nosocomial) infections. Hospitals, as witnessed during the SARS outbreak, have often become the main conduit for the spread of new and emerging infectious diseases. The PHAC-initiated, Canadian Nosocomial Infection Surveillance Program (CNISP) has helped develop Infection Control Guidelines for health care providers, governments and other institutions on how best to prevent and control infections during the provision of health care (PHAC, 2005k).

Provincial-led measures to reform Ontario's public health

In June 2004, Ontario's provincial government launched Operation Health Protection, a three-year action plan to revitalize the province's public health system. The plan addresses many of the recommendations made in Justice Campbell's first interim report on the 2003 SARS outbreak, as well as the Expert Panel on SARS and Infectious Disease Control (Walker report), and the NACSPH (Naylor report). Included in the reforms are a number of key changes intended to improve public health.

In respect of legislation, for example, amendments made to the Ontario Health Protection and Promotion Act increase the authority and independence of the chief medical officer of health (CMOH), (Canada Newswire, 2005; D'Cunha, 2004). In addition, the creation of a central Ministry of Health and Long-Term Care Emergency Management Unit (EMU) is intended to enhance the level of emergency preparedness along with the establishment of a provincial public health Epi-Centre to collect risk exposure and quarantine data on infected patients and manage a SARS database and produce daily epidemiological reports (OMHLTC, 2004b). Also, in order to address the perceived unfairness with which healthcare workers were treated during the SARS outbreak, legislation was passed that allowed eligible health-care workers to retroactively claim unemployment insurance benefits if they were excluded from the workplace during the SARS outbreak. (Lim et al., 2004)

In terms of investment, the provincial share of funding to local public health units has increased from 50 to 55 percent, and by 2007, it is set to rise to 75 percent. In terms of actual funding, this amounts to a provincial investment of $273 million Canadian (US$ 255 million) in 2004/05, and $469 million Canadian (US$ 442 million) by 2007/08 (OMHLTC, 2004a). The investment is intended for the delivery of screening programs such as vaccinations against major communicable diseases, health promotion prevention of sexually transmitted diseases including HIV/AIDS, and health protection measures in the areas of food and water safety, toxic waste handling and air pollution, public sanitation and spread of rabies (OMHLTC, 2004a).

To support these initiatives, infection control and occupational-health programs have received a considerable boost in both recognition and funding (Lim et al., 2004), and this has resulted in improved emergency department resources to better treat and protect patients with respiratory infections (OMHLTC, 2004b). For example, a further 180 infectious disease control staff have already been hired since these changes were made.

Increased funding has also been used to create an Emergency Medical Assistance Team (EMAT) to help Ontario's healthcare system respond swiftly to major health emergencies. EMAT is a well-equipped, mobile acute-care field unit consisting of twenty negative-pressure tents staffed by a team of healthcare professionals, medical equipment and supplies, a communications centre, electricity and water; it is on standby and is able to travel, set-up, and respond to emergencies in any Ontario location within 24 hours. (OMHLTC, 2004a and 2004b)

Further development has seen the establishment of Ontario's first scientific advisory committee, the Provincial Infectious Diseases Advisory Committee (PIDAC), comprised of experts in infectious disease, infection control, epidemiology and public health experts. Part of their mandate is to make recommendations to the CMOH on the prevention, surveillance and control of infectious diseases in Ontario. The Provincial Transfer Authorization Centre (PTAC) has been formalized as a provincial patient tracking system to facilitate surveillance of patients who are transferred between facilities or who are discharged and able to return home (OMHLTC, 2004b). The province is also developing a new Ontario Health Protection and Promotion Agency expected to be completed by 2006/07.

Operationally, Ontario hospitals have improved education programs, staff surveillance, and training, and all health care facilities are now subject to new and more rigorous standards and guidelines, especially during respiratory outbreaks (OMHLTC, 2004b). A registry of volunteer nurses and registered respiratory therapists who can assist in emergencies has been formalized and a protocol for emergency out-of-province recruitment and licensure is now in place (OMHLTC, 2004b). The Ministry is also developing a Health Pandemic Influenza Plan for Ontario and is in the process of collecting valuable feedback from health care partners to further refine the plan. To ensure that its plans are supported by an adequate supply of resources, the province is in the process of stockpiling protective equipment and clinical supplies and is developing a secure supply chain for their distribution during a crisis (OMHLTC, 2004b).

In an attempt to improve communication and coordination between provincial emergency responders and their federal counterparts, the province has started to cooperate with the federal government on reducing duplication and ambiguity in aspects of emergency management and response. Targets for reform include the development of a more streamlined quarantine surveillance system and the development of more effective channels of communication. Locally, the formation of Local Health Integration Networks (Ontario's version of regional health authorities), is intended to aid in future planning for similar emergencies and oversee the implementation of acute and chronic care, as well as public-health services for the region. (Lim et al., 2004).

### Think local, act global

Given the global scale and transmission of SARS, one of the key lessons from the GTA outbreak was that infectious disease prevention could no longer be conceived of as a local problem. Preventing and combating the spread of serious viral infection requires international coordination and support and, since the outbreak of SARS in Canada, the federal government has been taking steps to create and improve linkages between international and domestic health (PHAC, 2005c).

To this end, PHAC has been collaborating closely with the WHO, other UN bodies and various partners in the international community to improve global public health outcomes and contain the spread of disease (PHAC, 2005c and 2005g). For example, PHAC recently sent teams and equipment to Angola and Vietnam to help with diagnostic detection of the deadly Marburg virus and of the H5N1 strain of Avian influenza respectively. It also sent equipment to parts of tsunami-ravaged Asia to provide relief in the form of supplies for the purpose of treating the injured and ill and supporting team leaders (PHAC, 2005c, 2005g, 2005h, and 2005k). Significant federal contributions have also been made to combat some of the world's most contagious and deadly diseases, namely HIV/AIDS, TB, and malaria by approving the export of inexpensive generic drugs to developing countries, and providing more than $100-million Canadian (more than US$83 million) for prevention and treatment of HIV/AIDS in Africa (Druguid, 2005).

Ongoing collaborative efforts are also being made by the federal government to develop and enhance health capacity in a number of Asian countries. China and Canada, for instance, have recently agreed to exchange knowledge on pandemic planning and cooperate on a wide range of health issues, including health policies and regulations, public health emergencies such as emerging infectious disease outbreaks, blood safety and basic occupational health services (PHAC 2005e). Research training opportunities are also currently being developed in the form of public-private partnerships that aim to benefit both Canadians and citizens of developing countries (Canada Newswire, 2005b). The

CANADA-HOPE Scholarship Program, which falls under the CIHR/Canada's Research-Based Pharmaceutical Companies (RandD) Research Program, for example, enables promising young health researchers from developing countries to be mentored by prominent Canadian researchers. In addition, a national consortium of infectious disease research scientists was created: the Global Infectious Diseases Evidence and Analyses (also known as Global IDEA) (Canada Newswire, 2005b; Hunkin et al., 2004).

In addition, Canada has also been playing an active and significant role in the revision of the 1969 International Health Regulations (IHR); the aim of which is the establishment of a framework that clearly articulates minimum requirements of WHO member states for determining, monitoring, reporting and responding to public health emergencies of international concern. In the event of such an emergency, the WHO will then utilize the standardized data collected to issue recommendations regarding health and control measures (PHAC, 2005c and 2005j).

In the context of the much anticipated influenza pandemic, PHAC has also been collaborating with the WHO and members of the Global Health Security Action Group to expand preparedness and reduce uncertainty. In February 2004, this resulted in the Canadian Pandemic Influenza Plan (CPIP) which, amongst other things, clarifies the responsibilities for each order of government (PHAC, 2005k). To further improve preparedness, the PHAC recently committed to a \$34 million Canadian (US\$ 27 million), ten-year contract for pre-pandemic research on a mock vaccine. Until one is found, the federal government, in an attempt to provide short-term safeguards against an influenza pandemic, recently committed a further \$24 million Canadian (US\$ 19 million) to establish a national stockpile of antiviral drugs that would allow approximately one million Canadians to be treated during a pandemic (Kennedy, 2005a and 2005b).

More generally, positive health results should stem from the recent G-8 decision, for which Canada was partly responsible, to forgive \$40 billion Canadian (US\$ 34 billion) in debt for eighteen, and potentially another twenty, of the world's most highly indebted poor countries (CBC, 2005a and 2005b). Such efforts could have tremendous impact on efforts to improve global health, and subsequently the health of Canadians, as highly indebted nations are able to shift their efforts from paying off debt, to rebuilding and strengthening much needed health and education systems, infrastructure and capacity.

## What more needs to be done?

Public health in Canada will require commitments of long-term funding if strategic capacity and resources are to be built-up and sustained beyond the immediate aftermath of the SARS outbreak. In addition, a new governance framework, built around the PHAC, could be used to grant greater authority to the Minister of State for Public Health and re-align the reporting relationship of the

Chief Public Health Officer (CPHO) with the Minister of State for Public Health. Ultimately, the aim should be to institutionalize public health as a national priority and establish PHAC as an arms-length entity with enhanced federal powers. However, we agree with Campbell (2004) that direct authority and responsibility for the leadership and management of provincial and territorial public health should rest with the Chief Medical Officers of Health (CMOHs). Operational authority for public health labs, assessors, inspectors and enforcement could also be transferred from Ministers of Health (MOHs) to CMOHs.

We also agree with Campbell that the CPHO of Canada, the provincial and territorial CMOHs and local MOHs, should enjoy greater independence and freedom when "speaking out about local public health concerns without fear of reprisal, dismissal or other adverse employment consequences" (Campbell, 2004). The same principle should also be applied to healthcare workers and patients in the form of whistleblower legislation. However, privacy legislation, and concern for patient confidentiality, should not interfere with the necessary disclosure of personal health information to public health officials regarding cases of infectious disease (Campbell, 2004)

Another long-term priority must be to continue improving the relationships and trust between orders of government, NGOs, healthcare professionals, patients and other stakeholders. Improved communication and the sharing of knowledge and partnerships will play a key part in this and should be encouraged and facilitated through appropriate mechanisms that foster and promote horizontal integration. In addition to pursuing these domestic reforms, it is also essential that Canada, and other wealthy members of the OECD, maintain and develop an international focus and continue to work collaboratively with the World Health Organization, the World Bank, other multilateral organizations, NGOs, and civil society in less well off countries in the world, to build and improve public health systems in all countries. Not only is such intervention humanitarian, it is, as we have discussed, the first line of defense for Canadians and other developed countries in the fight against infectious diseases.

## *Conclusions*

The chapter addresses four key aims. First, it provides an overview of the SARS outbreak in Canada, in particular its epicenter in the GTA, and analyses attempts to manage and contain its spread. Second, it identifies many of the causes that contributed to the outbreak, spread and mismanagement of the virus, in spite of many reports warning of such an outbreak and identifying the serious limitations in Canada's ability to respond. In light of this evidence, Canadian politicians and health officials cannot plausibly claim that they were not warned, but it would appear that economic, political and other priorities took precedence over health and emergency preparedness in the years leading up to the SARS outbreak.

Third, the chapter identifies many of the key weaknesses, and strengths, in the GTA response to SARS. In this context, the lack of a coherent framework and collaborative relationships between the federal, provincial, and local orders of government in particular, helped create an ad hoc response to SARS but exacerbated the lack of healthcare capacity and strategic emergency preparedness. Fourth, the chapter maps out the major national and internationally focused reforms that have been undertaken in health and emergency response in the light of the inadequate and often inappropriate steps taken to combat SARS.

Although it is too early to know whether these reforms will produce a marked improvement in Canada's ability to prevent or cope with future outbreaks, we believe that more will have to be done in order to ensure that commensurate and lasting changes are achieved and maintained. Nevertheless, the direction and scope of the reforms currently being introduced by federal and provincial governments, and local public health units, does appear to demonstrate a degree of willingness on the part of politicians and healthcare officials to learn from the past and adapt accordingly for the future.

In many respects, it is the ability to learn and make effective changes that could provide the most crucial legacy of the SARS crisis. Given that SARS was only moderately infectious and potentially far more virulent pandemics threaten, the Canadian public will need to be reassured that appropriate measures are being put in place. The SARS experience and high levels of public concern have enabled politicians to make infectious disease control a top priority in Canada and channel considerable resources into this long neglected area of public health. Consequently, the political stakes in Canada have been raised significantly by SARS and the Canadian public is likely to be very critical of its governments if health emergencies are not prevented or handled more effectively in the future.

## *Notes*

1. Funding allocations in the 2004 Budget for public health, exclude $404 million in base funding for the Public Health Agency of Canada, an amount which was transferred from Health Canada's now defunct Population and Public Health Branch, along with its staff and expertise (PHAC, 2004b, 2004c, and 2004d).

2. The term "Pan-Canadian" is used instead of simply "Canadian" as a means to distinguish between federal and provincial efforts, in a country that is anything but unified. In other words, within the Canadian political context, the term "Canadian" often refers primarily to federal government effort without necessarily the buy-in from provinces and territories. Hence "Pan-Canadian" refers to a joint effort by all provinces and territories in conjunction with the federal government; it more accurately reflects a unified vision beyond the jurisdictional confines of the Canadian federal government alone.

## *References*

Bennett, Carolyn (2005) "Health in health care: System transformed into a 'sickness care'." *The Hill Times,* February 14-20: 14.

Binder, Sue, Alexandra M. Levitt, and James M. Hughes (1999) "Preventing emerging infectious diseases as we enter the twenty first century: CDC's strategy." *Public Health Report* 114(2): 130-4.

Bonnell, Greg (2003) "Young defends handling of SARS crisis amid allegations of draconian measures." *Canadian Press Newswire*, September 30.

Branswell, Helen (2003a) "Communications breakdowns, confusion and chaos heightened SARS risks: nurses." *Canadian Press Newswire,* November 17.

Branswell, Helen (2003b) "Sheer volume of SARS news coverage exacerbated the crisis, report says." *Canadian Press Newswire*, October 29.

Branswell, Helen (2005a) "Canadian health network launched." *The Gazette.* April 23: A15.

Branswell, Helen (2005b) "New pan-Canadian network makes public health unified system, not patchwork." *Canadian Press News Wire.* April 22.

Campbell, Archie (2004) "The SARS Commission Interim Report: SARS and Public Health in Ontario." *Biosecurity and Bioterrorism* 2(2): 118-26.

Canada Newswire (CN) (2003) "Report by SARS Expert Panel Calls on Province To Strengthen Public Health and Infection Control Capacity." *Canada Newswire,* December 15.

Canada Newswire (CN) (2005a) "Infoway Announces $100 million Public Health Surveillance Investment Strategy." *Canada Newswire*, March 3.

Canada Newswire (CN) (2005b) "New Health Research Initiatives to Improve Health in Developing Countries." *Canada Newswire* January 20.

Cash, Richard A., and Vasant Narasimhan (2000) "Impediments to global surveillance of infectious diseases: consequences of open reporting in a global economy." *Bulletin of the World Health Organization* 78(11): 1358-1367.

CBC News Online (2003a) "Timeline" *In Depth: SARS*. CBC News Online, December 15. Available at: http://www.cbc.ca/news/background/sars/timeline.html

CBC News Online (2003b) "Dead Silence." Disclosure. CBC, November 18.

CBC News Online (2004) "In Depth: SARS." *CBC News Online.* Available at: http://www.cbc.ca/news/background/sars/index.html

CBC News Online (2005a) "G-8 reaches deal on debt relief." June 11. Available at: http://www.cbc.ca/story/world/national/2005/06/11/g8-debt050611.html

CBC News Online (2005b) "U.S., Britain reach deal on debt relief for poor nations." June 10. Available at: http://www.cbc.ca/story/world/national/2005/06/10/african-debt 050610.html

Census 2001, "Canada's Ethnocultural Portrait: The Changing Mosaic." Statistics Canada (2003). Catalogue no.96F00XIE302001008.

CMAJ (2003) "Lessons from SARS." *CMAJ* 168(11): 1381.

Crowe, Kelly (2003) "Was Canada ready for SARS?" *In Depth: SARS*. CBC News Online April 30. Available at: http://www.cbc.ca/news/background/sars/crowe_ready. html

Crowe, Kelly and Stephanie Jenzer (2003) "Behind the mask." In Depth: SARS. CBC News Online, November 19. Available at: http://www.cbc.ca/news/background/sars/behindthemask.html

D'Cunha, C. (2004) "SARS: lessons learned from a provincial perspective." *Canadian Journal of Public Health* 95(1): 25-6.

Donovan, Kevin (2003) "SARS tracking deeply flawed." *Toronto Star*, October 1: A01.

Druguid, Terry (2005) "Global infectious disease and Canada's place in the world: Urging the PM to place infectious diseases at the centre of Canada's global commitment." *The Hill Times*, March 7-13: 52.

Frank, J and E. Di-Ruggiero (2003) "Public health in Canada: What are the real issues?" *Canadian Journal of Public Health* 94(3): 190-2.

Gandey, Allison (2003) "Canada's approach to public health must be reinvented: SARS report." *JAMC* 169(8): 824.

Hearne, Shelley A., Margaret A. Hamburg, and Laura Segal (2004) "SARS and Its Implications for U.S. Public Health Policy: 'We've Been Lucky." *Biosecurity and Bioterrorism* 2(2): 127-131.

Hunkin, John and Dominic D'Alessandro (2004) "We must stop the next SARS before it strikes." *National Post* September 27 [National Edition]: A12.

Kennedy, Mark (2005a) "Canada faces tough choices when next pandemic hits: Series: Killer Flu: Are We Prepared?" *Calgary Herald*, March 11: A7.

Kennedy, Mark (2005b) "Preparing for the inevitable." *The Ottawa Citizen*, March 11: A6.

Kombe, GC and DM Darrow (2001) "Revisiting emerging infectious diseases: The unfinished agenda." *Journal of Community Health* 26(2): 113-22.

Lim, Sue, Tom Closson, Gillian Howard, and Michael Gardam (2004) "Collatoral damage: The unforeseen effects of emergency outbreak policies." *Lancet Infectious Diseases* 4 (November): 697-703.

Lindsay, Colin (2007) "The Chinese Community in Canada." *Profiles of Ethnic Communities in Canada.* Statistics Canada, Government of Canada: Ottawa.

Mackay, Brad (2003) "SARS: "a domino effect through entire system." *JAMC* 168(10): 1308.

NACSPH (National Advisory Committee on SARS and Public Health) (2003) *Learning from SARS - Renewal of Public Health in Canada*. Health Canada, Government of Canada: Ottawa.

Nature (2003) "SARS: What have we learned?" *Nature* 424 (10 July): 121–126.

Naylor, C. David, Cyril Chantler and Sian Griffiths (2004) "Learning from SARS in Hong Kong and Toronto." *JAMA* 291(20): 2483-2487.

North Bay Nugget Editorial (2003) "Confusion heightened SARS risks–nurses." [Final Edition] *North Bay Nugget*, November 18: A5.

Ontario Ministry of Health and Long-Term Care OMHLTC (2003) "Diseases: SARS—Questions and Answers." Ministry of Health and Long Term Care, Province of Ontario. Available at: http://www.health.gov.on.ca/english/public/pub/disease/sars_4.html

Ontario Ministry of Health and Long-Term Care (OMHLTC) (2004a) "New provincial commitment to public health a positive change." News release, May 28.

Ontario Ministry of Health and Long-Term Care OMHLTC (2004b) "Ontario Government Commits to Action Plan on Public Health." News release, April 21.

Palmer, Karen (2003) "Doctor slams handling of SARS, blames crumbling public health system." *Canadian Press Newswire*, September 17.

Parashar, Umesh D., and Larry J. Anderson (2004a) "SARS preparedness and response planning." *Emerging Infectious Diseases* 10(2): 384-5.

PHAC (Public Health Agency of Canada) (2004a) "The Federal Strategy: A New Approach to Public Health in Canada." Available at: http://www.phac-aspc.gc.ca/about_apropos/federal_strategy_e.html

PHAC (2004b) "Government of Canada announces details of new Public Health Agency of Canada and appoints Chief Public Health Officer." News Release, May 17. Available at: http://www.phac-aspc.gc.ca/media/nr-rp/2004/2004_01_e.html

PHAC (2004c) "Frequently Asked Questions: Chief Public Health Officer of Canada/ Public Health Agency of Canada." September. Available at: http://www.phac-aspc.gc.ca/media/nr-rp/2004/faq_e.html

PHAC (2004d) "Strengthening the Pan-Canadian Public Health System: Key Concepts." Available at: http://www.phac-aspc.gc.ca/about_apropos/strengthening_e.html

PHAC (2005a) "Minister of State [Public Health] Announces Funding for Six National Collaborating Centers to Strengthen Public Health in Canada." News Release, April 22.

PHAC (2005b) "The National Collaborating Centres for Public Health." Fact Sheet.

PHAC (2005c) "Public Health Agency Responds to World Health Emergencies." News Release, April 21.

PHAC (2005d) "More Young Canadians Have Access to Disease-Fighting Vaccines." News Release, April 22.

PHAC (2005e) "Canada, China Sign Plan of Action on Health Cooperation." News Release, April 1

PHAC (2005f) "Public Health Goals Consultations." March.

PHAC (2005g) "Statement from the Chief Public Health Officer on the Crisis in Southeast Asia."

PHAC (2005h) "Public Health Agency/Health Canada Relief Effort Response, Including Emergency Stockpile Offer, for the Crisis in Southeast Asia." January 14.

PHAC (2005i) " 'Early Warning' System Tracks Global Public Health Threats 24/7." News Release, November 17.

PHAC (2005j) "International Health Regulations." News Release, November 3.

PHAC (2005k) *Report on Plans and Priorities 2005-2006*.

Rachlis, Michael M. (2004) "Moving Forward with Public Health in Canada." *Canadian Journal of Public Health* 95(6): 405.

Romanow, Roy J. (2002) "Building on Values: The Future of Health Care in Canada." Final Report. Commission on the Future of Health Care in Canada.

Talaga, Tanya and Kevin Donovan (2003a) "Why SARS alert was late." Toronto Star, September 22: A01.

Talaga, Tanya and Kevin Donovan (2003b) "SARS: The chain of errors." Toronto Star, September 20: A01.

Toronto District Health Council (2002) *Recommendation for Improved Response Coordination in Toronto's Health Sector.*

# Chapter 7

# The Morality of Quarantine in Ontario, Canada

Logan Atkinson

## *Introduction*

Quarantine represents one of the few legal instruments by which the Canadian state is authorized to detain a person without their consent, short of a criminal conviction. Otherwise it is only in cases of pre-trial detention for dangerous suspects in criminal law, involuntary committal under various mental health statutes, and the extraordinary suspension of civil liberties in situations of perceived insurrection that the state is entitled at law to deny a person certain constitutionally protected freedoms. As a result, quarantine is rarely employed, and then only when the state is left with no apparent efficacious alternative in defense of the public health.

As a matter of public policy, the decision to implement quarantine is necessarily heavily politicized, involving a difficult balancing act between the state's obligation to act in defense of the public health on the one hand, and the general insistence on the protection of fundamental civil liberties on the other. Because of the implications for the suspension of certain individual freedoms (of mobility, association and others) during the implementation of quarantine, it is often assumed that the decision to take this step is made only when the moral framework under which it is taken is beyond reproach. In other words, it is generally taken for granted that the risk of harm to the public good represented by a particular threat is understood to be significant enough to function as moral justification for the decision to impose a tough regulatory measure that suspends individual liberties thought to be basic to the functioning of a civil society.

The assumption of the moral justifiability of quarantine can function in the literature as a standard against which other forms of civil detention are measured. For example, in a debate between Michael Davis and Michael Corrado (Corrado, 1996a and 1996b; Davis, 1996a and 1996b) the question of the morality of quarantine was used to test detention in the criminal law for "dangerousness," that is, detention without conviction. The debate drew on an earlier paper by Ferdinand D. Schoeman (1979) in which Schoeman argued that, as a moral question, no more serious problems arise with civil preventive detention than arise with the "accepted" practice of quarantine, and further, that "[c]ivil preventive detention represents an assault on our notion of autonomous moral being only to the degree that quarantine does" (Ibid.: p. 27). Davis and Corrado drew on this analogy, and while they differed on the way in which we might reason through to a defense of civil preventive detention on moral grounds, they seemed to agree that, on certain conditions, quarantine is necessarily morally justifiable.

At first sight, Davis and Corrado appear to be correct in their assumption in this respect. Davis sets out three conditions on which quarantine might be morally defensible. First, quarantine must be necessary, that is, there must be no less intrusive alternatives available. Secondly, quarantine must generate significant net social benefit (i.e., if it succeeds, it would reduce harm substantially, and that reduction more than compensates for what we lose by detaining people who, left free, would do no harm). Thirdly, there must be a determination of the "probable effectiveness" of quarantine. Davis argues that this is an easy assessment to make in the case of quarantine, given that we know far more about tuberculosis, for example, than we know about the potential for criminal activity (Davis, 1996a). Corrado's defense of quarantine on moral grounds is perhaps less systematic than Davis's, but he does go so far as to say that there is little question of the morality of quarantine where the likelihood of committing harm is beyond the control of the confined person. In this way, we might justify the quarantine of a person with a disease that spreads irrespective of that person's intent (e.g., tuberculosis), but not where that person suffers from a disease the spread of which is within their means to control (e.g., AIDS). Davis's articulation of the conditions on which quarantine might be imposed was taken up by Stephen J. Morse in a later article (Morse, 1996 and 1999; Barnett, 1996). Morse suggested that "the state has an uncontroversial right to quarantine innocent, responsible agents if such agents have communicable diseases and no less intrusive intervention will prevent infection of others" (Morse, 1999:p 265, footnote 1).

The difficulty with Davis's conditions on which quarantine might legitimately be imposed lies in the fact that, to be met, the conditions themselves require previous moral deliberation. As history tells us, such deliberation leads to choices that are contested anew each and every time the decision is made to impose quarantine, meaning that the grounds on which Davis's conditions are generated are never free from doubt. Therefore, we can never be sure that the conditions are met in any absolute sense, and so can never be sure that the imposition of quarantine is a morally justifiable act. In connection with the first condition, we measure the level of intrusiveness of any particular measure through an assessment of the individual right or liberty to be violated by that measure. Some rights and liberties are more valuable to some members of the community than they are to others, such that an assessment of the depth of intrusiveness is necessarily subjective. Secondly, we evaluate success of a measure through its reduction of harm, but we define "harm" in different ways. Throughout history, it has been relatively clear that commercial lobbies, for example, value marketplace freedom more highly than conventional public health, meaning that a measure such as quarantine that interferes with the ordinary movement of people and goods cannot be understood to "reduce harm."[1] A healthy population is defined first by reference to a healthy economy, from this perspective. In the case of the third condition, choices must be made on the value of scientific opinion and other evidence, especially in the situation of new diseases, and it is not always clear the weight to be given such material. Perhaps the precautionary principle ought to compel the implementation of quarantine for minimal risk to the public; perhaps more conservative voices would suggest that a given threshold of scientific certainty must be met before jeopardizing ordinary social intercourse through the use of harsh regulatory measures. The point, then, is that we cannot get to the certainty expressed in Davis's three conditions without making a series of fundamental moral and political choices that are always contested, meaning that there is no certainty about the morality of quarantine at all.

In this chapter, I want to consider representations of the morality of quarantine during the SARS crisis in Ontario, Canada. By "quarantine" I mean three separate types of regulatory measure. First, the Canadian state has the power to stop and then isolate persons and goods at its international borders because those persons or goods represent a perceived threat to the public health. I shall refer to this power collectively as "border restrictions." Secondly, inside Canada the power exists to isolate persons perceived to be a threat to the public health, and I refer to this power as "domestic quarantine." Thirdly, the power to isolate particular locales (buildings or neighborhoods) can be employed when movement in and out of those locales is considered dangerous to the public health. This power I shall refer to as "site-specific quarantine." All three of these regulatory measures were employed during the SARS crisis in Ontario.

While it can be safely assumed that steps to implement quarantine are only undertaken when the regulator feels that the risk of catastrophe is significant enough to outweigh the infringement on individual liberties, it is also true that the success of quarantine depends on a widely shared consensus on its moral justifiability. As is always the case in a democratic society, an effective law is only achieved through a cooperative public, and the public's cooperation is ordinarily founded on a shared understanding of and commitment to the public good intended to be protected through that law. It is especially urgent that the moral framework in which the law is designed and employed is widely understood and shared where the infringement on important, central individual liberties is immediate and dramatic, as it is in the case of quarantine. The ability of the state to meet its obligations to protect the public health through the imposition of quarantine depends, then, on a public consensus about the extent of the risk faced by the public, the perceived relative inefficacy of alternatives to quarantine, and the need to sacrifice individual liberties for the sake of the whole community. In other words, the public policy variables relevant to the decision to implement quarantine must be considered by the regulator in a way that will appeal to a moral consensus that must be enlisted if quarantine is to function in the way it must to protect the public health.

The media play a prominent role in identifying both points of convergence and points of disagreement between the position of the regulator and the public's understanding of the moral framework in which quarantine is imposed. Therefore, the media are central to the ability of the state to meet its obligations respecting the protection of the public health through the implementation of measures consistent with moral consensus, or, alternatively, to the ability of the state to generate the moral consensus on which the successful implementation of quarantine depends. The media's role in this respect is performed both actively through functions of interpretation and the expression of opinion, and also more passively through the transmission of prepared communications. Therefore, it is not only as mere conduit that the media perform in this context. Rather, the media generate moral debate, and often direct that debate in editorial columns, guest columns and through the publication of readers' letters. As a result, the media play a central role in either generating the public moral concurrence necessary to assist the state in its enforcement of quarantine, or alternatively, in stimulating the outcry that often lies at the leading edge of civil disobedience.

In this chapter, representations of the morality of quarantine during the SARS crisis in Ontario, Canada, will be investigated through a review of four prominent newspapers. Two of those newspapers, the *National Post* and *The Globe and Mail*, are major national papers publishing in Toronto. The other two, the *Ottawa Citizen* and the *Toronto Star*, are the principal local papers publishing in Ontario's two largest urban centers. In each case, the period reviewed is March 1 to July 31, 2003. Conventional news items were surveyed to re-establish the chronology of events. Other frequently occurring categories of published material with a bearing on the subject of this chapter include editorial columns, guest columns, letters to the editor and state sponsored notices to the public. The review of this material generates three relevant observations. First, the SARS crisis in Ontario initiated debate similar to that which regularly occurs across Anglo-Canadian historical experience with epidemic disease. This observation gives credence to the argument that the morality of quarantine, as a starting point in the general discussion on the morality of civil detention, is not a safe assumption. In fact, this assumption may simply be wrong, if we measure not just the framework in which the state initially invokes quarantine, but also the broader context of the public's response to both the prospect and the reality of regulatory infringements on civil liberties.

Secondly, even if we can somehow resolve the question of the content of the public good respecting tensions between state perspectives and widespread public perception, there still remains the difficult problem of the individual case. In other words, as an intellectual exercise the predominant urge to the protection of the public health may be sufficient to justify the imposition of quarantine even though individual freedoms are dramatically affected. Yet this conclusion is regularly tested by the "hard cases," the (perhaps extraordinary) instances of individual suffering that inevitably challenge the moral consensus necessary for the efficacious imposition of tough regulatory measures.

Thirdly, we depend to a remarkable degree on the level of scientific certainty relative to regulatory responses to the etiology, method of transmission and treatment of disease. This dependency is particularly acute in the case of new or "emerging" diseases. Quarantine, then, is as much a medical prescription as it is a regulatory instrument, and the level of probability generated by scientific discourse makes a direct impact on the moral framework that lies beneath the bureaucratic decision to invoke quarantine. In turn, the development of a public consensus on the morality of the imposition of quarantine depends at once on a reasonable level of scientific certainty respecting the characteristics of the disease, and on a balanced, accessible description of that science in the popular press. In the case of Ontario's experience with SARS, the level of scientific uncertainty, especially early in the crisis, may have generated difficulties for state agencies in garnering the necessary public sympathy for and compliance with prophylactic measures.

Before investigating media representations of regulatory measures more carefully, however, I want to provide a brief summary of Canada's constitutional and legislative framework for the protection of the public health. That will be the subject of the next section of this chapter, to be followed by some reflections on media representations of the morality of quarantine, and a brief conclusion.

## *Canada's Constitutional and Legislative Framework*

As a federal state, Canada's legislative responsibilities are divided fully between the central government and the provincial governments (including Ontario) by virtue of sections 91 and 92 of the constitution (The Constitution Act, 1867). The powers of the federal government, although specifically enumerated in s. 91, also contain a residual power, meaning that any legislative topic not expressly assigned to the provinces pursuant to s. 92 will fall to the federal government. The residual power is to be exercised for the "peace, order and good government" of Canada. This is convenient, because "protection of the public health" is not one of the specifically enumerated topics in either s. 91 or s. 92. Legislative competence in the area, then, either must be implied in the various provincial powers in s. 92, or fall to the federal government pursuant to its residual power.

Provincial authority in the area of public health was discussed fairly comprehensively in the Supreme Court of Canada case, Schneider v. The Queen, [1982] 2 S.C.R. 112. There, it was unequivocally stated that the provinces have broad jurisdiction over matters of public health pursuant to s. 92(16) (purely local or private matters). Further, s. 92(7) specifically grants provincial legislative competence respecting hospitals. At the same time, however, s. 91(11) provides for federal competence in the area of quarantine, and the residual power is often interpreted to grant the federal government legislative jurisdiction in any situation where a matter of national concern is at stake, perhaps in the case of "an epidemic of pestilence" (*Toronto Electric Commissioners v. Snider*, 1925).[2] Therefore, general jurisdiction over public health is shared between the federal and provincial governments, depending on the nature of the difficulty to be addressed.

The federal government has acted on its legislative responsibility in the Canada Health Act, R.S.C. 1985, c. C-6, and the Quarantine Act, R.S.C. 1985, c. Q-1. In the former, the theory and structure of Canada's publicly funded medicare system are established, and the conditions of participation by the provinces are set out. This has but tangential relevance to this chapter. In the latter, however, we find the full procedural framework for the imposition of the sort of quarantine identified above as border restrictions. The Quarantine Act provides for the appointment of quarantine officers with specified powers respecting people, goods and conveyances either arriving in or leaving Canada. The powers of quarantine officers vary in some small ways depending on the disease under investigation. Included in a schedule to the Act is a list of "contagious and infectious" diseases, and in circumstances where the presence of one of these diseases is detected or at least suspected, quarantine officers have fairly extensive powers. Less extensive powers are vested in the quarantine officer in the case of the detection or suspicion of a "dangerous disease," defined by the quarantine officer (acting reasonably) as one that would "constitute a grave danger to public health" in Canada if introduced, even though not listed on the schedule. In the spring of 2003, SARS could only have been a "dangerous disease," although it was ultimately listed on the schedule to the Act as a "contagious or infectious disease," along with plague, cholera and others.

The Quarantine Act provides for two sets of powers for the quarantine officer in cases where the presence of a dangerous disease is detected or suspected. First, the combined effect of s. 5 and s. 7 gives the officer the power to stop, inspect and detain vehicles and other conveyances, their goods and cargo, and relevant documents. Detention may be as long as necessary to ensure compliance with the Act. If inspection discloses the presence of carriers or causative agents of either a dangerous disease or a contagious or infectious disease, then the officer may order the conveyance or cargo cleansed or removed from Canada. Secondly, according to s. 11, if a quarantine officer, acting reasonably, believes someone entering Canada may have or be the carrier of a dangerous disease, or may have been in close proximity to someone who has or is the carrier of a dangerous disease, then the officer may order that person to undergo a medical examination. If the person refuses to submit to the medical examination, or if the quarantine officer suspects the presence of a dangerous disease following completion of the medical examination, then the quarantine officer may either quarantine the person for up to fourteen days, or allow the person to proceed directly to their Canadian destination. In the latter case, the person must either sign an undertaking to report to a medical officer at their place of destination for the purpose of monitoring, submit to a vaccination, or both. In the case that a quarantine period of longer than forty eight hours is prescribed, then a series of procedural safeguards is implemented, including mandatory judicial review in most circumstances.

In the province of Ontario, the principal health protection framework is specified in the Health Protection and Promotion Act, R.S.O. 1990, c. H.7, as amended. It is in this statute that we find the requirements for the imposition of domestic quarantine and site-specific quarantine, as defined above. Much of the authority in this respect is delegated by the province to local Boards of Health, and they are given the sweeping responsibility for control of infectious disease in their locality. The Minister of Health for Ontario does reserve the ability to supervise Board activities, and to take extraordinary measures in investigating and directing Board activities where the Minister perceives a threat to the public health, but in the main the front-line responsibility in the cases of prevention of and reaction to threats to public health lies with Boards of Health.

For our purposes, the powers of the Boards lie in two significant areas, relating to jurisdiction over persons and jurisdiction over sites.[3] In both cases, the exercise of the Boards' powers represents significant encroachments on civil liberties, whether the constitutionally protected individual rights of mobility, association, and bodily integrity, or rights of property established in private law. Acting through medical officers of health, Boards have the power, by virtue of s. 22 and acting on reasonable and probable grounds that a communicable disease exists or may exist in a community, to order individual persons or classes of persons who have or may have that disease to be segregated from the community. In the event of non-compliance, and where the communicable disease is also a virulent disease, the Board may ask a judge for an order that the person be detained in custody. This is the basic provincial power respecting domestic quarantine. SARS was listed in the regulations to the statute virtually immediately as both a communicable disease and a virulent disease, meaning the extraordinary power of involuntary detention would lie in case of initial non-compliance.[4]

Section 22 also provides the basic power with respect to site-specific quarantine. An order under that section may require premises closed or disinfected, and may also require the posting of a placard advising the public of the closing of the premises. To facilitate the discovery of conditions necessary to support such orders, s. 41 provides a general right of entry for medical officers of health and their delegates. Co-incident with the power to enter are the powers to "make examinations, investigations, tests and inquiries," and to "make, take and remove . . . copies, samples or extracts" relating to such examinations. These powers may initially be exercised without a warrant, although they must be done "at reasonable times" and, in the case of a private residence, with the consent of the occupant. However, if the inspector encounters resistance, a warrant may be obtained under s. 41(11) and s. 43.

In general terms, then, these are the constitutional and legislative arrangements under which various forms of quarantine are implemented in Canada. The potential is strong for inter-governmental dispute, especially where, in the case of a disease originating outside of Canada, the province perceives that the federal government's implementation of border restrictions is weak. If the disease penetrates the defenses mounted by the federal government at points of entry into Canada and establishes itself inside provincial boundaries (as happened in the case of SARS), then responsibility for responding to the public health danger is squarely within provincial jurisdiction. In that case, the province must suffer not only the economic costs of responding to the disease, but also the potential political costs of implementing domestic and site-specific quarantine when the moral consensus on which it depends is in doubt.

## *Media Representations of the Morality of Quarantine*[5]

As might be predicted, media coverage of the emergence of SARS during the very early days of the problem, even after the disease first manifested itself in Canada, was speculative and confused. The speculation related both to the nature of the disease and its means of transmission, and the confusion arose through an admitted uncertainty on these questions on the part of both public health officials and the medical community. To the extent that the public justifiability of tough regulatory measures is connected to the level of scientific certainty on which decision-makers might rely, this early coverage gave the public some grounds on which to contest the implementation of an intrusive response. The conservative press, especially, downplayed the threat of SARS in the early days, suggesting that sensational reporting of minor problems served to sell papers and increase research budgets at North American universities. Excerpts from a column by Michael Fumento illustrate this type of reactionary position (Fumento, 28 March 2003):

> It's "an incident of unprecedented scope and magnitude," according to Toronto health officials. Ontario Health Minister Tony Clement has declared a 'health emergency.' The media have dubbed it the 'mysterious killer pneumonia' or 'super-pneumonia.
>
> But a bit of knowledge and perspective will kill this panic.
>
> The real questions are: How lethal, how transmissible, and how treatable is this strain? And the answers leave no grounds for excitement, much less panic.
>
> So why all the fuss over this one strain of pneumonia?

> First, never ignore the obvious: It does sell papers.[6]

This column appeared in March 2003 when, despite Fumento's cynicism, the etiology of SARS was just beginning to be explored in depth, and the ease of transmission of the disease was just beginning to be understood at all completely. Columnists intend to persuade, of course, and to the extent that they are successful in this respect there must of necessity be a skeptical response from the public toward more alarmist reporting, and, ultimately, an increased possibility of resistance to the enforcement of regulatory controls. This is especially the case when such cynicism is combined with the portrayal of a cautious, tough enforcement regime as an over-reaction and an unnecessary inconvenience to the innocent bystanders whose lives are disrupted as a result. One journalist told a story of a forty year old businessman who experienced problems when he was flying from Hong Kong to Vancouver (Martin, 29 March 2003).

> As the day-long flight progressed across the Pacific, cabin crew noticed he had developed a bad cough and high fever. They immediately isolated him in business class and, within minutes of landing in Vancouver, he'd been whisked away by ambulance. The two hundred passengers were shepherded into temporary quarantine until tests on the bewildered patient came back SARS negative and he was sent home to recover from the flu.
>
> And a loud rasping cough . . . is no longer just a loud rasping cough. It's potentially SARS.

While the author of this column does in fact encourage and support what he calls "professional action" designed to give the vulnerable sufficient comfort, the overall tone of his piece is to discourage over-reaction among officials and the general population. We must not be too concerned, he urges, about what appears to be a minor threat. "The numbers are unsettling given the speed SARS has struck Canada from out of the blue, but the day-over-day growth is not fast enough to suggest this is a bug you'll pick up by pushing an elevator button or extending a handshake" (Martin, 29 March 2003).

The media were quick to pounce on their colleagues for making more of the SARS outbreak than it allegedly deserved, further reinforcing the idea that there was little threat to be found in the latest new disease. One editorial column actually characterized the media as the fifth horseman of the apocalypse, doing more damage by sensational reporting of SARS than the disease itself. Referring to the author of the *Book of Revelations*, Jim Coyle wrote as follows (Coyle, 1 April 2003):

> The only thing the writer missed . . . was the fifth horseman. That, of course, would be the news media. For when it comes to apocalypse, nobody does it better.
>
> Other than sex, the SARS outbreak now bedeviling Greater Toronto has just about everything in the thriller writer's arsenal—rampant fear, a mystery killer, threats that flummox the brightest of experts, heroic efforts, a race against time, random danger, death and anguish.
>
> With such material to work with, it takes hardly any effort at all to turn a smallish, albeit deadly, viral outbreak into a potential Armageddon.

The media, then, play on our fears so as to whip up anxieties, and we ought not to allow ourselves to be so easily influenced, so the argument goes. The question remains, however, as to the bases on which the non-expert might make decisions about the appropriate level of precaution in a situation of virtually complete uncertainty. Co-incident with decisions in this respect are responses to the level of intrusiveness inherent in public health defenses. If an ordinary person is to be persuaded that the threat is not nearly as serious as certain of the media might suggest, such that wholesale changes in day-to-day patterns of activity ought to be avoided, then an enhanced level of skepticism about the moral and public policy justifications for quarantine in its various forms is a necessary, predictable result. Individual readers will react differently, of course, some believing that a precautionary approach to private decision-making based on the wildest predictions constitutes the safe and sure path, while others will prefer to minimize the risk in accordance with the skeptics and carry on as before. In any case, however, to the extent that this tension manifests itself in the public response to difficult regulatory measures, the moral justifiability of those measures is in issue and cannot be assumed. The ability of government to generate a reasonable level of compliance with voluntary quarantine, and to expect a compliant public when quarantine is imposed, is likewise placed in jeopardy. After all, unless one believes that a law is legitimate simply because it has been passed and enforced by the proper authority, respect for the rule of law and submission to its command is a product of a shared understanding of the justice of that law. This is a moral question, resolved to some important degree by reference to the very tests of reasonableness on which there appeared to be such disagreement in the press when the reaction to SARS was considered.

Given the tenuous hold on public perception enjoyed by policy makers, and given the uncertainty that must necessarily result when media coverage displays an urge to panic on the one hand and a cavalier nonchalance on the other, it is perhaps odd that public health and other government officials were among the most insistent of those who counseled little change in ordinary activities. At a time when the risk of contracting and the means of transmission of SARS were not thoroughly understood, the medical officer of health for the City of Toronto (Dr. Sheela Basrur), and Canada's Prime Minister were urging Ontarians to carry on their normal lives. In many newspaper accounts, the rhetoric of calm was perfectly juxtaposed with reports of the perplexities generated by SARS inside the medical community, giving the entire discussion a surrealistic air (Unsigned editorial, 2 April 2003).

> As the number of cases mount with each passing day, so too does the confusion and frustration of a population alarmed by a threat no one can dare say is under control.
>
> Prime Minister Jean Chrétien advised Canadians yesterday to remain calm . . . stressing that federal and Ontario provincial health officials are working together to control the outbreak.
>
> Those words were echoed by Dr. Sheela Basrur . . . 'The general public is not at risk,' she said. 'Go about your daily lives as best you can and try to remember that simple precautions will work.'

Despite the general tone of support for official efforts in this particular editorial in the *Toronto Star*, there is little question that most readers would immediately seize upon the ambiguity inherent in arguing at once that the disease is a mystery while at the same time suggesting that simple precautions will work. In light of such uncertainty, the justifiability of tough quarantine is doubly tested. First, medical authorities are unsure about the nature of the disease, which necessarily means they are unsure about the most efficacious reaction, from both legal and scientific perspectives. Secondly, the very decision-makers responsible for the design and implementation of the legal response are counseling but minor changes in day-to-day activities, holding out the prospect of a friendly continuation of the status quo while "the number of cases mount[s] with each passing day." To the extent that general moral approbation of an intrusive legal response depends on an unambiguous portrayal of each of the disease, the risk and the response, and to the extent that widespread instinctive compliance in turn relies on that moral approbation, both public health officials and politicians have the potential to undermine their own effectiveness.

The moral framework relative to the decision to impose the various forms of quarantine is made more blurry to the public through official insistence on a continuation of the status quo for the sake of the economy. Ontario's Premier, Ernie Eves, and other leading politicians were roundly criticized in the press for initially failing to assure the world that it was "business as usual" in Ontario, even given the mysteries associated with the appearance and spread of SARS (Saytar, 22 April 2003).

> Where is the leadership on this issue? Why are the mayor, provincial and federal politicians not appearing on American and European television news shows to reassure the world at large that life for the general population carries on normally in the Greater Toronto Area and that this region is safe to visit and conduct business?

Eves in particular was the target of the following letter appearing in the *Toronto Star* (Fyfe, 8 April 2003):

> Does Premier Ernie Eves feel he must shore up our friendship with America to protect our trade relationship, or just to protect his voter base? If he did care about trade, he wouldn't have dropped the ball over Ontario becoming a no-tourist zone because of SARS. Shouldn't he be on the phone reassuring conference organizers it is safe to come to Toronto? Shouldn't he organize a photo opportunity of himself, unmasked, circulating with people in hospitals and having a meal at College and Spadina?[7]

Criticism such as this did provoke responses from all three levels of government, perhaps most pointedly from the federal government and most passionately from Toronto's mayor, Mel Lastman. Lastman's tone of desperation indirectly suggested that the situation was actually out of control and, consequently, provided a hollow assurance of safety. The following comments made by Lastman regarding the negative media attention and its effect on the city's economy were widely reported (Benzie, 12 April 2003).

> 'It's the international press that are killing us—that are hurting us, hurting our restaurants and so on. I saw it on CNN and it made me sick,' said Mr. Lastman.
>
> 'There's not enough airplanes coming in, there's not enough people coming into Toronto. We're used to having 22 million visitors a year,' the mayor said.
>
> 'We've been on the phone . . . trying to get the province . . . [and Ottawa] so the moment we've got things under control we can start a great, big publicity campaign. Toronto is safe,' he said.

The ambiguity apparent in public pronouncements and reporting on the progress of and suggested individual response to SARS was evident in some letters to the editor. Jody Lanard pointed out the obvious when writing to the *National Post,* suggesting that the continuation of such ambiguity in official releases and interviews suggested a very unfortunate inexperience in the essentials of risk communication (Lanard, 31 March 2003).

> In risk communication terms, the most useful strategies at this point in a crisis are for officials to avoid over-reassurance, to acknowledge uncertainty, and to err on the alarming side at the start. It is a marvelous but well-established risk communication paradox that over-reassurance breeds outrage and doubt; and overconfidence leaves people alone with their fears. And despite how well established these principles are in communications terms, "experts" nearly always get it wrong in crises.

But then, such a precautionary impulse is undermined by potentially devastating criticism of the health establishment for over-reacting out of some ulterior motive (Corcoran, 3 April 2003).

> With so many unknowns, it is impossible to determine the seriousness of the global SARS outbreak.
>
> But whenever the inevitable strikes, it lands in the lap of health officials.
>
> It is a response . . . that can all too easily lead to system failure.
>
> The world health establishment . . . spends most of its time and money on self-aggrandizing campaigns against disease and illnesses that are often myths or are grossly overblown. When you spend billions preoccupied with and fighting non-disease, the sharpness of your ability to fight real threats to health and life are inevitably diminished.

At the same time as editorial writers were damning the public health bureaucracy for its preoccupations, respected medical professionals outside that bureaucracy were decrying the failure to explore all prevention and treatment alternatives, and implying that such failure related directly to the underlying selfish interests of those in positions of authority. The following is taken from a paid advertisement in the *National Post,* signed by respected researcher Matthias Rath. The argument begins by suggesting that viruses can be controlled through the use of appropriate natural remedies, such as Vitamin C and Vitamin A, and then continues as follows (Rath, 12 April 2003):

> The fact that the [WHO] is failing so seriously in disseminating live-saving [sic] information about natural, non-patentable health measures is no coincidence. It reflects the fact that WHO is not primarily serving the health interests of the people worldwide, but is apparently influenced by the interests of its largest corporate sponsors—the pharmaceutical industry. This investment industry profits from the sales of patentable synthetic drugs and the expansion of its "business with disease."

The credibility of public health officials and politicians is at least threatened by such criticism, and the confusion is only deepened when it is juxtaposed with pleas for a more sophisticated management of risk communication.

Predictably enough, disagreement among members of the public on the appropriate level of response manifested itself almost immediately. In general terms, letter writers offered support for tough border restrictions, but felt that regulations respecting site-specific quarantine had gone too far. In other words, citizens seemed to accept the alarmist's version of events when it came to considering the activities of potential immigrants and travelers, but paid greater heed to pleas for calm and tolerance when it came to their individual decisions and activities. It is possible, therefore, that the moral grounds on which the advisability of the various types of quarantine were judged by the general population were different, dependent on the nature of the regulation and the target population. This is not to say, however, that those who reportedly violated domestic quarantine were not condemned in letters to the editor, but it is to say that support for tough regulatory measures appeared to be more easily established when it came to border restrictions.

Popular support for strict border restrictions emerged very early in Ontario's SARS crisis. Almost all letter and editorial writers encouraged the government to mount a very aggressive, non-discretionary set of restrictions for those entering the country from "disease hot spots." The following letter is typical (Denbeigh, 4 April 2003):

> As I see it, there are two options: Ban all travel to and from infected areas (not terribly realistic), or quarantine all travelers returning from infected areas at the point of entry for the required ten days.
>
> Since individual provinces are responsible for their own health care, Health Canada will have to step up and take a leadership role. It may be costly and inconvenient, but it would be prudent. Trying to con-

> tain the disease while allowing more infected people to enter the country is simply pointless. Asking returning travelers to self-diagnose is equally pointless.[8]

*The Globe and Mail* reported on April 5, 2003, that "[s]ixty-six percent of Canadians believe everyone arriving from disease hot spots in the Far East should be quarantined or not let in, rather than simply screened" (Unsigned editorial, 5 April 2003). In other words, the moral consensus necessary to ensure public compliance with and sympathy for tough border restrictions seemed to have been established very early in the crisis, with little controversy.

Superficially at least, the same might be said of domestic quarantine. Incidents of violation of domestic quarantine were reported in all four newspapers reviewed for this chapter, with more or less prominence. The following excerpt, about a computer-company employee who went to work despite the fact that he had been ordered to stay home because of a SARS quarantine, in the *National* Post was typical (Blackwell, 11 April 2003).

> The office worker's flouting of the isolation order meant that almost two hundred of his colleagues at a Hewlett-Packard office in Markham were themselves ordered into quarantine at home.
>
> With "a great deal of regret," health authorities have asked police to investigate the situation and see whether charges are warranted, James Young, Ontario's commissioner of public safety, said.
>
> "This is not a direction we want to go," said Dr. Young. "But we have to clearly send the message that we cannot and will not tolerate people willingly breaching isolation. This puts everybody in the community at risk."[9]

A second breach of domestic quarantine at Albert Campbell Collegiate Institute in Scarborough was reported in *The Globe and Mail* on April 9 (Galloway and Abraham, 9 April 2003).

> Some students . . . are in quarantine after one of their classmates developed what is suspected to be SARS.
>
> "This is an individual who had been in household contact with a known case and, on the tenth day of the home quarantine, the individual attended class to write an exam," Dr. Basrur said.

> "Symptoms did develop late in the day once they had left the school. As a precaution, we have required that all of the classmate contacts, and any other course contacts in that school to be on home quarantine for a ten day period."[10]

Violations of domestic quarantine tend to suggest that there are some grounds on which individuals feel that the level of intrusiveness of the requirement cannot be justified relative to the individual need to continue with daily activities. Earning a wage or writing an exam may prove to be the simple motivation for denying the necessity, perhaps even the validity, of a quarantine order.

Despite the uncertainty evidenced by interviews with medical professionals, public health officials and politicians, letters to the editor in response to these and other reports of domestic quarantine violation were virtually unanimous in their condemnation. While there may be particular difficulties with living under a quarantine order sufficient to compel individual violation, public condemnation tends to suggest that the moral consensus necessary for the efficacious imposition of quarantine was already established. That in turn may counter the argument that the equivocation in both media representations of the severity of the disease and the level of intrusiveness necessary as a regulatory response tends to undermine the possibility of a compliant public. Following is a letter offering support for a tough response to violations of domestic quarantine (Van Gaal, 12 April 2003).

> The lack of any reasonable punishment associated with breaking a quarantine order is absolutely unacceptable. Recently, The Globe has published two stories about people breaking their quarantines.
>
> Both of these individuals were under quarantine, but selfishly placed their own interests ahead of the health of the people they came in contact with. This is utterly abhorrent, especially when there is very little to be gained. It is time to start recognizing these breaches of quarantine for what they are—inexcusably selfish acts that may kill others.

The moral judgment of this writer is obvious, by which the public good associated with conventional protections for the general health of the community overrides the writer's concern for the individual rights that must be sacrificed in service of that public good. At the same time, however, other letter writers continued the rhetoric suggesting that the crisis was exaggerated, undermining the force of the more communitarian argument. The following is one example:

> Based on Statistics Canada data, here are the top fifteen causes of death in Canada: cancers, diseases of the heart cerebrovascular diseases, chronic obstructive pulmonary diseases. . . .
>
> Note that all of them are far more likely to kill you than SARS. The meanest, cancer, kills nearly 60,000 Canadians each year, and HIV, number fifteen on the list, kills around 600 a year.
>
> While people are stocking up on respirators and canceling trips to Asia, they might also do well to remember to eat well, keep active, play safe and stay sane (Scott, 10 April 2003).

With respect to domestic quarantine at least, the issue is more or less joined. The moral impulse to self-sacrifice in defense of the community at large is a very real one, forming the basis on which those who would breach domestic quarantine are roundly condemned. However, some continuing skepticism is evident in those who, taking the risks of hubris, challenge their neighbors to continue daily activities as if the threat were minor.

While the rhetoric of the public good dominated the discussion of domestic quarantine, a marked shift in attitude can be detected when site-specific quarantine is the focus. The dominant moral consensus that appears in the condemnation of breaches of quarantine turns to sympathy when particularly difficult cases are discussed. For the most part, this sympathy was engendered through the site-specific quarantine of hospitals in Ontario. The quarantine orders in this respect were strictly enforced, meaning that seriously ill patients were sometimes prevented from receiving visitors. Virtually all of the comment on this situation urged that regulation had gone too far, and that public health authorities were doing more to damage the health of patients than they were promoting good health through erecting another impediment to the spread of SARS. The following letter to the editor of the *National Post* is typical (Marshman, 15 April 2003).

> My mother had a stroke shortly before the provincial ban on hospital visitors. Her speech, vision, and movement were severely affected, and in the first few days my sisters and I were at her hospital bedside constantly. Last Saturday, however, we were locked out . . . Doctors and nurses have told us the only thing that will help her is the stimulation of contact with her family. But we are stuck on the outside, looking in.
>
> The current restrictions could end up killing more people than the disease they're intended to stop.[11]

The message from this letter writer (and many others) is that the apparent moral consensus on which both the justifiability of quarantine is founded and the regulations themselves are enforced does have its breaking point. The writer would argue compassionate grounds (without recognizing explicitly that the order on which the quarantine of hospitals was based in fact transferred some discretion in that respect to hospital authorities).[12] Randall Denley, a popular city columnist with the *Ottawa Citizen*, provided perhaps the most stinging criticism in this respect, challenging provincial authorities and hospital personnel to justify the strict enforcement of site-specific quarantine in situations arguably crying out for compassion. Denley related the story of his former colleague, Harold Lundy, who was in the hospital for heart surgery and isolated from his family (Denley, 12 April 2003).

> Reducing risk is good, but the strategies need to stand up to reason. Based on what we've seen in Ottawa, the risk in [sic] infinitesimal, but the same precautions are being taken here as in Toronto, where there is a problem. The provincial government is behind that decision, not our hospitals.
>
> Health Ministry spokesman John Leatherby says the Ministry, too, understands people's frustration, but if rules are slackened and something happens, people will point their fingers at the Ministry.
>
> Better to prevent families from seeing sick patients than have the Ministry blamed for another SARS case.

Denley's concern appears to be the inflexibility in the way in which the site-specific quarantine orders were applied, that is, a blanket rejection of compassionate grounds on which exceptions might be made. This is his point, regardless of the actual grounds (compassionate, medical or otherwise) on which exceptions to the "no visitors" order might be made. The quarantine decision is based on a defense of the Ministry's reputation, he suggests, rather than a defense of the public health, meaning that the moral foundations on which the decision is made are weak and transparent.

## *Conclusion*

In an opinion column published in *The Globe and Mail* on 23 April 2003, Jocelyn Downie, one of Canada's leading health law academics, isolated the moral dilemmas inherent in the decision to impose quarantine, border restrictions, domestic quarantine, or site-specific quarantine. Downie wrote (23 April 2003):

> Because liberty is a keystone value in Canadian society, liberty-restricting methods to contain disease should only be contemplated in extraordinary circumstances. But they can be contemplated.
>
> To balance all these issues and interests in an ethical way, we need more information about risks of transmission and costs of alternative methods of reducing risk, about the potential harms involved as well as the potential benefits. Only then can we ascribe weights to the various values involved, and determine which methods that may restrict the liberties of our fellow citizens are ethically defensible.
>
> To act without such careful consideration is indefensible.

It is likely that Michael Davis's conditions (1996a: supra note 4) on which quarantine is morally justifiable can only be arrived through the type of thorough risk analysis and weighing of values and interests contemplated by Downie. But it cannot be overlooked that any process by which such analysis is completed is itself not value-neutral. Rather, such a process involves choices, and choices are necessarily made in a value-laden milieu, by which responsible people use their best judgment, relying on their experience and training, to make the appropriate decisions. There is no pure procedural justice here, by which we simply plug in the variables, apply the appropriate formula, and guarantee a just result. That attempt may give us grounds on which to defend particular decisions, but it does not generate absolute moral certainty. The difficulty is that our procedures are necessarily imperfect. Through the democratic process and the legislative process, we transfer responsibility for making tough decisions to our representatives, hoping all the while that the decisions they make will be wise and just. We know in advance, however, that our representatives will make mistakes, and we reserve the right to criticize.

To some extent, of course, the frailties inherent in the decision-making process constitute an impossible obstacle for decision-makers. Nevertheless, there can be no assumption that any decisions made in such circumstances are perfectly justifiable and defensible, either to the public at large or to any particular member of the public. The material isolated in this chapter from the *Toronto Star*, the *Ottawa Citizen*, *The Globe and Mail* and the *National Post* confirms that. Despite the apparent best efforts of bureaucrats, medical health professionals and politicians, crisis spawns extraordinary disagreement, such that the moral foundations on which decisions are made to impose quarantine are never unassailable.

## *Notes*

1. For a review of some of the implications of this position, see Logan Atkinson (2002: p. 288).

2. See also Hogg (1985).

3. Details in the case of both jurisdiction over persons and jurisdiction over sites are contained in Part IV of the Act, titled "Communicable Diseases." There are additional powers respecting jurisdiction over sites in Part V of the Act, titled "Rights of Entry and Appeals from Orders."

4. SARS was added to the lists of communicable and virulent diseases on 25 March 2003 by virtue of Ontario Regulation Nos. 97/03 and 95/03 respectively. In addition, on 5 May 2003, Royal Assent was given to the Ontario statute, the *SARS Assistance and Recovery Strategy Act, 2003*, S.O. 2003, c. 1. For us, the only provision relevant to the powers contained in the *Health Protection and Promotion Act* involves the ability of the medical officer of health to direct orders to classes of persons, as opposed to individuals, and to publish notice of such orders through the media. The intent is to avoid the delay attendant on individual notice and service, where such delay is likely to substantially increase the risk to the public health.

5. In the four newspapers considered for this chapter, there were many thousands of column inches devoted to the SARS crisis during the period under review. By necessity, I have been selective in the material I have chosen to cite. Readers ought not to assume that the pieces referred to in this chapter establish the sole portrayal of SARS in those papers, nor even the dominant portrayal. Rather, they are chosen so as to demonstrate the potential for the media to generate moral debate around the justification of tough regulatory measures, which in turn may raise doubts about any assumption of the morality of quarantine.

6. Fumento refers to Garrett (1994).

7. The intersection of College and Spadina is near the centre of commercial activity for Toronto's Chinese community.

8. While virtually all comment on border restrictions supported views similar to Denbeigh's, there was one flurry of articles and correspondence that argued against a strict enforcement of border restrictions in the case of Canadian families returning to Canada from China on adoption trips. See Duffy (3 April 2003) and Page (27 April 2003). In the Page article, the author argued passionately against the mandatory 10 day quarantine for all families returning from Chinese adoption trips. Her position was echoed by Julie Mason, Canadian grandmother to one of the adopted Chinese children. She wrote: "When we start arbitrarily shutting people away—even for ten days—just because we're scared, it isn't good science, it's moral panic, pandering to irrational fear. [Ottawa's medical officer of health] Dr. Cushman has a responsibility to oppose this, not encourage it" (Mason, 24 April 2003).

9. The incident was reported in Galloway (10 April 2003).

10. Gloria Galloway and Carolyn Abraham, "Hospitals adapting for the long term: Baffling new illness forces re-evaluation of how to contain infection in future." *The Globe and Mail*, 9 April 2003.

11. See also Berman (13 April 2003), Thompson (18 April 2003), and Avery (3 April 2003). Each of these items lamented the strictness of the order for the quarantine of hospitals, decrying the inhumanity of the consequences and pleading for reconsideration. In referring to the actions of Ottawa's medical officer of health, Robert Cushman, Thompson wrote: "Dr. Cushman should, for once, put himself in the everyday person's shoes (or slippers) and stop jeopardizing the well-being of the sick people he is supposed to care about."

12. See, for example, Ministry of Health and Long-Term Care (2004).

## *References*

Atkinson, Logan (2002) "Extending *La Longue Durée*: Commercial Impact in the Reform and Use of the Law of Quarantine." In *Law, Regulation, and Governance,* edited by Michael MacNeil, Neil Sargent and Peter Swan. Toronto: Oxford University Press, 288.

Avery, Simon (3 April 2003) "SARS forces son to leave ailing mother." *The Globe and Mail.*

Barnett, Randy E. (1996) "Getting Even: Restitution, Preventive Detention, and the Tort/Crime Distinction." 76 *Boston University Law Review,* 157-168.

Benzie, Robert (12 April 2003) "Everybody should feel safe in Toronto." *National Post.*

Berman, Hershl (13 April 2003) "SARS overreaction." Letters to the Editor, *The Globe and Mail.*

Blackwell, Tom (11 April 2003) "Police Probe Quarantine Breach: Employee Went to Work." *National Post.*

*The Constitution Act, 1867* (U.K.), 30 and 31 Vict., c. 3.

Corcoran, Terence (3 April 2003) "Never mind SARS, where's your cat?" *National Post.*

Corrado, Michael (1996a) "Punishment, Quarantine and Preventive Detention." *Criminal Justice Ethics*, Summer/Fall, p. 3-13.

Corrado, Michael (1996b) "Response to Michael Davis." *Criminal Justice Ethics,* Summer/Fall, p. 25-29.

Coyle, Jim (1 April 2003) "SARS is manna to media." *Toronto Star.*

Davis, Michael (1996a) "Preventive Detention, Corrado and Me." *Criminal Justice Ethics*, Summer/Fall, p. 13-24.

Davis, Michael (1996b) "Reply to Corrado." *Criminal Justice Ethics*, Summer/Fall, 29-33.

Denbeigh, Edward C. (4 April 2003) "Prevention plan must be more aggressive." Letters to the Editor, *Ottawa Citizen.*

Denley, Randall (12 April 2003) "Virus fight goes to ridiculous lengths: SARS strategy doesn't stand up to reason." *Ottawa Citizen.*

Downie, Jocelyn (23 April 2003) "How far should we go?" *The Globe and Mail.*

Duffy, Andrew (3 April 2003) "Love wins over SARS fear; adoption trip to China is on." *Ottawa Citizen.*

Fumento, Michael (28 March 2003) "Super-bug or super-scare?" *National Post.*

Fyfe, Peter (8 April 2003) "Eves dropped ball on SARS outbreak." Letters to the Editor, *Toronto Star.*

Galloway, Gloria (10 April 2003) "SARS virus empties out Ontario workplace." *The Globe and Mail.*

Galloway, Gloria and Carolyn Abraham (9 April 2003) "Hospitals adapting for the long term: Baffling new illness forces re-evaluation of how to contain infection in future." *The Globe and Mail.*

Garrett, Laurie (1994) *The Coming Plague: Newly Emerging Diseases in a World out of Balance.* New York: Penguin Books.

Hogg, Peter W. (1985) *Constitutional Law of Canada, 2nd Edition.* Toronto: The Carswell Company of Canada, 405-6.

Lanard, Jody (31 March 2003) "SARS is bad news." Letters to the Editor, *National Post.*

Marshman, Paul (15 April 2003) "SARS' human toll." Letters to the Editor, *National Post.*

Martin, Don (29 March 2003) "Hunkering down at the SARS wars battle station." *National Post.*

Mason, Julie (24 April 2003) "Irrational Fear." Letters to the Editor, *Ottawa Citizen.*

Ministry of Health and Long-term Care ( 2004). "Directive to all Ontario Non-Acute Care Facilities" SARS Provincial Operations Centre, Ontario Ministry of Health and Long-Term Care. Accessed on 12 December 2004. Available at: http://www.health.gov.on.ca/english/providers/program/pubhealth/sars/docs/new_normal/dir_non_acute_care.pdf

Morse, Stephen J. (1996) "Blame and Danger: An Essay on Preventive Detention." 76 *Boston University Law Review,* 113-155.

Morse, Stephen J. (1999) "Neither Desert Nor Disease." 5 *Legal Theory,* 265-309.

Page, Shelley (27 April 2003) "SARS mars adoption experience for Canadians." *Ottawa Citizen.*

Rath, Matthias (12 April 2003) "Vitamin C against SARS: What everyone should know—but what WHO won't tell you—about *natural* protection from the new epidemic." *National Post.*

SARS Provincial Operations Centre, Ontario Ministry of Health and Long-Term Care (Accessed 12 December 2004) "Directive to all Ontario Non-Acute Care Facilities." Available at: http://www.health.gov.on.ca/english/providers/program/pubhealth/sars/docs/new_normal/dir_non_acute_care.pdf

Saytar, Don (22 April 2003) "Face up to the crisis." Letters to the Editor, *Toronto Star.*

Schoeman, Ferdinand D. (1979) "On Incapacitating the Dangerous." 16/1 *American Philosophical Quarterly* 27-35.

Scott, Adam (10 April 2003) "Perspective on SARS." Letters to the Editor, *The Globe and Mail.*

Thompson, Nancy (18 April 2003) "Healing power." Letters to the Editor, *Ottawa Citizen.*

Toronto Electric Commissioners v. Snider, 1925. A.C. 396 at 412.

Unsigned editorial (2 April 2003) "SARS fight calls for calm, tolerance." *Toronto Star.*

Unsigned editorial (5 April 2003) "The danger of SARS." *The Globe and Mail.*

Van Gaal, Stephen (12 April 2003) "Can't be too cautious." Letters to the Editor, *The Globe and Mail.*

# Chapter 8

# Early International News Flow about SARS: Interconnected or Unconnected?

Joan Deppa, Andrew Seaberg, and Grace Han Yao

## *Introduction*

When Marshall McLuhan first spoke about the emerging "global village" and "world connectivity" in the1960s,[1] he could hardly have envisioned the strange test of his communications theories that would be created by SARS. The Canadian scholar believed electronic technology would change messages and their impact on audiences, turning individuals from isolated readers into tribes sharing experiences through movies, radio and television. The reality in early 2003, despite more and faster channels of communications, was quite different. The new disease came quickly and surreptitiously from Asia to Vancouver and Toronto—except for those who could read Chinese-language reports circulating on the Web and among ethnic communities around the world.

While a number of studies and articles have focused on communication about SARS after the World Health Organization announced its first global alert on March 12, 2003, we set out to understand when and how the news about this disease began to flow internationally. What we found raises basic questions: What were the barriers to rapid and accurate news flow? What steps have been taken to correct flaws in the system? Will those steps be sufficient to ensure timely news flow about future health threats?

Heymann and Rodier state that the Canadian Global Public Health Intelligence Network "picked up media reports of a suspected influenza outbreak in mainland China" in late November (2004: 173). These reports, however, reassured the Global Outbreak Alert and Response Network (GOARN) because they appeared to be normal both in number and type of influenza cases for that point in the flu season. Much later, Heymann and Rodier say, it would become clear that the disease known as SARS had been present already in November.[2] However, an in-depth report by the Canadian Broadcasting Corporation states WHO officials received clues on November 23, 2002, that an unusual respiratory disease was emerging in Guangdong province. The CBC quotes Dr. Klaus Stohr, head of the WHO influenza team, who recalled how a health official from the province spoke about a highly infectious respiratory disease that was causing deaths and making health care workers sick as well ("Dead Silence," 2003).

We were able to identify stories in Chinese news media originally published in early January 2003 and still available via the Internet in November 2004. One, which appeared in the daily newspaper for Heyuan City, reported that two people had been diagnosed with atypical pneumonia on December 15.

It said people in the city had begun to "crazily purchase" antibiotics because of rumors about the spreading of an unknown virus. The reporter checked with the city's Center for Disease Control and was reassured that there was no unknown virus (Huang, 3 January 2003). Two days later a reporter for the *New Express* in Guangzhou followed up by interviewing Dr. Yilong Wu, head of the No. 3 hospital of Zongshan University, who said that the atypical pneumonia was not infectious (Jinyang, 5 January 2003).

Such reports apparently failed to reassure the populace. In January, Chinese-language newspapers in Canada carried stories about the strange respiratory disease in China, and pharmacists in Vancouver reported customers buying surgical masks to send them to family members overseas ("Behind the Mask," 2003).

In February, cases increased and so did news stories, emerging for the first time in English-language wire service reports. Heymann cites unpublished WHO data that "a second wave of disease with amplified transmission to health workers began occurring during the first ten days of February" (Heymann and Rodier, 2004:173-174). On February 10, *Southern Metropolis Daily,* a business-oriented, Chinese-language newspaper published in Guangzhou, carried a story that was repeated in the *East China Times* the following day. It said the Guangdong committee of the Chinese Communist Party (CCP) and the Guangdong government had begun to pay close attention to cases of atypical pneumonia after learning the disease was spreading in Guangdong. Of 305 cases, the story said, 105 were medical staff; 5 of the cases had resulted in death and 59 had recovered. It quoted two leaders of the Communist party and the governor of the province, and said they had commanded health departments to send the best staff to investigate the cause and source of the epidemic in order to prevent it from spreading. They also indicated that medical staff should be well protected.[3]

The Associated Press transmitted a report from Beijing on February 10 (McDonald, 10 February 2003) announcing five deaths from an unidentified pneumonia virus that had left hundreds hospitalized in southern China. It echoed information carried by the *Southern Metropolis Daily*, including the fact that about one-third of those hospitalized were healthcare workers. It quoted unnamed health officials as stating that the outbreak "had been brought under control" and that rumors "of a surging death toll . . . had prompted residents to clear store shelves of antibiotics and pay inflated prices for white vinegar for use as disinfectant" (McDonald, 14 May 2003). The report mentioned that Hong Kong papers showed Guangdong residents wearing surgical masks. It added a paragraph that explained why the outbreak could be significant beyond the affected province:

> Southern China is a major source of new strains of flu and other viruses, which often are traced to the region's large poultry industry.

> An outbreak of bird flu in Hong Kong in 1997 killed six people and prompted health authorities to slaughter of all of the territory's 1.4 million chickens.

The story was distributed to AP clients in Europe, the Middle East, Africa and Asia. A longer story was moved to the same clients the next day, along with pictures from Guangzhou showing travelers, their faces covered with fabric masks, outside a train station (McDonald, 10 February 2003). An abbreviated version was transmitted the same day to American clients as the fourth of five items in an Asian news round-up.

The "under control" theme, carried in the second paragraph of the AP stories, was prominent in Chinese and English reports by Xinhua, the official China news service, which reported February 11 on a news conference in Guangzhou. The first two paragraphs read:

> The municipal people's government of Guangzhou says an outbreak of atypical pneumonia in the city in southern China is now under control.
>
> Plague and anthrax have been excluded as causes of the outbreak, according to a press conference held Tuesday by the Guangzhou government.

The "under control" theme continued in Xinhua dispatches about atypical pneumonia in Guandong province, even after the World Health Organization issued a global alert on March 12 and another on March 15, when cases had been reported in Hong Kong, Vietnam, Singapore, and Canada. It was not until March 26 that this theme in Xinhua dispatches began to change.[4]

We were also able to examine February dispatches from Agence France Presse and Deutsche Presse-Agentur that mentioned the cases in Guangdong. Reporting by wire services, however, does not mean that the information will be passed on to the public. We could find evidence of very few newspapers that gave AP or other reports space in February or early March.[5] Of the initial reports on February 10 and 11, in the United States only the *Desert News* in Salt Lake City carried the story, according to the Nexis search. That was as part of a world roundup credited to wire services. It followed up on February 15 with an AP article by Ted Anthony, headlined "China panics over deadly mystery illness."

Two other reports could be traced in U.S. media, both on television. WXIA in Atlanta carried a very brief report on February 11. The next day Wolf Blitzer on CNN, as part of an international roundup at the end of Wolf Blitzer Reports told audiences, "Mystery illness . . . The Chinese government says it's making headway against a mysterious illness that has many people wearing surgical masks in public. The illness, described as a form of pneumonia, is blamed for five deaths in southern China, but the government says the spread of the disease has been contained."

CNN did not mention the disease again until March 15, when CNN medical correspondent Elizabeth Cohen reported on a conference call and described what the World Health Organization and the U.S. Centers for Disease Control were saying about the disease. That was when most broadcasting outlets began reporting on the story, including Canadian television.

A Nexis search shows that on February 20 the *New York Times* did mention the mysterious pneumonia in Guangdong province relatively low in a Hong Kong story about bird flu cases (Altman and Bradsher, 15 March 2003). The paper's stories about SARS began March 15, when the World Health Organization issued the global alert to advise health officials of the illness and asking them to report cases that seemed to fit the symptoms. It finally made the front page of the *New York Times* on April 7 with over three thousand words prepared by seven reporters.

The *Washington Post* waited until March 14 to inform readers about the disease in Hong Kong and Hanoi; that report alluded to the cases in Guangdong province in mid-February. The following day the *Post* carried a front-page story on the WHO's global warning that the disease "posed a worldwide threat after spreading from Asia to Europe and North America" (Stein, 14 March 2003). Most other newspapers covering the story began to carry it at about the same time, including those in Canada.

Fortunately, some Canadians had other sources of information—the Chinese-language newspapers that served large immigrant communities from China and Hong Kong, concentrated in Toronto and Vancouver. Those papers were carrying the news about the epidemic in Guangdong and elsewhere. So, as Canadian Broadcasting Corporation would learn later, the arrival of a man who had come to the emergency ward of Scarborough Grace Hospital on March 7 after his mother died at their home triggered a memory for Nurse Agnes Wong. She recalled a story she had read in Toronto's *Sing Tao* newspaper. It told of a young family in Hong Kong who took a trip to mainland China. The father and then the daughter became ill and eventually two members of the family died. "So that is really sad and very unusual," Wong told the CBC. "That stayed with me" (Crowe and Jenzer, 2003).

The initial diagnosis of the Scarborough Grace patient had been tuberculosis (Donovan and Talaga, 2003). But Wong called the night nurse and asked her to check the mother's traveling history. She soon learned the mother had been to Hong Kong and came back ill. Wong urged the nursing staff to notify the physician. And that, according to the CBC and the *Toronto Star*, is how Canada's first SARS case was identified.

Information that might have alerted Canadian health professionals to the nature of the disease (particularly the risk it posed to medical personnel) had been transmitted to some health bureaucrats and hospital personnel but not, in most cases, to those who actually had to deal with patients suffering from the infection. Although Health Canada carried information about the Guangdong outbreak in its *Fluwatch Bulletin* that summarized influenza activity between February 9 and 15, the next week the same publication carried the assurance by Chinese authorities that the outbreak was "under control." Later that month e-mails and faxes were sent out by Health Canada concerning the mysterious respiratory disease in Guangdong and avian flu cases in Hong Kong.

The committee that investigated Canada's experience with SARS would hear from The Canadian Hospital Epidemiology Committee that the nation lacked a coordinated system for notifying hospitals of global health alerts and appropriate recommendations for managing possible cases ("Learning from SARS," 2003). So while the first patient seeking treatment was waiting to be placed in isolation at Scarborough Grace Hospital on March 7, he exposed many patients and staff. The significance of that exposure would become clear only after he died on March 13. Three days later another patient, who had been treated in an adjacent emergency ward bed, returned to the hospital with respiratory symptoms. But hospital personnel did not ask the second patient's wife, who had been with him in the emergency ward, if she had symptoms. Epidemiologists would determine that she infected seven visitors to the emergency ward, as well as six hospital staff, two patients, two paramedics, a firefighter and a housekeeper ("Learning from SARS," 2003).

Many Canadians apparently learned of the WHO alert about SARS and the cases in Toronto and Vancouver in the same stories. In Ontario, the *Toronto Star* based its front-page story on a March 14 news conference by the Ontario Ministry of Health and Long-Term Care and wire reports.[6] In British Columbia, the *Vancouver Sun* began extensive coverage on March 17. Apparently, the March 12 global alert from the WHO, which warned "Those at highest risk appear to be staff caring for the patients," was not published by Canadian news media. And while it was received by Health Canada, it was not passed along to medical personnel already facing the disease.

Ironically, the information flow in China's relatively closed society, which produced premature pronouncements that the disease was "under control," and the belated news flow and lack of public health leadership in Ontario's relatively open democracy had the same result: They failed to alert hospital staff to steps that could have protected themselves and patients seeking their help for other medical conditions.

## *Barriers to News Flow*

For the May 15, 2003, issue of the *New England Journal of Medicine*, the director of the U.S. Centers for Disease Control raised two important questions. Dr.

Julie Gerberding wrote:

> Speed of scientific discovery and speed of communication are hallmarks of the response to SARS and reflect amazing achievements in science, technology, and international collaboration. However, despite these advances, a very sobering question remains—are we fast enough? Can we prevent a global pandemic of SARS? (p. 2030)

The answer to Gerberding's question about preventing a global pandemic turned out to be "yes," thanks to the coordinated scientific energy used to identify and contain the disease—once the danger it posed was recognized. However, the answer to the "fast enough" question may be unclear until another unexpected biological threat emerges, either naturally or as a bioterrorist attack. Communications technology is in place, ready to speed information around the globe as fast as science can provide the answers and journalists can process them into messages understandable by the general public. This case history of communications about SARS highlights the weak link: The early phases of such an outbreak when symptoms—or their significance—may be hidden from scientists and journalists alike. Had SARS been more easily transmitted or had humans willfully spread it to other population centers the containable outbreak could have rapidly evolved into a global pandemic.

Identifying barriers to rapid, accurate transfer of information in the SARS outbreak may help to determine how similar obstacles might be removed or at least reduced in the face of future threats. The most obvious barriers do relate, of course, to language and political systems. It is incomprehensible that Canada's health intelligence system, working with the World Health Organization, had no capacity to translate Chinese messages from the Internet, especially given the role that Southeast Asia has played in recent disease outbreaks. Although that is being corrected through a grant from a foundation headed by CNN founder Ted Turner and former Senator Sam Nunn (Nuclear Threat Initiative, 2004), translation of messages into English will not guarantee that they will impel authorities to transmit rapid and credible information to the audiences that need it most. The fact that news about SARS languished for more than a month *after* news about the disease was reported in English makes that clear.

Governments, influenced by political or bureaucratic rationales, may see risk communications as inherently risky and hesitate while the opportunity for early intervention passes by. Such behavior does not seem to be confined to political ideologies to geographic areas; in some ways, the experiences of China and Ontario are more similar to one another (although possibly for different reasons) than they are to Vietnam, Vancouver and Singapore.

The significant barriers may be more related to failures of perception or cognition than to either language- or government-related obstacles. This analysis focuses on three such failures in the SARS experience that seem to cut across linguistic, governmental and geographic divides. All three could apply to scientific as well as journalistic failures, even though the three authors approach the issue from a communications perspective.

*Novelty*

News is often described as being focused on novelty[7] or deviance[8] but the reality is that very new phenomena may be ignored—or at least neglected—by news organizations until something or someone forces their attention on the novel occurrence. This was the case, for example, with such major stories as the AIDS epidemic and Islamic terrorism. Wright highlights a Kaiser Family Foundation study that shows how slow the news media were to report the story as the disease emerged in the early 1980s and then focused on "a series of big, attention-grabbing events" (2004). Parks (2002) argues that many news organizations were forced to play "catch-up" in the wake of the September 11 attacks because they had covered earlier attacks by radical Islamic fundamentalists only with episodic reporting that involved little follow-up or investigative effort, even when suspects were brought to trial. So it is hardly surprising, for instance, that the first *New York Times* article to mention the "atypical pneumonia" led off with avian flu cases and introduced the more novel phenomenon in the sixth paragraph (Bradsher, 20 February 2003).

What was especially novel about this respiratory disease, namely, its impact on healthcare workers and family members in close contact with the victims, became evident very early. But even the WHO seemed not to understand the urgency of sharing that information in a way that would gain the attention of those on the frontlines of medicine.

*"Under control"*

Although the version of the original *Southern Metropolis Daily* story available to us made no mention of the disease being "under control," most early reports used that term or a related theme to indicate the disease was no longer a threat—if it ever had been. The first English-language report, McDonald's dispatch for the AP on February 10, used the term in the second paragraph. The term "out of control" tends to describe a story of increasing news value while "under control" marks the end of a story's cycle as news. This role these terms play can be seen clearly in the coverage of major fires.

Chinese health officials' use of this term is hardly unique. In 2000, when pollution of the drinking water supply in Walkerton, Ontario, caused a lengthy outbreak of *E.coli* 0157:H7 that ultimately killed seven and affected more than 2,300 (O'Connor, 2002), the chief medical officer of health for Ontario said in the early days of the emergency, "I believe the outbreak is under control"

(Millar, 25 May 2000). In October 2001, when health authorities investigated the death of a photo editor in Florida and announced it had been caused by inhalation anthrax, the U.S. Secretary of Health and Human Services appeared at a White House briefing and asserted it was an "isolated event" (Weiss, p. A15). It soon became clear that case was not isolated, but the first of a series caused by anthrax mailed through the U.S. Postal Service. However, the confusion created by statements minimizing the dangers from *E.coli* and anthrax in North America was relatively temporary because Canadian and U.S. journalists operated in an open environment. They were able to seek other, more credible sources and pass that information on to their audiences. In China, the "under control" messages about the situation in Guangdong province and Beijing persisted in Xinhua and other Chinese media because of restrictions on the press that lasted well into April.

The second wave of SARS in Toronto provided another example of how categorizing phenomena as "under control" can have serious unintended consequences. As the national committee investigating SARS reported: "By mid-May, all levels of government were presenting a unified picture to the public that SARS had been contained" ("Learning from SARS," 2003, p. 38). Officials highlighted less dramatic numbers, such as the declining number of "active" cases and new cases, and Health Canada began issues weekly rather than daily bulletins. Infection control practices had begun to ease in late April, which turned out to be a tragic error. On May 23, health officials were forced to admit that they were battling a second wave of SARS. They instituted a new round of quarantines and ordered all hospitals in the Greater Toronto Area to reinstate infection-control procedures. The effect of this news can be seen by comparing the number of stories in the *Toronto Star* by comparison with Asian and U.S. news media. While the other newspapers continued to give attention to SARS-related stories, the *Star*'s coverage jumped to fifteen and then over twenty five in a two-day period.

*Misunderstanding of panic*

Beginning with the earliest reports, authorities in China seemed to assume that people in the regions affected by this new disease were behaving irrationally in response to rumors or would panic if they had more information. The news media, including those filing reports to English-speaking audiences, often took their cues from the authorities, playing up the idea that people were behaving "crazily" in their efforts to protect themselves. While there were instances in which precautions had tragic results, such as the two members of a family who died of coal fumes because vinegar was being boiled in a sealed apartment (Olesen, 17 March 2003), many activities represented logical responses to what could be learned through informal communications channels. The severity of the respiratory syndrome and the fact that a significant proportion of healthcare workers were "catching" the disease would be topics of interpersonal communications in the affected areas. Such basic measures against infectious disease as using masks and disinfectants were not only logical; in slightly different terms, they came close to "barrier nursing techniques" recommended by the WHO in its first news release about the disease (12 March 2003, para. 8).

This behavior is in keeping with a sizeable body of research into the way the public actually behaves in the face of disaster, which led The Working Group on "Governance Dilemmas" in Bioterrorism Response[9] to warn leaders against assumptions about panic:

> Decision-makers need to anticipate and tolerate their own emotional responses to crisis, taking care not to project their stress, fears and feelings of inadequacy onto the public. Leaders are often inclined to make reassuring statements prematurely, to avoid unnecessary alarm or a secondary "disaster" (e.g., people fleeing an area and clogging highways). Downplaying danger when its extent is not yet known tends to make a leader's or an agency's subsequent statements suspect, especially when the peril is real and even greater than anticipated. Though it is a fallacy to assume that all people act sensibly always, detailed study of population responses to actual disasters over the last five decades suggest that panic rarely occurs (2004).

*Professional experience*

For scientists and journalists, such a disease presents special problems: Few of the former are accustomed to communicating with the general public, especially about life-threatening phenomena that they themselves may not fully understand. Few of the latter, while experienced in communicating with the public, know what questions they need to ask or how to evaluate the answers they receive from scientists or public health professionals.

Under conditions of high uncertainty both groups are likely to fall back on past practices. Scientists, for example, may assume that it is sufficient to communicate with health care professionals. Journalists, including both those who gather news and those who process it, may treat a disease outbreak as "spot" news, that is, information about an event that can be immediately put into a news story and transmitted. Tuchman (1978) developed this and other categories of news from interviewing journalists about their work; typically, they used fires as examples of "spot" news, sometimes adding another event category such as a robbery, murder, accident, tornado, or earthquake. For reporters, their editors or the editors at news organizations receiving the wire service, the government statements that the disease was "under control" confirmed their judgment that the outbreak could be treated this way. So could the story element of panic since it is perceived as a sudden, fleeting behavior. It was not until March 12 that the Associated Press changed its approach to this story, coming closer to Tuchman's category of a "developing" story, one that lacks certain pieces of information that might prove vital in reporting the full picture. Meanwhile, the inattention of "gatekeepers" within news organizations to biological threats from distant places persisted in many news organizations, including Canada.

What journalists and scientists needed was a chance to clarify the issues. That was provided on March 17 when the U.S. Centers for Disease Control and Director Gerberding held a teleconference with journalists, several of them with science journalism training and/or experience. It started with the statement that there were no new developments to announce, but acknowledged the desire for information about SARS was pressing. This format benefited both sides, and ultimately the public. It is worth considering as one model to cut through the complexities and uncertainties of a biological threat.

## *Discussion*

Although some steps, such as translating news media reports in Chinese, Arabic and other languages, have been taken to correct flaws in the system, it remains to be seen whether those steps will ensure timely news flow about future health threats. That is partly because of the ways that key players in this "global village" share and process information—or fail to—about the health-threatening and life-threatening pathogens. The short list of barriers discussed here does not exhaust the subject, but it may help start the international dialogue necessary to help develop a truly interconnected system.

## *Notes*

1. McLuhan can still be heard making these predictions on a website of the Canadian Broadcasting System, http://archives.cbc.ca/400d.asp?id=1-74-342-1814 and http://archives.cbc.ca/IDC-1-74-342-1817/people/mcluhan/clip3.

2. This November report was forwarded to the WHO with an English header but was not translated ("Learning from SARS," 2003, p. 24).

3. This article was retrieved from the *East China Times* Website on November 23, 2004. *East China Times* is a subsidiary of *People's Daily*, and is published in Nanjing, Jiangsu Province, and daily distributed to Jiangsu Province, Zhejiang Province, and Shanghai.

4. The opening paragraph read: "The Health Bureau of south China's Guangdong Province announced Wednesday that notable progress had been made in controlling and treating atypical pneumonia." It also stated that by late February 680 cases of atypical pneumonia had been diagnosed and 24 had died in Guangzhoul. But the story quoted a

spokesman who "emphasized that there had been a drastic drop in the number of fresh cases . . . since the beginning of this month and patients suffering from atypical pneumonia had received timely and proper treatment."

5. Although some newspapers do not include wire service stories in the content they submit to Nexis and other databases, the number of stories that could be located in this time period was small by comparison with the number of stories, many of them wire stories, that appeared later.

6. The *Toronto Sun* carried a much smaller story that claimed the Toronto cases "may be linked to a massive outbreak of the disease in Asia" (15 May 2003, p.20).

7. An old saying provides a useful example: "When a dog bites a man that's not news, but when a man bites a dog that is news." Actually, dogs biting humans often make news, especially when the consequences of the biting involve serious injury or death. Nevertheless, the saying is often repeated in journalism texts.

8. See for example Shoemaker, Chang, and Brendlinger (1986).

9. The first author was a member of the Working Group.

## *References*

Altman, Lawrence and Keith Bradsher (15 March 2003) "Mysterious Respiratory Illness Afflicts Hundreds Globally." *New York Times.*

Anthony, Ted (15 February 2003) "China panics over deadly mystery illness." *Associated Press.*

Bradsher, K. (20 February 2003) "Man's Death Of 'Bird Flu' In Hong Kong Raises Fears." *New York Times*, p. A9. Accessed on 30 November 2004 from Nexis.

Crowe, K., and S. Jenzer (19 November 2003) "Behind the Mask." Canadian Broadcasting Corporation. Accessed on 22 November 2004. Available at: http://www.cbc.ca/news/background/sars/behindthemask.html

"Dead Silence" (18 November 2003) Canadian Broadcasting Corporation. Accessed 22 November 2004. Available at: http://www.cbc.ca/disclosure/archives/031118_sars/main.html

Donovan, K., and T. Talaga (20 September 2003) "SARS: The chain of errors." Accessed 30 November 2004.

Eysenbach, Gunter (6 June 2003) "SARS and Population Health Technology." *Journal of Medical Internet Research.* Accessed 26 November 2004. Available at: http://www.jmir.org/2003/2/e14/

Gerberding , J.L. (15 May 2003) "Faster. . . . but Fast Enough? Responding to the Epidemic of Severe Acute Respiratory Syndrome." *New England Journal of Medicine.* Accessed 26 November 2004. Available at: http://content.nejm.org/cgi/content/full/348/20/2030

Gerberding, J.L. (17 March 2003) "Telebriefing: CDC's Response to Severe Acute Respiratory Syndrome." Accessed 5 December 2004. Available at http://www.cdc.gov/od/oc/media/transcripts/t030317.htm

Heymann, David and Guénaël Rodier (2004) "Global surveillance, national surveillance, and SARS." *Emerging Infectious Diseases,* 10:173-5.

Huang, Liqi (3 January 2003) "Incident Resulting from Rumors of an Unknown Virus,

Heyuan City Citizens Fight to Buy Antibiotics." *Jinyang Net* (the online version of the Yangcheng Evening News).

*Jinyang Net* (the online version of the Yangcheng Evening News) (5 January 2003) "Heyuan City Citizens go to Guangzhou in Panic Buying of Antibiotics."

Lanard, Jody and Peter Sandman (6 May 2003) "SARS Communication: What Singapore is doing right." *The* (Singapore) *Straits Times*. Accessed 26 November 2004. Available at http://www.psandman.com/articles/sars-3.htm.

"Learning from SARS: Renewal of Public Health in Canada" (2003) Report of the National Advisory Committee on SARS and Public Health. Accessed 3 December 2004. Available at: http://www.hc-sc.gc.ca/english/protection/warnings/sars/learning.html.

McDonald, Joe (10 February 2003) "Unidentified Illness Kills 5 in China." Available at: http://www.freerepublic.com/focus/f-news/840711/posts

McDonald, Joe (14 May 2003) "China Cracks Down on High-Tech SARS Rumors." *Associated Press, AP Online.*

Millar, Cal (25 May 2000) "An outbreak of bacteria." *Toronto Star*. Accessed 2 December 2004 from Nexis.

Nuclear Threat Initiative (17 November 2004) "New Tool Launched in Fight Against Infectious Disease Outbreaks." Press Release. Accessed 4 December 2004. Available at: http://nti.org/index.html

Oh, David C., and Wanfeng Zhou (2004) "Framing SARS in Toronto: A comparative analysis of the World Journal and the Toronto Star." Paper presented at the Mass Communication and Society Division, Association for Education in Journalism and Mass Communication.

Olesen, Alexa (17 March 2003) "Travelers arriving in southern China wear face masks, fearing deadly flu." Associated Press. Accessed 5 December 2004 from Nexis.

Parks, Michael (2002) "Beyond Afghanistan—Foreign News: What's Next?" *Columbia Journalism Review*. Accessed 2 December 2004. Available at: http://www.cjr.org/issues/2002/1/foreign-parks.asp.

O'Connor, D. (2002) "Walkerton Commission of Inquiry into the contamination of the Walkerton water supply and into the safety of Ontario's drinking water." Accessed 2 December 2004. Available at: http://www.attorneygeneral.jus.gov.on.ca/english/about/pubs/walkerton/

"Shaping the future." (2003) *SARS: Lessons from a new disease.* The World Health Report. Available at: http://www.who.int/whr/2003/chapter5/en/print.html.

Shoemaker, P., T.K. Chang, and N. Brendlinger (1986). "Deviance as a predictor of newsworthiness: Coverage of international events in the U.S. media." In *Communication Yearbook*, edited by M.L. McLaughlin. Vol. 10., p. 348-365. Beverly Hills, CA: Sage.

Stein, Rob (14 March 2003) "Experts Sent to Probe Asian Disease Outbreak; Pneumonia-Like Illness Fatal in 1 Case." *Washington Post.*

Tuchman, G. (1978) "Making News: Time and Typifications." New York: *The Free Press.*

Weiss, Rick (5 October 2001) "Fla. Anthrax Case Not a Result of Terrorism, Officials Say." *Washington Post.* Accessed 2 December 2004 from Nexis.

The Working Group on 'Governance Dilemmas' in Bioterrorism Response (January 2004) Leading during Bioattacks and Epidemics with the Public's Trust and Help. *Biosecurity and Bioterrorism: Biodefense Strategy, Practice, and Science,* Vol. 2, No. 1: 25-40.

Wright, Kai (2004) AIDS: Hiding in Plain Sight. *Columbia Journalism Review.* Accessed 2 December 2004. Available at: http://www.cjr.org/issues/2004/2/wright-aids.asp

Xupei, Sun (2004) "Freedom of the Chinese Press vs. Keeping State Secrets in Light of the SARS Case." Presented at the Association of American Law Schools. Accessed 27 November 2004. Available at: http://www.aals.org/am2004/Xupei2004.pdf.

# Chapter 9

# China and SARS: Crisis Management in a Legitimacy Vacuum[1]

Stephanie Buus and Eva-Karin Olsson

## *Introduction*

According to most epidemiological accounts, Severe Acute Respiratory Disorder (SARS) first emerged in southern China in late 2002 and proceeded to spread to over two dozen countries worldwide, infecting more than eight thousand people and killing approximately nine hundred before subsiding in July 2003.[2] Described by the World Health Organization (WHO) as "the first severe and readily transmissible new disease to emerge in the twenty-first century,"[3] the first wave of the SARS pandemic was naturally the object of a surge of international media attention—attention that has since turned elsewhere in the wake of other events and other diseases, most notably a virulent strain of avian influenza (H5N1) that spread across Asia "like wildfire" in January 2004 and threatened to become "a global pandemic far worse than the SARS outbreak" ("Averting a global plague," *Economist*, 2004).

As identified as the epicenter of the SARS contagion by most national and international epidemiological accounts of the disease, China clearly occupied a central role in Western media coverage of the first wave of the pandemic.[4] A quick survey of the news stories and headlines produced during the first wave of the SARS outbreak suggests that the "why" and "how" of SARS were intrinsically linked to China. China was consistently identified as the origin of the SARS pandemic, with southern China—the initial site of transmission—described as a "notorious crucible of infection" in one *Economist* article and a "breeding ground for new diseases" in another.[5] Moreover, headlines such as "China Syndrome—SARS hits Canada," "Please lie less—SARS in China," and "WHO assails China for faltering on SARS" all suggest China's conspicuous role in the initial wave of the SARS pandemic and its responsibility for the spread of SARS to other countries. Indeed, during the period in question, the media sources studied are quite preoccupied with China's ethical as well as instrumental relationship to SARS and the media coverage examined consists of a sustained and often quite harsh critique of the country's view of and approach to managing the SARS epidemic. It suggests that the media can be seen as a play ground for what media scholars tend to refer to as "blame-game." The term includes a representational struggle over how to make sense of the event, involving all kinds of actors (such as governments, policy makers, affected communities and various organizations), all affected by or trying to handle the crisis. Further, the media itself should not only be seen as merely a platform for various actors but also as an actor in its own right (Schudson, 1995; Edelman, 1977; Brändström and Kuipers, 2003).

The aim of this chapter is to return to the initial media accounts of the first global disease of the twenty-first century and to look more closely at how a number of Western media sources portrayed the SARS pandemic during its initial (and largest) wave of transmission in relation to China. For the reasons stated above, the study focuses on China as a crisis management actor and the ways in which the coverage of SARS were framed so as to attribute accountability and responsibility for the disease and its spread in China and globally as well as the symbolic textual devices used to indicate the presence of such a "responsibility frame."[6] In order to illustrate the blame game and how responsibility was depicted in relation to SARS and China, three major international newspapers (*The Economist*, *Financial Times*, and *International Herald Tribune*) were chosen for this study.[7] All three newspapers can be said to have a large international, primarily Western elite, readership and reputation for in-depth analysis of global affairs.

## *SARS: An Overview*

On February 14, 2003, the WHO wrote in a press release that they had received tests for laboratory analysis from health officials in China taken from patients living in the Guangdong province who were suffering from an unidentified form of acute respiratory syndrome. According to the WHO a total of 305 cases including 5 deaths were reported between November 16, 2002, and February 9, 2003 (WHO press release, 14 February 2003). The next press release from the WHO came almost a month after, on March 12, stating "that the Department of Health in Hong Kong has reported on an outbreak of respiratory illness in one of its public hospitals." The outbreak in Guangdong was mentioned in the same release but no links were established, thus far, between the two of them (WHO press release, 12 March 2003). Two days later the WHO released travel warnings to the infected areas since "This syndrome, SARS, is now a worldwide health threat" (WHO press release, 15 March 2003). Two days later the WHO confirmed the outbreak of SARS in China and the Chinese government requested help from a WHO team (WHO press release, 17 March 2003). The first official statement on SARS from the Chinese came from the Minister of Health, Zhang Wenkang, on April 3, 2003, in response to WHO's travel warnings to Southern China. He claimed, "It is perfectly safe to come to China to work, travel and hold business meetings" (Forney, 21 April 2003). On April 4, China started daily electronic reporting of the SARS infection and death count. On April 17, the Standing Committee of the Politoburo demanded accurate and honest reporting on SARS (Huang, 2003). On June 24, Beijing was removed from the list of affected areas, leaving only Taiwan and Toronto subject to WHO's travel advisories (WHO press release, 24 June 2003). By July 2003,

WHO officials considered the SARS threat under control and lifted all remaining travel advisories. At that point, 8,099 people in thirty two countries had been infected by SARS and 744 people had died.

## *Mass Media, Crisis, Blaming and Framing*

Many scholars have argued that there exists a fundamental link between crises and the media, since the media plays a crucial role in the process, not only by documenting crises but also by creating or constructing them ('t Hart, 1993:39). Although crises are seldom planned, it has been argued that the media is often very quick to frame a crisis event in a particular way (Perse, 2001:63). As part of this process, news journalists often attempt to squeeze the incoming information into already-existing media frames in much the same way as people in general tend to deal with new information—based on what they already know (Wolfsfeld, 1997:34). As a result, such media "frames" construct a reality that is already familiar to us in a number of ways; thereby "helping" us to understand that reality in certain ways. For these reasons, the public is largely dependent on the mass media for information and interpretation when a "crisis" occurs. This dependency results in the fact that the mass media naturally becomes a vital actor, not only by disseminating information about crises but also more generally by defining what we consider dangers and risks (Perse, 2001).

Notions of a "frame" and "framing" are derived from a large and diverse body of literature in media studies on the role of news in the representation of social phenomena (see Robertson, 2001; Bardhan, 2001; Hallahan, 1999). Our use of the term "frame" in this chapter refers to the central organizing of ideas or storylines as well as the symbolic framing devices (as metaphors, catchphrases, visual images etc) (frames) to signify the presence of one or more frames (Pan and Kosicki, 1993). In short, the different linguistic ways in which the major newspapers (included in this study) tried to make sense of SARS in connection to responsibility. Various media scholars have argued that the activity of framing inevitably entails acts of attribution—operations of diagnosis and prognosis in which the problem and the entity responsible for it are identified and one or more solutions to the problem implicitly and explicitly proposed (Robertson, 2001:68; Hallahan, 1999: 219; 't Hart, 1993; Kelly, 1967). In particular, once an event has been framed as a crisis, questions of accountability inevitably appear in the media coverage. The attribution of blame, and what often subsequently develops into a "blame-game" between different media and policy actors, is thus an inexorable part of the crisis process ('t Hart, 1993; Brändström and Kuipers, 2003). From a communicative and symbolic perspective, a crisis can be defined as "a breakdown of familiar symbolic frameworks legitimating the pre-existing socio-political order" ('t Hart, 1993:39). The process of legitimization, delegitimization, and re-legitimization is thus a fundamental component of crises

(Lull and Hinderman, 1997; 't Hart, 1993) and the main venue for this is the media.

Legitimacy can, therefore, be seen as the capital that actors have when handling a crisis, which can both increase and decrease depending on how the crisis management is portrayed in the media. Inherent in a crisis is thus the capacity to undermine legitimization, which actors fight over, and what Thompson refers to as symbolic power, defined as the "struggles over symbolic power in which reputation and trust are at stake" (Thompson, 2000:245). A commonly used concept for the process in which media mediates in the struggle over symbolic power is "status conferral." Here the media legitimize or de-legitimize actors by connecting them with certain issues and values (Simonson, 1999). As explained by Simonson, "Via the status conferral function, media contribute to the social process of confidence by boosting the public standing of the ideas, institutions, and people they portray. Media give these social objects a metaphorical aura that recommends them as a ground for public confidence" (Simonson, 1999:109). Media thus has the power through the act of framing both to legitimize and de-legitimize involved actors. As we argue in what follows, SARS was clearly framed as an institutional failure for China in the three major newspapers we examined. This was done, in part, by publishing stories of personal tragedy and impassioned metaphors aimed at conveying this central idea. How this was done is the focus of our analysis.

## *Analysis*

We conducted an online database search in Factiva with the search parameters, "SARS and China" and "China and pneumonia." Since our intent was to examine Western international media coverage of SARS and China during the first and most substantial wave of SARS transmission, we selected a time frame of March 1, 2003-July 30, 2003.[8] Every article with a length of 500 words or more was selected. The number of articles coded was as follows: *Financial Times*, 109 articles; *International Herald Tribune,* 225 articles; and *The Economist*, 20 articles.

The framing analysis in this study was conducted at two different levels: one macro and one micro. At the macro level, we coded for a number of broadly-conceived categories aimed at identifying the kinds of subjects covered in relationship to SARS and China as well as the types of actors/institutions named or cited in relation to SARS and China. The intent of the macro analysis pursued in this paper was to provide an overall picture of the general substance of SARS coverage vis-à-vis China in the news sources examined during the period in question. The questions asked were the following; 1) what is the main subject of each article, 2) which actors are "active" or "taking action" in each article, 3) which actors are quoted in each article? The micro level, in turn, consisted of a content analysis in which we undertook closer textual readings of a sample of the news accounts examined. As outlined in the introduction, this part of the analysis attempted to identify the nature of the "responsibility frame" at work in the depictions of SARS in relation to China as well as those symbolic devices (metaphors, key words, exemplars, depictions, etc.) indicating the presence of a particular "responsibility frame" in the accounts examined.

*A quantitative overview*

The first question asked was which topics were covered in the articles studied. The articles were coded according to their overall content. In those cases in which there was equal focus on two subjects, both were coded. The disease/crisis management (CM) category included articles focused on SARS itself (for example, the spread of the disease and/or the measures taken to curb its spread). The politics category consisted of articles dealing with issues related to political activities (for example, relations between other countries and China or within China on the national level) which are not related to actions taken in order to directly curb the SARS outbreak. The economy category included articles dealing with the concrete economic impact of SARS (for example, the stock market or the tourist industry). The findings are illustrated in Figure 1.

**Figure 1: Subject categories for articles included in the study**

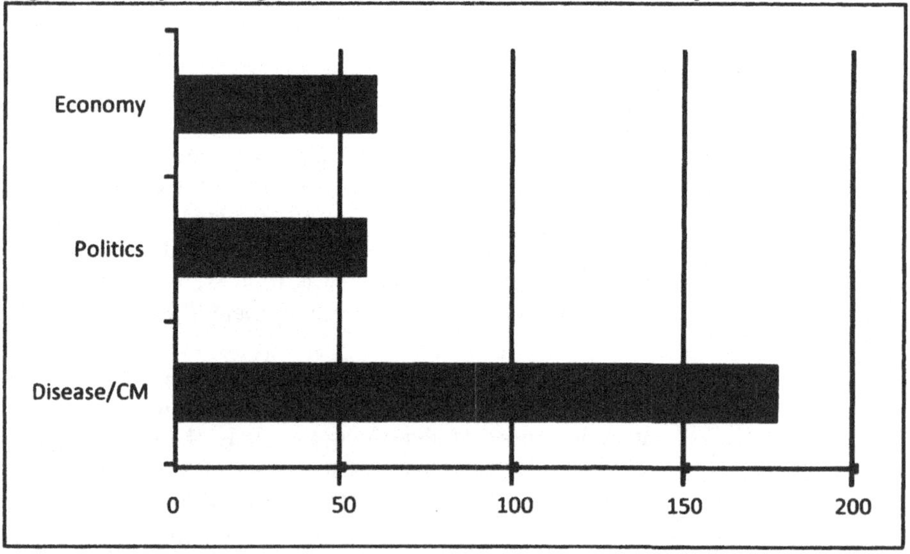


The results revealed that all three of the newspapers focused on the disease itself and the measures taken to curb it. Economic and political issues were reported to a lesser extent, nearly as often.

Firstly, actors described as "taking action" or "doing something" were coded when being described in relation to one or more verbs (i.e., "the Chinese government decided to. . . ."). Each actor was coded every time he or she was indicated as doing something. Therefore, the same actor could be coded several times in the same article. Secondly, actors were coded when they were quoted or cited, or in some way their opinions expressed. Moreover, the actors coded were always concrete entities (never, for example, "the propaganda machine," "some people," etc.). Actors that were coded less than four times were not included in the final results. The findings from all three newspapers are summarized in Figure 2.

**Figure 2: Distribution of the main actors described as "taking action" or "doing something"**

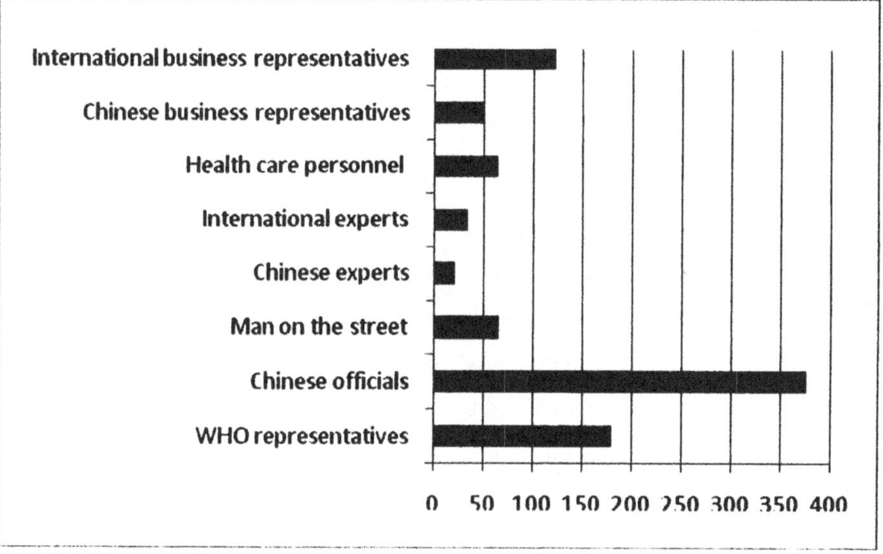


What we observe from Figure 2 is that the Chinese authorities are the ones most frequently depicted as "taking action" or "doing something." Since we selected only those articles dealing with SARS in mainland China, this should not come as a surprise. More unexpected is the large presence of WHO in the news articles, appearing as the second actor most frequently depicted as "taking action." The WHO was given a large proportion of news attention and was often portrayed as an active crisis management actor from the very beginning of the SARS outbreak despite the fact that the organization was not given permission by the Chinese authorities to enter the country during the initial outbreak. This helps to illustrate the tension that was created between China and the international community. The WHO was described as being "active" while China was described as being reluctant to co-operate and, in general, unable to handle the situation. Further, it should be noted that the number of business actors described as "active" appeared as the third largest group; an observation that makes sense given the general focus and market liberalist ideology of the newspapers (in particular, *The Economist* and *Financial Times*) and the focus on China as the largest expanding economic area in the world.

The second category focused on the actors who were quoted or cited, or in some way their opinions were expressed in the text either in the form of a direct quote or where it was clear that a statement referred to a particular actor. Furthermore, in order to be coded, the actors had to be identified by name. Every statement made by a particular actor was counted as one statement. Thus, there are times when we coded multiple statements by one particular actor in any given article.

**Figure 3: Distribution of main actors quoted or cited, or in some way their opinions were expressed**

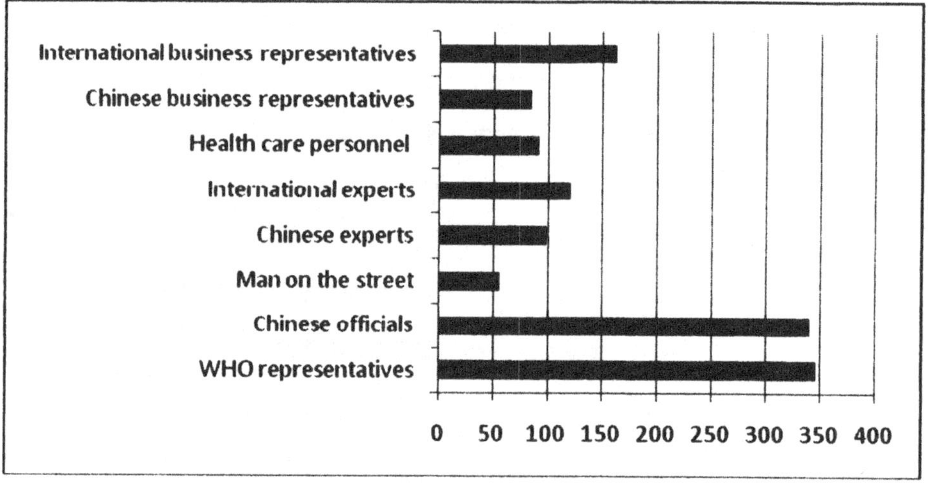


The results revealed that the main actors quoted/cited were WHO and Chinese officials. If considered together with Figure 2, Figure 3 clearly reinforced the strong presence of the Chinese officials and the fact that they were one of the most frequently mentioned in the newspaper articles. This may not be surprising, given the practical constraints facing the WHO in its efforts to actively address the first outbreak of SARS. China's repeated refusal to allow WHO researchers and scientists to travel to China until the end of March 2003 effectively left the WHO in a passive position. It could merely speculate about the nature and scope of SARS and issue a few warnings and advisories, but it was largely unable to act to combat the spread of the new disease. The third largest category was "international business representatives" which indicates that the international health community did not have the exclusive right on behalf of the international community to comment on SARS. The power of judgment to a large extent laid within the international community, for most part the WHO.

*Covering a new pandemic in an old country: A qualitative view*

Our quantitative analysis highlighted the tensions and symbolic struggle regarding which actor(s) had the "right" to deal with the SARS crisis and how that it should be done in the most effective way. The majority of the discussion centered around the conflict of whether or not the SARS outbreak was purely a domestic issue for China or whether China should open up for international cooperation. In an attempt to look more closely at how this symbolic struggle was played out in the three newspapers we analyzed, a discourse analysis was conducted on a sample of the articles. From the analysis, we identified three predominant themes related to issues of accountability in overlapping ways. All three of these themes were related to expressions of a "responsibility frame" focused mainly on systemic, or structural, factors rather than the deeds—or misdeeds—of specific individuals within Chinese society. Three themes identified are as follows:

- The cover-up and the lone hero
- China's ability to manage SARS
- The economic impact of SARS

*The cover up and the lone hero*

A predominant theme found in the news accounts studied involved China's secretive attitude when it came to releasing information about SARS. China was not telling the whole truth—either to its own people or to the international community. Alternately, China was not telling the truth at all, a sentiment forcefully expressed in the headline of *The Economist* entitled, "Please lie less—SARS in China" (12 April 2003). China's perceived inability or unwillingness to release information—to come clean about SARS—was in turn linked in many of the accounts examined to the purported "personality" of the Chinese system and its "habit" of avoiding sensitive or negative issues. One interesting feature of the reporting was the number of references made to China's political culture and earlier historical events.

While individual motives for a Chinese SARS cover-up were occasionally mentioned, most of the accounts studied clearly proposed that China's failure to "talk SARS" was directly attributable to systemic factors, one of which being China's political legacy. "Old habits die hard and China's secretive attitude on sensitive health matters stems, in part, from its longstanding emphasis on not wanting to cause panic among citizens or allow chaos in society. Therefore statistics are often massaged or collected half-heartedly if the results are likely to be negative" (*International Herald Tribune,* 7 April 2003). Several accounts, too, ascribed China's inscrutability about SARS to a historical legacy of suffering in China that later assumed institutional expression—a sort of Chinese "collective repression" of those events that might be harmful on a large scale. Such a legacy, the news accounts argued, was forged in the wake of Mao Zedong's leadership with the Great Leap Forward and other mass tragedies that, by virtue of their ruthless drive towards collectivization, resulted in the death of many Chinese.

> Once again, China's penchant for burying bad news and manipulating statistics for political ends has increased human suffering. In the late 1950s and early 60s, historians estimate that tens of millions of farmers starved in the aftermath of Mao Zedong's disastrous experiment in collectivized agriculture during the Great Leap Forward (*International Herald Tribune*, 7 April 2003).

It is interesting to note that the news accounts we examined increasingly became somewhat more positive after April 9, 2003—the day that the Chinese officials presented their first detailed briefing on the SARS outbreak in China (*International Herald Tribune*, 9 April 2003). From this time onward, there was a small but persistent focus on the Chinese efforts to provide information and the Chinese government's issuance of "stringent new rules requiring local officials to report epidemics of disease to Beijing immediately" (*International Herald Tribune*, 15 May 2003). The change in China's policy on releasing information and the official apology for having kept quiet so long was subsequently described in metaphorical terms as "China's political u-turn on openness," since the country's "dismissals [of certain public officials], self-criticism and mea culpas represent a level of public accountability not seen from China's generally secretive leadership since 1989's massacre of pro-democracy demonstrators in central Beijing" (*Financial Times,* 22 April 2003). In most cases, however, issues of accountability were framed in systemic terms; the driver of the car making the "u-turn" was not an individual but a government, a system. In contrast, coverage in the news sources regarding the motives underlying the Chinese "u-turn" from silence to more openness actually focused often on individual foreign actors and groups, including "pressure from Asian neighbors, international organizations and foreign investors" (*International Herald Tribune*, 30 April 2003).

In addition to international pressure, a senior retired military physician was depicted as the most important factor within China for the change of policy. This was the second theme in the cover-up reports which consisted of a story of a single, brave individual who alone challenged the corrupt system. The lone hero in this case was Dr. Jiang Yanyong who publicly accused the Chinese Health

Ministry of lying about the number of SARS patients in Beijing. The official figures only reported twelve cases and three dead in Beijing when in fact the number of SARS patients in just the military hospitals was "up to one hundred." After hearing about the official statement, Yanyong described the doctors at the military hospitals as "furious." He wrote, "As a doctor who cares about people's lives and health, I have the responsibility to aid international and local efforts to prevent the spread of this disease" (*International Herald Tribune*, 12 April 2003). On June 2 the doctor was described by *International Herald Tribune* as "playing a key role in exposing the official cover-up of SARS." Yet his heroic efforts were not appreciated by Gao Qiang, Executive Minister of Health, since;

> Jiang was not been punished for speaking out and has recently won praise from a few newspapers, but he was also ordered by military superiors to stop speaking to the press. I don't know why people are so interested in Dr Jiang, Gao said when asked about the man considered by many people to be the real hero (*International Herald Tribune*, 2 June 2003).

The story of the lone hero changing the corrupt system is often frequently portrayed in the media, and here it reinforced the notion of the brutal Chinese system, which repressed the lone hero instead of appreciating his courage.

There are two main metaphors that were frequently employed in relationship to the cover-up theme, both of which are strongly systemic in focus. In addition to the metaphor of "the u-turn" mentioned above, the second most frequent metaphor employed in the news accounts we studied equated the SARS crisis in China to the 1986 Chernobyl disaster in the Soviet Union. In terms of the cover-up theme and China's failure to "speak SARS," this metaphor clearly links the former Soviet response to the nuclear disaster at Chernobyl (initial denial and silence) to the Chinese response to the epidemiological "disaster" in Guangdong Province and beyond (initial denial and silence). The logic of this metaphor states that China failed to tell the truth to its own citizens or the citizens of other countries, just as the former USSR failed to tell the truth and act in a properly and timely fashion in the wake of Chernobyl, despite the fact that both phenomena had "spread" across national borders. The Chernobyl metaphor worked to illustrate the long cultural tradition in China of failure or indifference to protecting its own citizens. The inability to deal with a new disease (such as SARS) was more or less expected since the Chinese system was "sick." Still, even if the system itself was sick, there were still individuals with the capacity to change it, like the military surgeon described in the articles, which gave hope for the future.

*China's ability to manage SARS*

This theme deals with China's ability to handle the SARS outbreak, where the main focus is on China's unwillingness to cooperate with the WHO (especially in the beginning of the outbreak) as well as the implications for not doing that. China's handling of this new pandemic was compared to its handling of another recent pandemic, AIDS, following a pattern of "denial . . . reluctant acknowledgement and hesitant mobilization of resources to combat the epidemic" (*International Herald Tribune*, 22 April 2003). This was a nightmare situation for the WHO, which constantly had to fight to get information as well as access to and within the country. The struggle did not only take place in the physical sense, but also on a more symbolic level regarding who should have the final say about SARS in China—whether SARS was even in China and to what extent. The WHO finally won this representational fight, since China was in a weak position when it came to confidence. Accordingly, many of the statements issued by the Chinese officials included some type of repudiation to the information being reported by the WHO. For example, when the Chinese officials claimed that SARS had been brought under control but that "such reassurance contrasts sharply with the unprecedented warning against travel to Guangdong issued by the WHO this week" (*Financial Times*, 5 April 2003). This could be seen in line with what was said about status conferral and legitimization. Since, whenever the Chinese authorities gained access to speak in the media, their statements sharply contrasted those issued by the WHO. The WHO and the international community were assigned the role of good guys who are fighting to save the world from the SARS infection, and one of their main obstacles, besides the infection itself, was China and its reluctance to cooperate.

Even though China's "political u-turn" improved its relationship with the WHO (*International Herald Tribune*, 15 April 2003), according to our findings it did not help China win the representational struggle over how SARS was to be defined in the longer term (should it be primarily approached as an economic issue? or primarily a health issue? or a mixture of both?). In other words, the country's actions and motives were still heavily questioned in the news accounts we examined. For example, when the May Day holiday was cancelled by the Chinese authorities, the newspaper accounts we examined construed this measure anything but humanitarian. According to one *Economist*'s headline, the cancellation was, "Not out of concern for public health, to be sure . . ." (26 April 2003). The change in China's policy attitude was thus portrayed as mostly cosmetic, since this was about saving face and not about renewing the Chinese system itself. In the opinion of the *International Herald Tribune*, it was purely a case of "altered attitudes on an operational level" (2 June 2003). In order for China to become a sound—and morally responsible—partner in the international community, the country needed to adjust its norms and standards to suit an international, rather than a national, yardstick. The Chinese system must become a profoundly new—and profoundly global—system.

This theme also touched upon China's internal ability to cope with SARS, and two aspects in particular were emphasized. First, the newspaper articles we studied stressed that China had in fact managed to implement strong measures to prevent further outbreaks of SARS by creating, for example, "provincial response teams, disease monitoring systems and better training for medical workers" (*Financial Times*, 8 May 2003) as well as the use of "extreme measures" like large-scale quarantines to stem the tide of the epidemic (*Financial Times*, 7 May 2003). As the *Financial Times* observed, the entire Chinese society had been mobilized in the fight against SARS and the "long tentacles of the Chinese Communist Party" had finally begun "to grapple with the deadly virus" (30 April 2003). In a seemingly positive sense, then, SARS "has thrown China's capital to its old reflexes. The machinery of grassroots control has been dusted off, and the retired people who staff the street committees seem to be enjoying life in the limelight again" (*Financial Times*, 3 May 2003). However, while the octopus-like, or Medusa-like, reach of the Chinese system was suddenly praised for its all-encompassing approach to containing SARS, the success of this approach had paradoxically made those "long tentacles of the Chinese Communist Party" more visible, and in a number of cases more tangible for a domestic as well as an international audience. As "China's rusting machinery of totalitarian control is being pressed back into service" to block the further spread of SARS, the contours of that hidden or dormant machinery were being revealed (*The Economist*, 3 May 2003). While the Chinese system was portrayed in a number of accounts as possessing certain qualities uniquely suited to managing the spread of an epidemic, the types of metaphors actually employed to convey the nature of these qualities (e.g., "long tentacles" and "rusting machinery") suggest a frail core—and possibly sinister. Again, the thematic frame was strong where responsibility was assigned to the system as such.

The other aspect stressed in relation to China's internal capacity to cope with SARS was the dire medical situation in rural China, which was seen to be the result of the longstanding and destructive Chinese health policy. As a headline from the *Financial Times* read, "Rural hospitals struggle to cope with the virus—decades of underinvestment have left disease prevention measures in Chinese villages severely lacking" (*Financial Times*, 26 April 2003). China's focus on economic prosperity "now threatened by SARS is paradoxically what has allowed the virus to proliferate. China's economic reforms have brought the country's rural health care system to the brink of collapse" (*Financial Times*, 8 May 2003). The reason for these problems was the irresponsible medical policy of the Chinese government derived from the government's refusal, or inability, to see health in a larger—and by implication—more inherently moral sense; that is, to see the economic progress of a country as directly linked to progressive health policies that place a premium on the physical well-being of its citizens. "The Ministry of Finance was never ever interested in the theories about health and economic development" (*Financial Times*, 8 May 2003). The state of the Chinese health care system was in turn exemplified by the description of a young man running a "roadside clinic" in the Chinese countryside. "Zhan Yansheng´s main qualifications for a role on the front lines of Chinese medicine are a high-school diploma, a collection of health magazines and a counter well-stocked with cold remedies and cheap antibiotics" (*Financial Times*, 8 May 2003). Such a description hardly presented a reassuring picture of the medical situation in China. The figure of Zhan Yansheng later became a figure or symbol of the Chinese health care system in the same article. "While there is no doubting the good intentions of the sleepy-eyed twenty-four year-old who runs a roadside clinic in northern Herbei province, Mr Zhan's lack of training and focus on medicine-peddling are potent reminders of the weakness that plague China's health system (*Financial Times*, 8 May 2003).

Again, it is not one or more individuals, but the very system itself in China that stood out as the world's Achilles heel in the fight against SARS in our newspaper analysis. China was depicted in the newspaper accounts as an "old" country using traditional outdated methods to deal with "new" and modern threats. Even if the Chinese system helped stop SARS, thanks to a tradition of mass mobilization, this same system was hampering the fight against SARS because it could not "see" the actual state of health of the masses it was mobilizing. Instead of individual bodies, the Chinese system "saw" Yen signs. This lack of vision proved to be fatal. Many of the news accounts we studied seemed to suggest that China's failure to view health as a moral imperative—a basic human right that enables economic development—resulted in the dangerous commodification of healthcare in the country, a state of affairs that medicine-peddling health product entrepreneurs like Zhan Yansheng epitomize.

The issue of China's ability to cope with SARS was also explored in the "SARS is China's Chernobyl" metaphor discussed earlier in this chapter. In an article by Wei Jingsheng in the *International Herald Tribune*, the "Chernobyl" metaphor was invoked to explore the notion that SARS may present a "capacity watershed" for China—the crisis that would "break" the current Chinese system just as the events of the Chernobyl nuclear power plant accident helped "break" the Soviet regime in the late 1980's. Jingsheng expressed some reservations to this theory and cited China's history as an indicator of how applicable the Chernobyl metaphor ultimately would be in the case of SARS:

> Almost no one expects SARS alone to challenge or to force basic changes in the one-party rule or to end political control of the media. Even the official candor, while involving an outpouring of facts, has been carefully scripted from above, and the voluminous news reports

> have been shaped to flatter the leaders and present a society unified in heroic struggle (*International Herald Tribune*, 14 May 2003).

Moreover, Jinsheng suggested that it may be impossible to compare an outcome during the Cold War period to a forecast in the post-Cold War period. "Times are different now," he wrote, and 1986 can only cautiously—or only partially—be compared to 2003 (*International Herald Tribune,* 14 May 2003). Among other things, the West needed China's support in dealing with Iraq and North Korea in a post-Cold War era, which is more fluid and more global than that of the Soviet Cold War period, making "China's leaders accountable to their own people and to the world at large" (*International Herald Tribune*, 2 May 2003).

## *The Economic Impact of SARS*

The economic theme deals with how SARS affects China, and the rest of the world, by the actual risk of SARS disturbing economic growth. The focus is both on the actual concrete consequences (for example, tourism and air traffic) but also on the fear of a possible worst case scenario in which the SARS causes long term economic disturbance.

The economic effects of SARS are threatening the economy since they risk hampering the economic boom, which not only the Chinese economy is depending on, but also the world economy. Besides the risk of real effects, SARS highlights systematic problems within the Chinese system, which runs the risk of effecting economic growth in the long run. The most pressing one is "the lack of information and transparency" since it creates problems of confidence for China, as one business representative puts it; "If a government can't tell you there is an epidemic on, what is the value of the accounts of Chinese companies?" (*Financial Times*, 1 April 2003). It is said that "China must take emergency measures in order to restore investor trust" (*Financial Times,* 5 April 2003) since the "lack of transparency over SARS . . . has already hurt Beijing's reputation with international investors" (*Financial Times*, 17 April 2003). Another systematic problem exposed by SARS is the lack of structural foundations highlighted by the "difficulties to mobilize the population" (*Financial Times,* 14 April 2003) and the difficulties with enforcing rules. Due to its economic strength, China is a part of the global economy, even though it still drags on with systematic weakness from a non-capitalist system. The handling over SARS is risking "the trust of the rest of the world, which had come to believe that China was beginning to understand the need to play by international rules, could take far longer to repair" (*The Economist,* 26 April 2003).

The news accounts shifted when the first uncertainty vanished, and more optimistic voices were heard, forecasting that that SARS might not have the feared devastating effects. Voices from a business community, being depicted as not easily scared, cried "place business health ahead of threat from SARS" (*Fi-*

*nancial Times,* 16 April 2003). For these companies "it would take more than a health scare to stop them answering the call of the world's most attractive market" (*Financial Times,* 16 April 2003). SARS might have had an effect, but not in the long run, since "the alarming SARS reports are short-term dislocations, and we are not going to be distracted by them . . . we have a long tradition of sitting tight" (*International Herald Tribune*, 23 April 2003). The alarming prognoses offered in the beginning of the outbreak were revisited and claims that the effects might not be as bad as expected "if the authorities make headway in controlling SARS, the economy should continue to prosper as it improves the quality of its growth" (*Financial Times,* 6 May 2003). The incitement to stay in China was so strong, that much more was needed to scare off the international companies and to get them out of the market since "there is much potential and excitement for investors. Little wonder foreign fund managers are knocking at the door and are being allowed to trickle in" (*Financial Times,* 14 April 2003). In one way, China was demanded to transform its system in order to be a respected global business partner. On the other hand, even if China did not change, the business community would still be there doing business with the Chinese since they are dependent on the Chinese market despite its flaws.

## *Conclusions*

As noted at the beginning of this chapter, the media are likely to play a particularly important defining role in times of confusion and uncertainty—in this case a looming pandemic—since the public and even policy makers often find themselves particularly reliant on information and turn as a result to various forms of media for information and explanation (Robinson, 2001: 533; Perse, 2001; Cook, 2001). This was clearly the case during the SARS outbreak. SARS was by all accounts a new disease with clearly global ramifications: the apparent source, China, continued to classify the epidemic as a state secret; the WHO was long refused entry into the county; the Chinese media continued to play as a mouthpiece for the Chinese government; and the Western media was historically viewed as one-sided and even hostile in its portrayals of the Chinese Government and Chinese people (Saich, 2003:5-6; Sun Yu, 2003:92-93; Robertson, 2001: 65). The aim of this chapter has been to look more closely at what was actually written in three international newspapers (*The Economist, Financial Times* and *International Herald Tribune*) in terms of how China was portrayed as a reliable crisis management actor.

For a start, the quantitative study revealed that Chinese officials were the ones most often depicted as active or doing something in our newspaper analysis, indicating that they were the main actors responsible for dealing with the crisis. The second most commonly mentioned main actor, described as active or doing something in the text, was the WHO although only half as often as the Chinese officials. Looking at Figure 3 regarding the actors who were quoted or cited in the text, the WHO representatives and the Chinese officials were almost cited equally. In short, the Chinese authorities were presented more often as "actors" (i.e., doing something) in the newspaper articles than as speakers (i.e., cited, quoted or have their opinions expressed). This implies that the actions taken by the Chinese authorities to a large extent were described, interpreted and framed by other actors in the reporting. These actors then had the "status conferral" power to describe Chinese policies and actions as legitimate or not. The Chinese authorities had also, on a more concrete level, problems with controlling the media reporting, as suggested by the military surgeon Dr. Jiang Yanyong's suspicions about the Chinese media cover-up concerning the reported number of people infected by SARS in China. As scholars from various fields have also pointed out, the increasing inability of the Chinese government to control or to "frame" the flow of information on SARS, both within China as well as between China and the rest of the world, suggests not only the growing interpretative power of the media and media technologies within China and globally, but also the central role that the media and media technologies already play in the world's understanding of infectious diseases and their management (Saich, 2003: 17-18).[9]

In the qualitative analysis, we studied some of the ways in which the coverage of the SARS crisis in 2003 was framed so as to attribute accountability for the disease and its (mis)management to China, and in particular, the Chinese socio-political system. Along these lines, we identified three themes prevalent in the newspaper articles that clearly expressed a responsibility frame, which from different angles focused on a systematic failure. The most evident frame was thus the one which focused on the Chinese system as such. Media reporting was characterized by a systematic rather than an actor-based perspective on SARS in relation to China and attributed the evolution of the SARS pandemic to the lack of evolution in the Chinese Communist system. SARS had not come from God or Mother Nature, or even from the flawed actions of a few individual Chinese authorities; rather the system was responsible for the creation of the pandemic—an obsolete, isolationist and idiosyncratic system. SARS itself was consequently depicted in these accounts largely as a socio-economic issue rather than a biomedical issue—an illness that to a large extent had been perpetuated, if not created, by structural inequalities in the Chinese system rather than individualized "risk behaviors" of the Chinese people.[10] It should be said that the very same system, with its absurd characteristics, was also portrayed as an asset when using its "long tentacles" to combat SARS in every village in the enormous country. Against this monumental system stood the military surgeon Dr Jiang Yanyong; the scenario represented a classic David and Goliath struggle. Here was a brave individual who because of his moral responsibility spoke up against a corrupt system. Symbolically, it was portrayed that the Chinese communist collective system could only be changed by individuals with the moral power to fight against it.

The second underlying idea in the newspaper reports was the systematic failure frame. A system that does not function is portrayed as a system that either needs to change—or to die? Change was needed, and hoped for, if China was to be able to live up to its global responsibility. Although the newspaper articles invoked a number of "systematic" images as a means of shaping the readers' understanding of who was responsible for the SARS crisis, one key metaphor was pushed forward; that is, comparing the SARS crisis in China to the 1986 Chernobyl disaster in the former Soviet Union. On the one hand, this comparison suggested notions of contagion and the uncontrollable spread of harmful agents across borders (corona virus in one case and radioactive particles in the other). The beleaguered Soviet Union initially failed to interpret the 1986 Chernobyl nuclear disaster as a global problem and consequently resulted in increased frustration which challenged the Soviet communist system and eventually helped to usher in a new political and economic system. Several articles on the SARS disaster in China suggest that China's failure to approach SARS as a global problem—to successfully manage both the local "explosion" and the global "fall-out" of SARS—might likewise provide the "chain-reaction" needed to produce the transformation of another ailing communist system ("China's Chernobyl? China and SARS," 26 April, 2003).

Thirdly, a frame of global responsibility was evident in the newspaper articles. As was the case with Chernobyl, SARS was not only a national problem but also crossed national boundaries and had a global effect. The SARS disease was constructed in the newspaper accounts as a global phenomenon with Chinese origins, although China itself was portrayed in the same regard as generally incapable of, or unwilling to, accept this global set of problems. Responsibility in a globalized world with a global set of problems means that crisis management capacity in one country creates effects far beyond its own borders. In the newspaper analysis, the story of SARS in China was often portrayed as the story of a new disease in an old system—a system incapable of facing up to and managing the domestic as well as global effects unleashed by a modern disease (Saich, 2003:2). First and foremost, SARS was consistently depicted as a fluid disease wreaking havoc on and in a static system—a system deemed incapable of controlling either the dissemination of the disease beyond all manner of borders (local, regional, national) or the dissemination of information about the disease (via the Internet, cell phones, etc.) beyond the same borders (Yu, 2003:92; Saich, 2003:16; Erni, 2003). By treating the epidemic as a state secret and treating SARS as a local phenomenon, the Chinese system was therefore in a number of newspaper articles deemed "guilty" of failing to conceive the disease as a global phenomena, to see the world as a single entity, and to assume its rightful, global responsibility for the disease. China needed to be "educated" by the older members of the international community. Despite the fact that China was depicted as an unwitting and recalcitrant global partner (for example, in its relations to the WHO), international pressure eventually succeeded in "forcing" China to adopt a more "globalist" view of, and responsibility for, SARS. An important aspect of this globalized world is the interconnected world market, and a large portion of the media coverage on SARS and China was devoted to economic issues. There was clearly a global economic discourse underlying each of the newspaper accounts we studied that assumed a mutual interdependence between China and the West, if not the fundamental dependence of the West on China. In short, China must be able to stop the spread of deadly diseases from the East to the West, so that fewer people became ill and the world economy can continue to prosper. Not surprisingly, business representatives were considered important actors in all three newspapers (both in our "active/doing something" category and our "quoted/cited/opinion expressed" category). China's key global role and its responsibility for and to the world market were never questioned.

What can these frames tell us about how China was depicted as a crisis management actor? According to 't Hart (1993), a crisis can be seen as a dynamic process of legitimization and de-legitimization, where trust is the main capital for successful crisis management. Our study indicated that there was little trust in the ability of China's political system to deal with SARS. It also illustrated that even though the Chinese authorities tried to deal with the crisis, their actions and policies were to a large extent interpreted and framed by other stakeholders throughout the crisis. One way for the Chinese authorities to regain trust was to make a u-turn, after it was evident that they had lost a significant amount of trust in the beginning of the outbreak by not telling the truth. The newspaper articles also suggested that the lack of legitimacy was much deeper than originally thought, and references were made to China's historical and cultural traditions of putting its citizens' health and wellbeing before political objectives. The use of the metaphor "u-turn" emphasizes that China was adopting a totally new type of policy—by telling the truth. The change in policy was often described as cosmetic, and claims were made that the same old sick system was still in operation. This old Chinese system stood in contrast to the effective Western way of dealing with an epidemic (i.e., through an international organization such as the WHO). In conclusion, it seems like China's political system had a historical deficit concerning legitimization from the very beginning of the SARS outbreak, which did not change, but perhaps just got worse, despite its efforts to handle the crisis. In contrast to this stands China's economic system, where legitimization seems to be much easily restored. Some may say that legitimization and confidence are more easily restored when we want something from the other party and therefore "need" to trust them.

## Notes

1 The empirical data used in this chapter are also available in an earlier article published in *the Journal of Contingencies and Crisis Management* (Buus and Olsson, 2006).

2. The brief chronology offered here was taken from WHO's website.

3. See WHO report (16-17 May 2003).

4. See for example the WHO and CDC websites.

5. "The Shock of the new—A mysterious new disease," *The Economist*, 22 March 2003 as well as "After the Outbreak," *The Economist*, 5 April 2003. It is interesting to note that the latter article also identifies China more generally as a main origin of global infection—the source of several previous and devastating epidemics such as the influenza epidemic of 1918-1919 that killed "tens of millions."

6. For a more thorough discussion of "responsibility frames," see Valkenburg et al., 1999.

7. *The Economist* is circulated to over 830,000 people, more than four-fifths of them outside Britain. The American circulation accounts for a third of the total. The *Financial Times* has a daily circulation of more than 435,000 copies, more than one million readers and is available in 140 countries (Sources: *The Economist* homepage and *Financial Times* homepage).

8. Although the first outbreak of SARS apparently occurred in southern China as early as November 2003, Western and non-Western media coverage of SARS first appeared in earnest after WHO officer Dr. Carlo Urbani reported to the WHO the appearance of a new pneumonia-like illness among patients in Vietnam in early March 2003. The WHO officially declared the chain of SARS transmission broken on July 5, 2003 (See "Updates" on the WHO website).

9. It is, perhaps, not surprising in this context to note that the WHO regularly "scours" the Internet for the latest information on possible emerging diseases in the world, roughly 40 percent of which are in fact identified through this Internet scouring process (Prescott, 2003: 220).

10. Nilanjana Bardhan makes a similar point about transnational wire service coverage of HIV/AIDS (2001: 298). According to Bardhan, media coverage of HIV/AIDS in developed regions of the world focused significantly more on biomedical issues, whereas coverage in developing regions of the world focused far more on socio-economic themes. See also Saich on SARS in China (2003: 2).

## References

Aronowitz, R.A. (1998) "Making Sense of Illness." *Science, Society, and Disease*. Cambridge: Cambridge University Press.

Bardhan, N. (2001) "Transnational AIDS-HIV News Narratives: A Critical Exploration of Overarching Frames." *Mass Communication and Society*. 4(3): 283-309.

BBC, homepage (24 June 2003) "China's SARS triumph." Jill McGivering.

Brändström, A. and S. Kuipers (2003) "From 'Normal Incidents' to Political Crises: Understanding the Selective Politicization of Policy Failures." *Government and Opposition.* 38(3): 279-305.

Buus, S. and E-K Olsson (2006) "The SARS Crisis: Was Anybody Responsible?" *Journal of Contingencies and Crisis Management.* Vol. 14: 2: pp. 71- 81.

"China's Chernobyl? China and SARS" (26 April, 2003) *The Economist.*

Cook, E. T. (2001) "The Future of the Institutional Media." In *Mediated politics: Communication in the future of democracy,* edited by L. Bennett and R. Entman. Cambridge: Cambridge University Press.

Coombs, W. T. (1999) *Ongoing Crisis Communication: Planning, Managing and Responding.* Sage Publications, Thousand Oaks, CA.

De Vreese, C. (2001) "Europe in the News: A Cross-National Comparative Study of the News Coverage of Key EU events." *European Union Politics,* vol 2 (3) 283-307. London: Sage Publications.

*Economist, The* (26 April 2003 and 3 May 2003) Available at: www.economist.com

Edelman, M. (1977) *Political Language: Words that Succeed and Policies that Fail.* New York: Academic Press.

Edelman, M. (1988) *Constructing the Political Spectacle.* Chicago: University of Chicago Press.

Entman, R. (1993) "Framing: Toward Clarification of a Fractured Paradigm." *Journal of Communication.* 43(4):51-58. Philadelphia, Pennsylvania: Annenberg School.

Erni, J. N. (2003) "SARS and 'Global' Reporting." Accessed on 2 July 2004. Available at: http://www.rthk.org.hk/mediadigest/20031017_76_107244.html

Fairclough, N. (1995) *Media Discourse.* New York: St. Martin.

Farnham, B. R. (1997) *Roosevelt and the Munich Crisis: A study of political decision-making.* Princeton, NJ: Princeton University Press.

Featherstone, M. (1995) *Undoing Culture. Globalization, Postmodernism and Identity.* London:Sage.

*Financial Times* (1 April 2003, 5 April 2003, 14 April 2003, 16 April 2003, 17 April 2003, 22 April 2003, 26 April 2003, 30 April 2003, 3 May 2003,6 May 2003, 7 May 2003,. and 8 May 2003) Available at: www.ft.com

Forney, Matthew (21 April 2003) "Silent for too long: Beijing is calling for an end to the SARS cover-up, but the damage to China´s credibility has been done." *Time Magazine.*

Gutteling, J. M. and O. Wiegman (1996) *Exploring Risk Communication.* Dordrecht: Kluwer.

Hansén, D. and E. Stern (2001) "From Crisis to Trauma: The Palme assassination Case." In *Managing Crises: Threats, Dilemmas, Opportunities,* edited by U. Rosenthal, A. Boin, and L. Comfort. Springfield, Illinois: Charles C Thomas.

Hallahan, K. (1999) "Seven models of framing: Implications for public relations." *Journal of Public Relations Research.* 11(3), 205-242.

't Hart, P. (1993) "Symbols, Rituals and Power: The Lost Dimension of Crisis Management." *Journal of Contingencies and Crisis Management,* Vol 1, No 1:36-50.

't Hart, P. (2001) "Institutional Crisis and reforms in Policy Sectors: The Case of refugee Policy in Europe." *Journal of European Public Policy,* 8, 2, pp 286-306.

't Hart, P. and P. D. Gray (1998) *Policy Disasters in Europe: A Comparative Exploration.* London: Routledge.

Huang, Y. (2003) "Implications of SARS Epidemic for China's Public Health Infrastructure and Political System" Prepared Statement dated May 12, 2003, pp. 33-41 in *Dangerous Secrets—SARS and China's Healthcare System*, Roundtable Before the Congressional Executive Commission on China, 108th Congress, 1st Session,

*International Herald Tribune* (7 April 2003, 9 April 2003, 12 April 2003, 15 April 2003, 22 April 2003, 23 April 2003, 30 April 2003, 14, May 2003, 15 May 2003, and 2 June 2003) Available at: www.global.nytimes.com

Iyengar, S. (1993) "Television News and Citizens Explanations of National Affairs." In *Media Power in Politics,* edited by D.A. Graber. Washington, D.C.: CQ Press.

Iyengar, S. (1996) "Framing Responsibility for Political Issues." *Annals*, AAPPSS 546: 59-70.

Iyengar, S. (1991) *Is Anyone Responsible? How Television Frames Political Issues.* Chicago: Chicago University Press.

Kelley, H. H. (1967) "Attribution in Social Psychology." In *Nebraska Symposium on Motivation,* edited by D. Levin, pp. 192-240. Lincoln, Nebraska: University of Nebraska Press.

Lerbinger, O. (1997) *The Crisis Manager: Facing Risk and Responsibility.* Mahwah, N.J.: Lawrence Erlbaum Associates.

Luke, T. W. (1993) "Chernobyl: The Packaging of Transnational Ecological Disaster." In *Media Power in Politics,* edited by D.A. Graber. Washington, D.C.: CQ Press.

Lull, J. and S. Hinderman, Eds. (1997) *Media Scandals: Morality and Desire in the Popular Culture Marketplace.* New York: Columbia University Press.

McCoy, T. S. (1993) *Voices of Difference: Studies in Critical Philosophy and Mass Communication.* Cresskill, N.J.: Hampton.

Moeller, S D (1999) *Compassion and Fatigue: How the Media Sell Disease, Famine, War and Death.* London: Routledge.

Neuman, W., M. Just, and A. Crigler (1992) *Common Knowledge: News and the Construction of Political Meaning.* Chicago: University of Chicago Press.

Norris, P. (1995) "Restless Searchlight: Network News Framing of the Post-Cold War World." *Political Communication.* 12:4.

Pan, Z. and G. M. Kosicki (1993) *Framing analysis: An approach to news discourse. Political Communication.* Vol 10, 59-79.

Perse, E. M. (2001) *Media effects and society.* Mahwah, NJ.: L. Erlbaum Associates.

Prescott, L. M. (2003) "SARS: A Warning." *Survival, International Institute of Strategic Studies.* 45(3): 207–226. London.

Price, M. (1995) *Television, the Public Sphere and National Identity.* Oxford: Clarendon Press.

Price, V., D. Tewksbury, and E. Powers (1997) "Switching trains of thought: The impact of news frames on readers' cognitive responses." *Communication Research,* 24:481-506.

Robertson, A. (2001) "Mediated Threats." In *Threat Politics. New perspectives on security, risk and crisis management,* edited by J. Eriksson, pp. 61-83. Aldershot: Ashgate.

Robinson, P. (2001) "Theorizing the Influence of Media on World Politics." *European Journal of Communication,* 16(4): 524-544.
Roosvall, A. (2005) Utrikesjournalistikens antropologi, nationalitet, etnicitet och kön i svenska tidningar [Foreign journalism's anthropology, nationality, ethnicity and gender in Swedish newspapers]. Akademitryck AB, Edsbruk.
Rosenberg, C. (1987) "Disease in History: Frames and Framers." *Millbank Quarterly,* 67, suppl. 1: 1-15.
Saich, T. (2003) "SARS: China's Chernobyl or Much Ado About Nothing?" Paper presented at workshop on SARS in China: Economic, Political, and Social Consequences at Cambridge University.
Schlesinger, P. (1997) "From cultural defence to political culture: Media, politics and collective identity in the European Union." *Media, Culture and Society,* 19:369-391.
Schudson, M. (1995) *The Power of News.* Cambridge, MA: Harvard University Press.
Scott, E. M. (2003) "SARS: A Warning." *Survival,* 45(3): 207-226.
Silver, R. and E. Thoman (1992) "Media Culture: Why We Can't 'Just Say No'." *Media and Values,* 57.
Simonson, P. (1999) "Mediated Sources of Public Confidence: Lazarfeldt and Merton." *Journal of Communication,* Spring 1999, 49:2:109-122. Philadelphia, Pennsylvania: Annenberg School Press.
Sontag, S. (1977) *Illness as Metaphor.* New York: Picador.
Thompson, John Brookshire (2000) *Political scandal: power and visibility in the media age.* Cambridge: University of Cambridge.
Tjernström, V. (2001) Europa norrifrån: en nordisk komparativ studie av europeisk politisk kommunikation [Europe from the north: A Nordic comparative study of European political communications]. Umeå University.
Valkenberg, P. M., H. Semetko, and C. de Vreese (1999) "The Effects of News Frames on Readers." *Communication Research,* 26(5): 550-569.
WHO Press Release (14 February 2003) Acute Respiratory Syndrome Being Monitored in Guangdong.
WHO Press Release (12 March 2003) Who Issues a Global Alert About Cases of Atypical Pneumonia.
WHO Press Release (15 March 2003) WHO Issues Emergency Travel Advisory.
WHO Press Release (17 March 2003) WHO coordinates International Effort to Identify and Treat SARS.
WHO Press Release (24 June 2003) WHO lifts SARS travel advisory against Beijing.
WHO report (16-17 May 2003) Consensus document on the epidemiology of severe acute respiratory syndrome (SARS). Accessed 1 July 2004. Available at: http://www.who.int/csr/SARS/en/WHOconsensus.pdf
WHO website (2003-2005) Available at: http://www.who.int/csr/SARS/en/
Wolfsfeld, G. (1997) *Media and Political Conflict: News from the Middle East.* Cambridge: Cambridge University.
Yu, S. (2003) "Lessons from SARS coverage." *Nieman Reports.* Winter.

# Chapter 10

# Transboundary Crisis Management: Implications for Research and Practice

Eva-Karin Olsson and Kaibin Zhong

## *Introduction*

SARS will be remembered for being the closest the world has been in the twenty first century to a real outbreak of a deadly disease at the global level. In connection to the 2009 outbreak of the A/H1N1 pandemic flu, SARS functioned as a point of reference from which lessons can be learned on how to handle a pandemic from a crisis management perspective. In order to contribute to such knowledge, this concluding chapter aims to single out findings from the chapters included in this book for understanding and improving governments' and international organizations' ability to respond to potentially global pandemics and transmitted infectious diseases in the future. From a crisis management perspective, yet without losing sight of the important findings from a national perspective, the transnational character of the crisis is of particular interest due to the lack of previous research in this area. In drawing upon the findings from the chapters included in this book, we aim to contribute to the growing concern among crisis management scholars on how to understand crises that move across geographical boundaries and therefore require the involvement of a variety of actors from different political levels and systems.

Therefore, the management of SARS has to be understood against the backdrop of globalization where today's frequent traveling fueled the spread of the disease and made it harder to contain. A UNWTO study roughly estimated that in 2005 of the total number of tourists some 750 million were international and 4,000 million domestic. Of the latter almost half takes place in developing countries, the other half in developed (the IPCC OECD90) countries (UNWTO-UNEP-WMO, 2008). The roles of air travel in the modern epidemiology of influenza and its impact on the spread of the disease have been examined in a substantial body of work. For example, Eric Lofgren et al. (2007) demonstrate that, "A constantly exposed population that becomes vulnerable to infection triggered by seasonal changes in virus biology, immunocompetence, or social habits is vastly different from a population which, due to the rapid flow of people and diseases across the globe, is periodically bombarded by new viral strains in a short period of time over a wide geographic area." According to an OECD report released in 2003, in the context of globalization, "novel risk situations might be met with excessive inertia or inappropriate institutional responses" (OECD, 2003, p. 48). On the other hand, other aspects of globalization such as new information technologies helped facilitate the crisis response by enabling information-sharing beyond national borders. Globalization can then be understood as a double edged sword in both constraining and enabling crisis management efforts at the global level. Yet empirical knowledge about the management of transboundary crises is still sparse (Lagadec, 2009; Quarantelli et al., 2006).

Even if empirical research addressing crisis management from a transnational perspective is yet limited, there is a growing awareness amongst crisis management scholars that the nature of crises, and the corresponding implications for political crisis management, are changing and bound to continue to do so even more in the future. For example, building on the traditional notion of crisis with its core conceptual elements of threat, urgency, and uncertainty, Arjen Boin and Mark Rhinard (2008) use the concept of "transboundary threats" to define threats with the potential to cross geographic and functional boundaries. What sets this concept apart from the more traditional definition is its emphasis on the tightly woven web of critical infrastructures that characterizes modern society, and as a result challenge the structures of nation states that were built for more "classical threats." Later, Arjen Boin (2009) broadens and summarizes key characteristics defining transboundary crises as the crossing of geographical boundaries, functional boundaries, and time boundaries. In focusing on the intersection between ecological crises and institutional responses, Galaz et al. (2010) use the term "cascading" for crises characterized by complex causality, nonlinear change, recombination potential, and cross-scale cascading dynamics. From a political leader perspective, Arjen Boin and Paul 't Hart (2003), in drawing upon Ulrich Beck's notion of "risk society," argue that leaders today face substantial challenges due to the mismatch between global threats and national political institutions. "The risk society is characterized by a substantial gap between citizen expectations and leadership efforts in preventing and containing crises. It nurtures a culture of concern in which political and bureaucratic leaders do not seem to measure up to the increasingly urgent demand for effective crisis prevention, preparedness, and response" (p. 546). According to Quarantelli et al. (2006), SARS provides a good example of what they refer to as "trans-system social ruptures" since: it jumped between international and national/political governmental boundaries; it quickly spread across the globe; no known central point of origin; it had an inherent potential to claim a large number of victims; and the local community solutions were unable to tackle it and therefore evoked informal social networks (p. 26-27).

Keeping the transboundary dimension in mind, this chapter will examine the management of SARS in the respective countries, the WHO and the media through the lenses of early warning, acute crisis management, communication, and after phase processes.

## Managing early warning

Previous research on early warning in national settings has shown how cognitive-psychological, bureau-organizational, and agenda-political influences affect nation states' ability to pool together and eventually make sense of incoming information (Parker and Stern, 2002). It is no wonder that it is even harder to detect and coordinate information signals on the global level considering the increasing number of actors and institutions. In the case of SARS, early warning became even more intricate due to the lack of initial knowledge about the origin and potential effects. As stressed by Zhong (chapter 2 in this book), the Chinese Government missed out on the initial phase of SARS due to problems with identification, information collection, risk assessment and isolation. In the following section, we will examine the mechanisms for early warning impacting on the crisis management of SARS focusing on media and institutional aspects.

## Institutional and cognitive aspects

The most obvious obstacle to crisis prevention and mitigation in the SARS case was the initial denial and cover-up by the Chinese authorities, whether it did so on purpose or not. When in early March 2003, it was clear that the disease was a serious threat. The medical staff at Beijing's hospital was briefed about the outbreak but was told not to go public with the information for fear of jeopardizing the ongoing National People's Congress meeting in Beijing, which is the most important annual political event in China. On March 12, the WHO issued a global alert and three days later they named the new disease the "Severe Acute Respiratory Syndrome" (SARS) and issued a travel advisory. On April 2, a travel advisory was also issued for Hong Kong and Guandong. The Chinese government remained quiet until April 9, when the retired military physician Jiang Yanyong bravely released a written statement to several news organizations revealing that the numbers at Beijing's No. 309 People's Liberation Army hospital were much higher than previously reported. The cover-up meant that there was little reliable information available from the official Chinese government sources and as a result this delayed the initial efforts at curbing the outbreak in China as well as hampered the work of the WHO. This was the single most severe obstacle to the initial attempts to curb SARS.

However, due to new information technologies and globalization, the cover-up also illustrates that public officials do not longer have information monopoly. According to Galaz (2009), despite the difficultness related to information collection and sharing, much of WHO's success the last decade has been due to technological developments in new information technologies, which has created an independence from official reports. In relation to the SARS outbreak,

Zhu (chapter 3 in this book) demonstrates that new information technologies such as the Internet and mobile phones enabled the Chinese public to access information from other sources than official ones. In the early stages of the outbreak, Short Message Service (SMS) played a vital role for information exchange in the Guangzhou area. The numbers of SMS[1] exploded after the Chinese New Year Holiday on February 8 when 126 million text messages were exchanged over the period of three days. Due to the lack of official information personal networks became essential for people trying to confirm the information received by text messages (Tai and Sun, 2007: p. 998).[2] In contrast, the internet played a marginal role in the initial stage of the outbreak and only gained momentum when the disease spread to other areas in Mainland China, and in particular to Hong Kong (ibid, p. 999). However, it should be noted that unofficial information, that is denied or not confirmed by authorities, has its own problems. In this case, the fragmented information from the internet as well as personal SMS's in combination with the Chinese government's official information (which was incomplete and sometimes even inaccurate) caused the spread of rumors (Zhu, chapter 3 in this book). Consequently, this lack of trust for the information provided by the Chinese government meant there were no reliable, trustworthy and credible information sources to which the public could turn. This is particularly troublesome in the context of infectious diseases since when people have to rely upon unofficial information sources, there is a major risk that the information presented is incorrect which in the worst case will have contra effects in facilitating further spread of the disease. According to Ma (2008), the massive amount of rumors transmitted in Mainland China during the SARS outbreak can be explained by a unique combination of the collective Chinese culture, the restricted media environment, and the use of new information technologies.

It was not only deliberate attempts to conceal information that added to the problems in the initial stage of the outbreak but also a lack of suitable institutional arrangements and structures for dealing with the initial phase. This was evident in for example the Hong Kong Special Administrative Region (HKSAR), which due to the lack of a formal surveillance system forced the Government to rely upon reports from healthcare providers, a procedure that hampered the early warning phase. The lack of institutional structures did not only affect the initial responses at the national level but also had effects on the transborder and transnational level. Even though there was already an agreement in place between several cities located in the Pearl River Delta of Guangdong (including the exchange of monthly statistics and information on specific infectious diseases), the system was unable to detect the SARS outbreak. According to Shen (chapter 4 in this book), the failure to track down the disease can be attributed to two major facts. Firstly, the system did not allow for an exchange of information about diseases that were not already listed in the system, which naturally did not include SARS. This finding corresponds to previous research stating that one of the main reasons for why most organizations fail in detecting non-routine signals is that they were not designed to search for information that goes beyond their everyday mandate (Boin et al, 2005: p. 21; Simon, 1976; Cyert et al., 1963). Secondly, it was difficult to acquire information from other cities and provinces, which were not participating in the agreement, since there was no exchange of information between the HKSAR and mainland China's other cities and provinces outside this regional agreement. When the HKSAR received the first alarm from the media on February 10, they tried to get information from the health authorities in Guangzhou, but the latter did not reply. The HKSAR was unable to obtain any information until they contacted the Ministry of Health in Beijing (Shen, chapter 4 in this book). This made the HKSAR Government initially repeat the reassurances from the Chinese Government to the public in stating that the epidemic was isolated and brought under control. As a result, no public warning was issued on cross-border traveling in relation to the WHO announcement on the 10th of February stating that 350 cases had been found in Guangdong (Lee, 2007).

As noted by Parker and Stern (2002), another hampering effect on early warning is over-crowded policy agendas referring to decision makers being caught up in every day work which make them miss out on potential risks. This was yet another reason for why the three governmental actors included in this study (Mainland China, the HKSAR and Canada) were caught off guard. For example, chapter 6 in this book by Markel and Stoney shows how the Canadian government's ambition in downsizing, restructuring and reengineering, tax reductions, and health sector spending steered its focus away from measures aimed at strengthening pandemic preparedness. The ambitious political agenda at hand resulted in the fact that the Government missed the warning signs coming from various sources about a potential pandemic outbreak. Given this background, it should come as no surprise that Ontario's public health system was caught by surprise and lacked both crisis plans as well as professional expertise to deal with the SARS outbreak. It thus seems like the parties involved in combating the first and critical outbreak of the disease were all suffering from a lack of mental awareness and, as a result of this, subsequently institutional preparedness.

Yet another aspect contributing to the shortcomings in the initial phase was optimism and overconfidence in existing plans and procedures. The main cognitive challenge for crisis managers is to make sense of incoming signals and to size up the situation. In chapter 3 of this book written by Zhu, we learn that the Beijing municipalities were not only lacking institutional preparedness but also mental awareness. According to Zhu, the lack of mental vigilance could at least partly be explained by an overconfident attitude towards the Government's capacity for crisis management. The same tendency can be seen at the HKSAR level. What is particularly interesting here is that even though the HKSARG had previously experienced the avian flu in 1997, which killed six people and prompted the Government to slaughter all the territory's 1.5 million poultry, there were still no plans in place in 2003 for coping with a pandemic. According to Shen, this can be explained by an overconfident approach based on previous successful handling—where the Government managed to contain the disease without the help of a crisis plan. These findings correspond to Janis's and Mann's (1977) argument that complacency encourages decision makers to ignore information on potential risks, and as a result they do not reflect upon a new situation but rather follow past policies, so called "unconflicted adherence." The risk with organizational overconfidence in responding to changes in the external environment has been replicated by other crisis management and organizational scholars (Weick, 2001; Kets de Vries, Manfred and Miller, 1984; Hambrick et al., 1993; Pauchant and Mitroff, 1992).

The institutional aspects contributing to the quick spread of SARS is summed up by Markel and Stoney (chapter 6 of this book). Firstly, the Chinese denial and cover-up negatively impacted the effectiveness of the initial response. Secondly, the initial symptoms of SARS are non-specific and therefore resemble those of many other respiratory infections (such as the common cold), which made it hard to detect. Thirdly, public health measures (such as infection control, isolation and transmission precautions) were virtually non-existent in Canada as well as in China. Another aspect hampering early warning was overcrowded political agendas within Canada, Mainland China and HKSAR which made actors focus on the here-and-now issues instead of the looming outbreak of SARS (cf. Parker and Stern, 2002). The overly confident attitude added to the problem, where decision makers did not search for additional information nor question the existing procedures in place to deal with the outbreak. Further, there were not enough elaborated systems on the transnational level able to share information across borders. As can be seen from the list above, there were both conscious attempts to cover up information as well as more systematic institutional and cognitive aspects hampering early warning in the case of SARS. In the next section we will examine how the media functioned in terms of early warning.

## *The media and early warning*

The media plays an important role in connection to early warning. In contrast to other actors such as governmental agencies, the media is often praised for its ability to pick up signals and contribute to information spreading across borders and nations. However, the chapters in the book demonstrate that the so-called "media logic" is operating also in connection to initial reporting on infectious diseases—which impedes on media's function as a mechanism for early warning. The media logic was first coined by Altheide and Snow (1979) and refers to the media's tendency to report news in a dramatic, spectacular, entertaining, simplified narrative fitting with a conventional values manner.

The chapter by Deppa, Seaberg and Yao (chapter 8 of this book) identifies four aspects of media performance, in line with the notion of media logic that had a hampering effect on the media's ability to function as a whistle blower. According to the authors, the media's modes of production produce four main barriers summed up as: novelty, "under control," misunderstanding of panic and professional experience. In terms of early warning, media are in general ill-suited to pick up on new phenomenon, until something is happening that steer their attention in that direction. Further, the media's format is poorly adapted to reporting complex news events, and as a result, journalists have a hard time adjusting their communicative techniques when dealing with a life-threatening disease, such as SARS. Adding to the problem is also media's inherent need for official sources to recognize new problems which tend to make them hostages of the official rhetoric. This is in itself a paradox since the established news sources (such as governmental representatives) tend to emphasize the "under control" frame. The tendency for media to rely upon official sources in times of crises, the so-called "command post" tendency, has also been noticed in relation to media's reporting on natural disasters (Scanlon, 2007, p. 83; Quarantelli, 1996; Quarantelli, 2002). We can see this pattern in all three countries/regions included in the book. For example, the Canadian media's initial reporting relied heavily upon official sources, since the media thought alarmist reporting might lead to panic and that people were behaving irrationally. Consequently, it was reported in April that according to the Canadian Government the situation was under control, yet this news was quickly followed by a second wave of outbreaks in May (Deppa et al., chapter 8 in this book). Further, the problem with conflicting information was not only limited to Hong Kong and Mainland China but also occurred in Canada. Markel and Stoney highlighted how new information technologies with the possibility to publish 24/7 led to incorrect information and rumor spreading. The pressure of continuous publishing in combination with a myriad of actors, who commented regularly on the media coverage, led to confusion concerning fundamental issues: such as if SARS was contagious or not, how it was spread, and whether or not it was under control. Again, this is problematic given how important reliable information is for stopping the spread of rumors. In the end, the inability of the Canadian authorities to communicate the crisis properly fuelled confusion and panic among the citizens since they did not know how dangerous the disease was or how it was spread. In chapter 7 written by Atkinson, we learn that foremost the conservative press in Canada initially downplayed the threat of SARS by arguing that the sensationalist reporting only served increased university budgets and news managers. Atkinson also points to an important distinction between columnists and ordinary news coverage when speaking about mass media coverage where the columnists were urging for a skeptical stance towards the alarmist media coverage. These two modes of media reporting further added to the confusion. As stated by Atkinson, "There is little question that most readers would immediately seize upon the ambiguity inherent in arguing at once that the disease is a mystery while at the same time suggesting that simple precautions will work" (see chapter 7 of this book). This reminds us that journalism is not a uniform profession but rather that journalists reporting in crises might take on different type of roles such as traditional journalists, experts and social commentators (Reynolds and Barnett, 2003; Riegert and Olsson, 2007).[3] The chapter by Atkinson also stresses that precautionary measures such as quarantines, disinfection, basic hygiene, and some surgical procedures, are in democratic societies ultimately a moral matter that needs to be discussed amongst the citizens. Media is then not only a potential whistle-blower, information source and scrutinizer of political actors but also as an actor providing a public sphere in which matters of freedom and ethics are to be discussed.

Taken together, the chapters in the book stress the need for a realistic understanding of the media when it comes to its capacity for reporting in an accurate and speedy way, and in doing so compensate for slow information gathering and sharing within various governmental bodies.

## *Managing the crisis—Leadership and coordination*

### *Institutional aspects*

One of the main problems identified in crisis management at the national level is the issue of coordination and cooperation. If cooperation in crises is difficult within the boundaries of single nation states, it becomes ultimately complex in a crisis such as SARS, involving several individual nation-states and one international coordinating actor (WHO). Not surprisingly, coordination and leadership problems in relation to the management of SARS were evident in several of the chapters in this book. Furthermore, institutional problems at the national level often cascaded to the transnational and international level further complicating coordination and leadership. Starting with the institutional structure that hampered the Chinese response, Zhong (chapter 2 of this book) points to the fact that the Chinese lacked a unified national body for crisis management when SARS suddenly broke out in southern China at the end of 2002. Since they lacked clear leadership, the Chinese authorities were caught off guard when faced with an unfamiliar and unwelcoming phenomenon such as SARS. Instead of one leading agency with a clear mandate, the response at the central level became characterized by ad-hoc solutions. The crisis response was handled in accordance to the existing legal framework, which was characterized by a strict division of labor and responsibility between several central agencies affected by the crisis. There were then no legal possibilities to create a central unit that could handle the necessary strategic planning. Instead, the government had to adjust the response in accordance to the existing plans and practices originally developed for general social security. However, the ad-hoc character of the response fitted well into the Government's general tendency to rely upon ad-hoc solutions in times of threats or crises, arguing that it "sharpens its spears at the last moment" (Zhong, 2007). Somewhat paradoxically the Government's practice in relying upon an ad-hoc style of management resulted in less flexibility and a compromised improvisational capacity when handling the SARS outbreak. The tendency for decision makers to act in a rigid fashion, and to fall back into previous dominant modes of thoughts and actions rather than being innovative and vigilant in times of crises has been stressed by other management scholars (Roux-Dufort and Vidallet, 2003; Staw et al., 1981: p. 502). From a public administration perspective, one main obstacle in times of crises is that bureaucracies tend not to be designed for improvisation which makes them rely upon organizational cultures and procedures that foster routine responses (Boin et al, 2005: p. 55-56).

The lack of clear leadership did not only impact on the ability for strategic planning but did also contribute to the lack of clear roles and mandates hampering cooperation between Chinese agencies, as for example between the Beijing municipality level and the central government. Eventually the situation led to bureau-political infighting which had a negative effect on the SARS reporting system. Also local responses such as the Beijing response were hampered by the lack of a national coordinating body with the muscles to coordinate Beijing's response with those of other municipalities, the central government, the army, and relevant international organizations (Zhu, chapter 3 in this book). The Beijing municipality only gained momentum for a response once internal coordination was organized. It was not until April 23 that the state council, China's cabinet led by Premier Wen Jiabo, decided to set up the SARS Control and Prevention Headquarters with the Vice-Premier Wu Yi as its Commander-in-Chief. This solution led to that China finally got a central unifying command system able to integrate various national institutions of importance to combat the outbreak. However, as emphasized by Zhu, the command centre was depending upon the high leaders of the country, which eventually led to too much centralization and politicization. This can be seen as an example of the so-called "upscaling dilemma," which relates to that centralization is often necessary to accomplish co-ordination between governmental agencies and levels in the first place; however, centralization tends to create other sets of problems related to central and operational levels (Boin et al., 2005: p. 56-57).

Bureau-political infighting was not only a setback in China. Even though the HKSARG set up a central body soon after the Prince Wales outbreak on

March 14, not all decision-making power was centralized to the task force (even though its role grew with time). On March 25 yet another body was set up, namely the Chief Executive's Steering Committee (CESC). In addition, the Government set up the Interdepartmental Action Coordinating Group aimed at coordinating the implementation of decisions. Altogether there were three ad-hoc bodies within the government dealing with the issue which led to a crisis management response heavily influenced by bureau-politics. A similar fragmented institutional setting was prevalent in Canada's public health authority, which was multi-leveled and complex. At the time of SARS, Ontario was the only province lacking a regional health authority to coordinate efforts for a major outbreak. Further, the division of responsibility between the local and provincial powers led to dual roles and responsibilities. In sum, cooperation between the municipal, provincial and federal levels was characterized by confusion, conflict, duplication, and inconsistency. The degree of complexity and fragmentation is evident by the fact that ultimate responsibility for the management of SARS was never clarified in Canada.

Looking at the international level, one can see the effects caused by institutional weakness at the national levels. According to the WHO, it was obvious that Mainland China was simply not prepared for managing a crisis of this proportion. The institutional fragmentation and the lack of leadership caused difficulties in receiving information from China. Throughout the crisis, the WHO received data from two sources: the epidemiological department at the Chinese Ministry of Health (MOH) and the Chinese Center for Disease Control and Prevention (CDC). Adding to the problem was the fact that information flows within the Chinese CDC were organized into central, provincial and city and municipality levels so there was no overview or summary of the entire situation. Not only was the international response plagued by coordination problems at the national level, but also the WHO lacked a clear mandate for taking a leadership role. In practice this meant that crisis management had to be organized on an informal basis, where personal contacts and networks played an important role. In chapter 5, Deverell stressed how personal contacts between the WHO experts and Chinese authorities played a crucial role in managing the event and where personal characteristics (such as creating trust, mutual understanding and respect) were vital for the response work. The WHO had a delicate task in China since it had the mission of determining whether or not China was able to contain the outbreak on its own. At the same time, the WHO had to convince the Chinese authorities that it was also there to assist them.

### *Interpersonal crisis management*

After having discussed the institutional framework for handling SARS we will now turn to some of the more personalized aspects of crisis management by discussing the interaction between mainly Mainland China and WHO inspired by the concept of epistemological communities (Haas, 1992). In the following we stress the importance of the interaction between lower level experts in the system for building trust and eventually solve the problem. The importance of these kinds of epistemological communities for crisis management has also been demonstrated in the dioxin scandal in Belgium in 1999, where Belgian and EU-Commission civil servants after the acute phase started working together in persuading the political actors within the EU system that Belgium could be trusted (Olsson, 2005). In the case of SARS, there were in general two types of meetings held between Chinese and WHO officials: formal and informal. Whereas the formal meetings were highly politicized and had a tough tone to them, the informal meetings between experts had more of a friendly character which substantially improved cooperation between the two parties.[4] In a similar manner to the dioxin scandal, the SARS crises shows how trust between actors at the expert level was built through intense and close cooperation. This should come as no surprise since social processes tend to be process of convergence where "imitation, compromising, and bargaining, for example, are all processes that tend to reduce differences among people" (March, 1994: p. 118).

Due to the cover-up, China started the process with a huge trust deficit, which affected the way WHO handled the process and the amount of control they felt was needed in order to make sure that China was following their obligations. An example of this was told by a WHO representative with the Beijing team. The WHO members from the central level urged the Chinese authorities to hand over all the numbers they had regarding SARS so that the WHO could do a proper analysis. This greatly upset the local WHO team members situated in Beijing, since it was obvious that the WHO central level distrusted the information they had already been supplied. What is interesting here is that also the WHO representative on the Beijing team was frustrated by the skeptical attitude that the WHO central level had towards the assessments made in Beijing, even though the WHO Beijing team was actually sitting on all of the first hand data. Accusations were also made that some WHO consultants in Beijing were unwilling to deliver all of their data since they wanted to save some of it for future scientific publications (Deverell, chapter 5 in this book).

In the case of health crises, scientific data are an essential part of situation assessment. As has been noted by scholars of crisis management and communication, one of the most important assets in crisis management is credibility (Boin et al., 2005: p.78). This means that in a public health crisis, scientific data do not only need to be available but the producer of the data in question also needs to be trustworthy. As expressed by March (1994: p. 125) "In such a world, counting sample size becomes less important than determining the credibility of information sources and the plausibility of their information." A telling example of producing credibility was the fact that the WHO consultant in Beijing helped the Chinese civil servants prepare their presentations since he had knowledge of what the WHO wanted to see prior to the visit of the central WHO team (led by Heymann). Throughout the preparation phase, the WHO representative worked closely with the Chinese civil servants on their presentations. One illuminating detail was when the WHO representative urged the representatives from each of the affected regions to design their presentations in slightly different ways to disguise his own involvement in the process and in doing so increase the credibility of the presentations. "Therefore some differences in the various provinces' presentations, in terms of layout but also in terms of certain aspects that were important in one province but maybe not in another, were required. So, although the basic contents were the same, different provinces gave somewhat different presentations. The message was that they had been thinking and investigating independently and that they understood what they were doing" (Deverell, chapter 5 in this book). The observation underlines that actors who do not behave in accordance to the demands and needs initially risk having to spend a lot of time on trust-building measures later on in the process.

When trying to understand transboundary crisis management, cultural differences have to be taken into account. As Shen underlines in chapter 4, the lack of cooperation between the HKSAR and Mainland China was not only due to the lack of institutional structures but also the result of cultural differences and a lack of willingness to communicate with unknown organizations. The tendency for crisis actors to prefer working with people and organizations already known to them is a general feature in crisis management research (Quarantelli, 1998: p. 373-385; Drabek, 1986). However, the chance that actors might know one another is even far less likely in a transnational context than in a national one and consequently these kinds of problems will most likely become even more frequent in the future. The WHO representative working in Beijing described how he with time learned about the Chinese culture; for example, the reluctance of admitting that data were missing was not due to bad intentions but rather a face-saving mechanism (Deverell, chapter 5 in this book). Even though this might be regarded as mere details, such knowledge played a part in the crisis management.

In sum, the section illustrates how hard it is to build trust once it is lost. The chapter by Deverell stresses the importance of personal contacts in order to re-build credibility. This primarily took place between experts and civil servants working at the non-political level. The roles these contacts play as a form of trust-building mechanism in responding to transnational crises is one important lesson for further research in transnational crisis management. It is also equally important to notice the dynamic inherent in the center-field relations where collaboration efforts were not only problematic from time to time between the WHO and China, but also between WHO representatives at the local and central levels.

*Managing communication in crisis*

In addition to fulfilling an important role in the initial crisis phase, the media continues to perform a vital role in the acute crisis management phase. In times of crisis the demands for information tend to be insatiable where the media plays a key role in providing information not only to the public but also to the authorities. Research in the field of communication in connection to infectious diseases unanimously points to the importance of speedy and accurate communication in order to raise awareness among the public on how to behave in order to reduce the risk of spreading (Reynolds and Quinn, 2008). The urge for information means that there is an information void to be filled, and when responsible authorities keep silent, it will be filled by other actors making authorities lose control over both concrete factual information as well as the overall framing of the crisis (Coombs, 1999; Strömbäck and Nord, 2006). As a way of gaining at least some control over the media reporting, it is vital for actors to as quick as possible tell their story of what happened, why it happened and how to resolve the situation (Boin et al., 2005: p. 69-70). In this section we will discuss the management of SARS from a crisis communication perspective.

As stated by Zhong in chapter 2, the main problem with China's response was not the lack of understanding within the medical community but rather the delay in public information which enabled the disease to spread across the country as well as internationally. The Chinese authorities initially thought the outbreak could be handled by applying their usual PR strategy, referred to as "internal vigilance and outward calmness (Neijin Waisong)"; that is, they tried to mask the problem. Due to the traditional authoritative political system and its tradition of secrecy, censorship and manipulation, the Chinese authorities tried to cover up the facts for fear of damaging the image of the country and the flow of visitors and investors to the Canton Export Fair. As noted by 't Hart (1993), masking is a risky strategy which, if revealed, most probably will have serious backlash effects. In this case, due to today's diversity in communication techniques, it turned out that such an approach is no longer possible and the Chinese citizens were able to obtain information from cell phones as well as from the internet, where international news agencies played an important role.

The chapter written by Buus and Olsson demonstrates the reactions of the international press to China's management of SARS. The authors conclude that even though China's initial cover-up of the information made big headlines and was one of the three most important themes found in the overall reporting of SARS, the lack of trust in China was even deeper. Besides the obvious lies told in the beginning of the outbreak, the international press (e.g., *International Herald Tribune, Financial Times*, and *The Economist*) stressed the impact of China's historical and cultural traditions of placing political objectives in front of the well being of its citizens. The story being told was one of a new disease in an old system, which is described as obsolete, isolationistic and idiosyncratic where new facts were interpreted in the light of old stereotypes. The findings reveal how devastating a crisis can be for a country's image. Yet the reporting was not one sided but rather complex given China's strong role in the world economy. Thus, there was a big difference between depicting China as a crisis manager versus an economic actor, where the latter emphasized the vital role China performs in the world economy and how the West is actually dependent upon China. The chapter also demonstrates the dominant role played by the WHO representatives in describing the situation and how their statements were depicted as the most credible news sources.

That the WHO was seen as the most trustworthy actor in the international media discourse made China depend on their statements and assessments in reassuring the rest of the world that the disease was under control. In juxtaposing what we learned in Deverell's chapter on the WHO, we can understand parts of this dynamic relationship between China and WHO and its effect on international media reporting. As mentioned in the section "Managing the crisis" in this chapter, the WHO consultant team in Beijing helped the Chinese civil servants prepare presentations that ought to convince WHO that the situation was under control. At the same time they were working on their presentations, they could read how Heymann quoted in various media outlets said that he did not trust the Chinese numbers. It is interesting to note that Heymann's tone changed considerably in the international media, after having listened to the presentations given by the Chinese civil servants. In fact, he even stated that the SARS disease had finally been contained in China and he also praised China's efforts (CNN, 12 June 2003). This underlines the fact that trust-building measures are very much a matter of personal relations even at the transnational level. Certain individuals (such as the WHO expert in this case) can function as trust mediators between conflicting actors (such as China and the top-managers at WHO) and can successfully reestablish trust needed for effective crisis communication. It can be argued that trust building at the personal level is even be more important at the transnational level, considering that distance and different modes of communication in general tend to undermine communication.

The chapters in this book revealed that communication was not only a challenge at the international level but also for national actors. As already mentioned, China broke with one of the golden rules in crisis communication, that is, telling the truth immediately which resulted in that they initially lost credibility as a communicator. As a way of repairing this damage, since April 20, the Beijing government changed its communication policies after the initial cover-up and started to communicate with the public and the media via telephone hot lines and press conferences. In the chapter by Shen, we read how the majority of criticism from the Hong Kong residents was the Hong Kong administration's inability to issue the same information to the public. In the beginning of the crisis, mid March, the silence from the HKSARG made the media take on the role as crisis managers by providing a forum for ventilating public anxiety but also in initiating community campaigns. At times they even took on the practical task of delivering support to health personnel and affected citizens (Hayllar, 2007: p. 49). According to Shen, the main reason for the initial confusion was the fact that different governmental bodies were in charge of managing the crisis, which resulted in conflicting information. Yet, this changed on April 19, when the Hong Kong Hospital Authority (HA) and Department of Health (DH) as a response to such criticism started to hold joint press conferences.

One "best practice" in the crisis communication literature is to provide as much access to key spokespersons as possible (Seeger, 2006: p. 240). However, accessibility demands careful strategic planning, if not, organizations run the risk of overburdening their operational crisis management (Deverell and Olsson, 2010). In line with this, Markel and Stoney (chapter 6 in this book) stress the problems with intensive media pressure and how it took valuable time and energy from those people who were directly dealing with the crisis. Health personnel felt pressure to respond to the media at the same time they were trying to deal with patients. As a result, the constant demand for new information affected the ability of the already overworked health care staff to do their jobs.

The conclusions to be drawn from this are the complexity of information at all levels in the system, cascading from one level to another. The cases of Mainland China, the HKSAR and Canada all accentuate the power of communication management in the wake of a crisis. Actually, in the initial phase of crisis, information asymmetry appears to be the rule rather than the exception, particularly in facing those non-routine and unpredictable catastrophic disasters like SARS in 2003. In dealing with those familiar and routine disasters that happen with a degree of regularity, decision makers and relevant government agencies are allowed to anticipate and prepare for them accordingly. However, when faced with unfamiliar crisis or the so-called "virgin risk/crisis" (Kousky et al., 2010), which decision-makers have not experienced before nor thought much about and require mangers to learn new techniques, the core problem is to recognize and react to novelty, and to develop skills in problem diagnosis, improvisation, communication, and collaborative action.

## *Managing the after phase: Accountability and learning*

In the literature on learning and reform, crises are often seen as triggers and opportunities since they open up the system for criticism (Sabatier, 1999; Kingdon, 1995; Hansén, 2007; Nohrstedt, 2005; Nohrstedt, 2008). Crises tend in general to give birth to longer term dynamic processes of accountability and learning which are characterized by official investigations, blame games, political maneuvering, media scrutiny and crisis exploitation (Boin et al., 2008). The chapters in the book provide many illustrative examples of such processes and dynamics. As Zhong notes in his chapter, even though the effects of SARS on the Chinese system should not be overstated due to the Chinese political system, the event still had significant implications for the structuring of China's crisis management system. In general, SARS was an important alarm bell for the Chinese authorities in that it revealed the weakness of the traditional way of coping with crises, underlying the need for openness in contrast to secrecy. This is certainly the case if China wants to be a full member of the international trade community. Likewise, the SARS crisis pointed out the social imbalances in China which have not been addressed enough in order to keep pace with the recent economic developments.

In terms of learning, the Beijing government implemented lessons on both general and specific levels, as Zhu examines. The first round of implementations was focused on preventing another wave of SARS infections in the country. Consequently, every prevention and control center was required to install a SARS reporting system, which was operational on 24/7 basis. Another lesson learned was the importance of communicating with the public, which led to that more press conferences were held. Further, the system was reorganized in accordance to the principle "one mechanism" (the establishment of one uniform and authoritative command system) and "four systems" (disease prevention and control system, public health emergency treatment system, public health information system, and public health supervision system).

Within the Hong Kong administration, Shen describes how a SARS expert committee was set up in order to review the outbreak. The committee ended up giving recommendations on how to enhance the efficiency of the health care system and to prevent further outbreaks. Shen concludes that the Committee was successful in providing and implementing recommendations, but failed when it came to assigning responsibility to the officials who had dealt with the response. To the public, the committee appeared untrustworthy in assigning responsibility since it had been appointed by the Chief Executive. Therefore, the Legislative Council published its own report on accountability and set up an independent committee in response to the refusal to do so by the HKSARG. In the report published on July 5, it was concluded that various officials from the Health, Welfare and Food Bureau (HWFB), the Hospital Authority (HA), and the Department of Health (DH) were responsible for enabling the SARS outbreak. However, these officials were not required to resign from their positions as they were not responsible or accountable to the Legislative Council under the existing system. Nevertheless, due to public pressure in response to the report published by the Legislative Council, the Chairman of the HA (Dr. Leong Che Hung) and the Secretary for Health, Welfare and Food (Dr. Yeoh Eng Kiong) were forced to resign (Shen, chapter 4 in this book). The dissatisfaction with the

Government's handling of SARS led to an all time low in opinion polls for Chief Executive Tung Chee Hwa in April 2003 and also become one of the driving forces behind a massive protest in 1 July 2003 (Lee, 2007: p. 202).[5]

Not only were the HKSAR government officials forced to leave their positions due to poor performance in handling the SARS epidemics, but also their Chinese counterparts. In fact, two senior officials in Mainland China were forced to resign since they did not properly deal with the SARS epidemic in a timely fashion. Zhang Wen Kang was removed from his position as Minister of Health by the Standing Committee of the National People's Congress (NPC). Meng Xuenong was dismissed as Deputy Secretary of the Communist Party of China (CPC) in the Beijing Municipal Committee and later he resigned from his position as Mayor of Beijing. Zhang was blamed for not being adequately prepared for a public health crisis, while Meng was blamed for failing to provide timely and accurate reports on the progress of the disease. Although these officials left their offices in Hong Kong and Mainland China due to the SARS epidemic, the timing and approaches used were different and thus people's reactions varied in the two places. In Mainland China, the two senior officials were removed in April 2004, at the time when the country was still facing the SARS crisis. Part of the reason might well have been China's initial crisis of confidence and the country's desire to restore its tarnished reputation. Thus, this action was thought to be used as a window of opportunity for image-restoration in the wake of the international criticism against the management of the disease. However, according to Shen, the resignations in the HKSAR did not manage to curb people's uneasy feelings since they came too late and were done voluntarily, giving the impression that the HKSAR Government would not punish officials who had made mistakes.

Public anger was also aroused in Canada due to the fact that SARS claimed lives and took up to four months to contain. The criticism resulted in a political blame game that eventually led to serious inquires. The Canadian reforms in the wake of SARS have been many with the aim of improving procedures at the local, regional as well as national levels. As mentioned in the chapter written by Markel and Stoney, national efforts in Canada have also been aimed at strengthening its presence and work on the international level when it comes to cooperation with international organizations (such as the WHO) as well as with specific countries.

For WHO that operated to be front-line defense against epidemics during the SARS near-pandemic in 2002/2003, many lessons were learned that can be applied to the potential operational risks from H5N1 avian influenza and A(H1N1) pandemic influenza. SARS have shown that while infectious diseases may be local in origin, they can pose an imminent and ongoing global threat. During the SARS crisis, WHO has been coordinating the international response to provide the epidemiological, laboratory, clinical and logistic requirements needed to contain this disease. Since the SARS crisis, WHO dramatically stepped up its international disease surveillance and response (IDSR), and much has been invested heavily in new laboratory equipment and collaborative training. A major framework in the fight against emerging diseases is the newly revised International Health Regulations (2005), adopted by the World Health Assembly (WHA) in May 2005, which call on Member States to build, strengthen and maintain their core capacities for surveillance and response. At the early stage of the Influenza A(H1N1), WHO Director-General, Dr Margaret Chan, stated in April 2009, "On the positive side, the world is better prepared for an influenza pandemic than at any time in history," and she also stressed that "the international community should treat this as a window of opportunity to ramp up preparedness and response" (WHO, 29 April 2009). Compared with the SARS outbreak in 2002/2003, in facing the H5N1 avian influenza and A(H1N1) pandemic influenza, the world including countries and organizations like WHO is better prepared and its capability has been improved to respond to future pandemics and to future large-scale global public health events.

## *Conclusions*

Effective and legitimate crisis management is becoming an important aspect of the public policy agendas of nations as well as those of international organizations. This comes as no surprise given the fact that a crisis is the ultimate test for the resilience of political systems and societies (Boin at al., 2005). The emergence of SARS in southern China at the end of 2002 and its subsequent spread from east to west demonstrated that McLuhan's thesis of an increasingly integrated and interdependent global community is ever more tangible in times of crisis (McLuhan, 1964). By drawing upon a comparative case study approach based on cases from the worst affected SARS areas such as Mainland China, Hong Kong, and Canada as well at the WHO, this book found that one important set of lessons to be learned from the SARS outbreak relate to its transboundary character—an area of crisis management that has so far been underresearched.

By examining the SARS crisis from a transboundary perspective, this book addresses the growing concern amongst crisis management scholars advocating the need for the development of theories with the potential to grasp transboundary crises, which is defined as the crossing of geographical boundaries, functional boundaries, and time boundaries. Being the first global pandemic of the twenty-first century, SARS demanded the attention of national and international leaders as well as the public worldwide to the overwhelming importance of transboundary crisis management. Its emergence and subsequent spread justifies the tendency of crises to spill over national boundaries and an increasingly politically, economically, socially and not least ecologically interdependent world. The management of this new transnational crisis tested the mettle of leaders and the robustness of institutions in both developed and developing countries. Local, regional, national, as well as international responses to the SARS crisis in turn revealed a number of political and institutional frailties at all levels of the traditional crisis management system in these countries. This calls for the necessity to direct the attention of national and international leaders to consider ways of peaceful negotiation and respectful understanding among nations and peoples. Accordingly, the governance of transboundary crises demands the establishment of appropriate and adequate legal instruments, institutions and management tools from a transboundary perspective.

## *Notes*

1. The massive transmission of text messages has been pointed out as an important reason for why the Chinese Government decided to lift the censorship on SARS related information (Ma, 2008; Tai and Sun, 2007).

2. According to Thornton (2009), the text messages sent between February 8-10, 2003, contained the brief message "deadly flu outbreak in Guangzhou" and prompt local officials to break their stonewalling temporarily. On February 11, Guangdong officials held a press conference stating that 305 cases had been reported, admitting the lack of known treatment and the uncertainty about whether the outbreak had been contained or not. Due to orders from the provincial Party official on February 23 the brief period of openness came to an end which lasted through the running up of the National People's Congress in March (p. 32).

3. For example, due to a higher degree of press freedom, online sites in Hong Kong acted as "interactive crisis managers" whereas the news sites in Mainland China, due to press restriction, served rather as "online agents of contamination" (Lee, 2008).

4. This same pattern could be seen in the dioxin scandal where official meetings with member state representatives and political officials within the EU-Commission continued to be politicized even after the acute phase of the crisis, whereas trust and mutual understanding was fostered at informal expert meetings between the Belgian and EU Commission civil servants (Olsson, 2005).

5. According to Lee (2007), the reasons for the protests against the HKSAR Government can be summed up as following: failure to alert; judgment error in treating SARS as a public health issue; lack of containment policy, absence of figure head related to Tung's absence for two weeks in the beginning of the outbreak; absence of media spokesperson related to no one designated a spokesperson role within the Government Information Service; poor inter-bureaucratic communication and coordination; inconsistent message about the wearing of masks; denial of the seriousness of the outbreak in March 2003; slow and reactive response in implementing isolation policies and poor media management (including defensive attitude and apathetic manner).

## *References*

Altheide, David L. and Snow, Robert P. (1979) *Media logic*. Beverly Hills, CA: Sage Publications.

Boin, A. (2009) "The New World of Crises and Crisis Management: Implications for Policymaking and Research." *Review of Policy Research*. 26(4): 367-377.

Boin, Arjen and Paul 't Hart (2003) "Public Leadership in Times of Crisis: Mission Impossible?" *Public Administration Review*. 63(5): 544-553.

Boin, Arjen, Paul 't Hart, Eric Stern, and Bengt Sundelius (2005) *The Politics of Crisis Management: Public Leadership under Pressure*. Cambridge, UK: Cambridge University Press.

Boin, A., A. McConnell, and P. 't Hart, Eds. (2008) *Governing after Crisis: The Politics of Investigation, Accountability and Learning*. Cambridge University Press.

Boin, A. and M. Rhinard (2008) "Managing Transboundary Crises: What Role for the European Union?" *International Studies Review*. 10(1): 1-26.

CNN (12 June 2003) "SARS under control in China: WHO." Downloaded on 6 May 2004. Available at www.cnn.com/2003/HEALTH/06/12/sars.wrap/index.html

Coombs, W. T. (1999) *Ongoing Crisis Communication: Planning, Managing, and Responding*. Thousand Oaks, CA: Sage.

Cyert, R. M., March, J. G., and Clarkson, G. P. E. (1963) *A Behavioral Theory of the Firm*. Englewood Cliffs: Prentice-Hall.

Deverell, E., and Olsson, E-K. (2010) "Organizational Culture Effects on Strategy and Adaptability in Crisis Management." *Risk Management*. 12(2):116-134.

Drabek, T. E. (1986) "Managing the Emergency Response. *Public Administration Review*. 45: 85-92.

Galaz, Victor (2009) "Pandemic 2.0: Can Information Technology Help Save the Planet?" *Environment: Science and Policy for Sustainable Development*. 51(6): 20-28.

Galaz, Victor, Fredrik Moberg, Eva-Karin Olsson, Eric Paglia, and Charles Parker (2011) "The institutional and political leadership dimensions of cascading ecological crises." *Journal of Public Administration*.

Grönvall, J. (2001) "Mad Cow Disease: The Role Of Experts And European Crisis Management." In *Managing Crises: Threats, Dilemmas, Opportunities*, edited by U. Rosenthal, A. Boin, and L. Comfort. pp. 159-176. Springfield, IL: Charles C Thomas.

Haas, P. (1992) "Introduction: Epistemic Communities and International Policy Coordination." *International Organisation*. 46(1):1-36.

Hambrick, D., M. Geletkanycz, and J. Fredrickson (1993) "Top Management Team Commitment to the Status Quo: Some Tests of Its Determinants." *Strategic Management Journal*. 14: 401-418.

Hansén, Dan (2007) *Crisis and Perspectives on Policy Change: Swedish Counter-terrorism Policymaking*. Doctoral thesis, Utrecht University: Utrecht, Netherlands. CRISMART Volume 34.

't Hart, Paul (1993) "Symbols, Rituals and Power: The Lost Dimensions of Crisis Management." *Journal of Contingencies and Crisis Management*. 1(1): 36-50.

't Hart, Paul (1993) "Symbols, Rituals and Power: The Lost Dimensions of Crisis Management." *Journal of Contingencies and Crisis Management.* 1(1): 36-50.

Hayllar, Mark (2007) "Governance and Community Engagement n Managing SARS in Hong Kong." *Asian Journal of Political Science.* Vol. 15: Issue 1, April, pp 39 - 67.

Janis, I. and L. Mann. (1977) *Decision Making: A Psychological Analysis of Conflict, Choice, and Commitment.* New York: Free Press.

Kets de Vries, F. R. Manfred, and D. Miller (1984) *The Neurotic Organization: Diagnosing and Changing Counterproductive Styles of Management.* San Francisco: Jossey-Bass Inc.

Kingdon, J. W. (1995) *Agendas, Alternatives, and Public Policies.* 2nd ed. New York: Harper Collins.

Kousky, K., J. Pratt, and R. Zeckhauser (2010) "Virgin versus Experienced Risks." In *The Irrational Economist: Making Decisions in a Dangerous World,* edited by E. Michel-Kerjan and P. Slovic. pp. 99-106. New York: Public Affairs Books.

Lagadec, P. (2009) "A New Cosmology of Risks and Crises: Time for A Radical Shift in Paradigm and Practice." *Review of Policy Research.* 26(4): 473-486.

Lee, A. Y. L. (2008) "Internet Press Freedom and Online Crisis Reporting." In *The Social Construct of SARS: Studies on A Health Communication Crisis,* edited by J. H. Powers and X. Xiao. Philadelphia: John Benjamins Pub.

Lee, B. K. (2007) "The HKSR Government's PR Sense and Sensibility: Analysis of Its SARS Crisis Management." *Asian Journal of Communication.* 17(2): 201-214.

Lofgren, E., N. H. Fefferman, Y. N. Naumov, J. Gorski, and E. N. Naumova (2007) "Influenza Seasonality: Underlying Causes and Modeling Theories." *Journal of Virology.* 81(11): 5429-5436.

Ma, R. (2008) "Spread of SARS and War-Related Rumors through New Media in China." *Communication Quarterly.* 56(4): 376-391.

March, J. G. (1994) *A Primer on Decision Making: How Decisions Happen.* New York: The Free Press.

March, J. G. (1991) "Exploration and Exploitation in Organizational Learning." *Organization Science.* 2(1): 71-87.

McLuhan, M. (1964) *Understanding Media: The Extension of Man.* New York: McGraw Hill.

Nohrstedt, D. (2005) "External Shocks and Policy Change: Three Mile Island and Swedish Nuclear Energy Policy." *Journal of European Public Policy.*12(6): 1041-1059.

Nohrstedt, D. (2008) "The Politics of Crisis Policymaking: Chernobyl and Swedish Nuclear Energy Policy." *Policy Studies Journal.* 36(2): 257-278.

OECD (Organization For Economic Cooperation and Development) (2003) *Emerging Risks in the Twenty First Century: An Agenda for Action.* Paris:OECD.

Olsson, E–K. (2005) "The Dioxin Scandal." In *Crisis Decision Making in the European Union,* edited by S. Larsson, E-K. Olsson, and B. Ramberg. Stockholm: Swedish National Defense College.

Pan, Z. and G. M. Kosicki (1993) *Framing analysis: An approach to news discourse. Political Communication.* Vol 10, 59-79.

Parker, C., and E. Stern (2002) "Blindsided? September 11 and the Origins of Strategic Surprise." *Political Psychology.* 23(3):601-630.

Pauchant, T. C., and I. I. Mitroff (1992) *Transforming the Crisis-Prone Organization: Preventing Individual, Organizational, and Environmental Tragedies.* San Francisco, CA: Jossey-Bass Publishers.

Quarantelli E. L. (1998) "Where We Have Been and Where We Might Go," In *What Is a Disaster?,* edited by E. L. Quarantelli. pp.146-159. London: Routledge.

Quarantelli, E. L. (1996) "Local Mass Media Operations in Disasters in the USA." *Disaster Prevention and Management: An International Journal.* 5(5): 5-10.

Quarantelli, E. L. (2002) "The Role of the Mass Communication System in Natural and Technological Disasters and Possible Extrapolation to Terrorism Situations." *Risk Management.* 4(4): 7-21.

Quarantelli, E. L., P. Lagadec, and A. Boin (2006) "A Heuristic Approach to Future Disasters and Crises: New, Old and In-Between Types." In *Handbook of Disaster Research,* edited by H. Rodriguez, E. L. Quarantelli, and R. Dynes. pp.16-41. New York: Springer.

Reynolds, A., and B. Barnett (2003) "This Just in. . . . How National TV News Handled the Breaking 'Live' Coverage Of September 11." *Journalism and Mass Communication Quarterly.* 80(3): 689-703.

Reynolds, B., and S. C. Quinn (2008) "Effective Communication During an Influenza Pandemic:The Value of Using a Crisis and Emergency Risk Communication Framework." *Health Promotion Practice.* 9(4): 135-139.

Riegert, K., and E-K. Olsson (2007) "The Importance of Ritual in Crisis Journalism." *Journalism Practice,* 1(2): 143-158.

Roux-Dufort, C., and B. Vidaillet (2003) "The Difficulties of Improvising in a Crisis Situation: A Case Study." *International Studies of Management and Organizations.* 33(1): 86-115.

Sabatier, P. A., Ed. (1999) *Theories of the Policy Process.* Boulder: Westview Press.

Scanlon, J. (2006) "Potential Problem and Potential Ally: The Mass Media in Crisis and Disaster." In *Handbook of Disaster Research,* edited by H. Rodríguez, E. L. Quarantelli, and R. R. Dynes. pp. 413-429. New York: Springer Science Business and Business Media.

Scanlon, J. (2007) "Research about the Mass Media and Disaster: Never (Well Hardly Ever) the Twain Shall Meet." In *Disciplines, Disasters, and Emergency Management: The Convergence and Divergence of Concepts, Issues and Trends from the Research Literature,* edited by D A. McEntire. pp: 75-94. Springfield, Ill: Charles C Thomas.

Seeger, M. W. (2006) "Best Practices in Crisis Communication: An Expert Panel Process." *Journal of Applied Communication Research.* 34(3): 232-244.

Simon, H. A. (1976) *Administrative Behavior: A Study of Decision Making Processes in Administrative Organisations.* New York: The Free Press.

Staw, B. M., J. L. Sandelands, and J. E. Dutton (1981) "Threat Rigidity Effects in Organizational Behavior: A Multilevel Analysis." *Administrative Science Quarterly.* 26(4): 501-524.

Strömbäck, J., and L. W. Nord (2006) "Mismanagement, Mistrust and Missed Opportunities: A Study of the 2004 Tsunami and Swedish Political Communication." *Media Culture Society.* 28(5): 789-800.

Tai, Z., and T. Sun (2007) "Media Dependencies in a Changing Media Environment: The Case of the SARS epidemic in China." *New Media and Society*. 9(6):987-1009.

Thornton, P. M. (2009) "Crisis and Governance: SARS and the Resilience of the Chinese Body Politic." *The China Journal*. 61: 23-48.

UNWTO/UNEP/WMO (2008) *Climate Change and Tourism—Responding to Global Challenges*. Madrid, Spain: World Tourism Organization and United Nations Environment Program.

Weick, K. E. (2001) *Making Sense of the Organization*. Oxford: Blackwell Publishers.

WHO (World Heath Organization) (29 April 2009) Statement by the Director-General of WHO, Dr Margaret Chan. Available at http://www.who.int/mediacentre/news /statements/2009/h1n1_20090429/en/index.html

Zhong, K. (2007) "Crisis Management in China." *China Security*. 3(1): 90-109.

# About the Contributors

**Logan Atkinson** is an Associate Professor in the Department of Law at Carleton University in Ottawa, Canada. His principal research interest lies in the interdisciplinary intersection of law, medicine, theology and literature in history. In addition to the current piece on SARS, he has published on London's Great Plague of 1665 and Upper Canada's cholera epidemics of the 1830s. Dr. Atkinson holds a B.A. from Mount Allison University in Sackville, New Brunswick; an LL.B. from the University of New Brunswick; an M. Phil. from Memorial University of Newfoundland; an M.A. from Carleton University; and an LL.D. from the University of Ottawa. He is also a former University Secretary at Carleton University, and is a Fellow of the Institute of Chartered Secretaries.

**Stephanie Buus** is a Research Fellow at the Swedish Institute of International Affairs. Her research interests include the cultural study of threats, nationalism, travel and tourism studies, Scandinavian studies, and translation studies. She has previously been affiliated with the Centre for European Studies at Aarhus University and the National Centre for Crisis Management Research and Training at the Swedish National Defense College. She holds a B.A. from the University of Michigan, Ann Arbor and received her M.A. and Ph.D. in Scandinavian Languages and Literatures at the University of California, Berkeley. Her current research project is entitled "Chernobyl to September 11: Culture, Threat, and State in the Popular Imagination" and is funded by the Swedish Emergency Management Agency (SEMA).

**Joan Deppa** is Associate Professor at the S.I. Newhouse School of Public Communications at Syracuse University. She earned her Ph.D. from Michigan State University in 1981. She teaches courses in news writing, reporting, critical perspectives on news, communicating with computers (interactive multimedia), electronic publishing (print and websites), and computer-assisted investigative reporting. She has also studied communication failures and successes surrounding Hurricane Katrina and the coverage of climate change in newspapers on three continents since 1997. She is the principal author of "The Media and Disasters: Pan Am 103," and has a strong interest in ethical issues relating to journalism, including international media ethics.

**Edward Deverell** is the Director of Analysis and Studies and a Senior Analyst at CRISMART. In addition, he is a research fellow and lecturer at the Swedish National Defense College. His research focuses on crisis management on the organizational level, decision making under stressful conditions, and organizational crisis-induced learning. He defended his PhD dissertation "Crisis-induced learning in public sector organizations" at Utrecht University in the Netherlands in 2010. He also holds a Master's Degree from Uppsala University's Program of International Studies and a Bachelor's Degree in Political Science from Stockholm University. In 2006-2007, he was Seconded Expert Advisor on crisis management issues at the Government Offices of Sweden.

**Dan Markel** is a policy analyst with Public Health Agency Canada. He holds an MA from the School of Public Policy and Administration, and a BA Honours, summa cum laude in Social Anthropology from Carleton University in Ottawa. At the time of writing this chapter, his research interests focused on public health policy, and in particular, infectious disease prevention and control, and emergency preparedness and disaster management.

**Eva-Karin Olsson** holds a Master's degree in Political Science from Stockholm University, and a PhD from the Institute of Journalism, Media and Communication at Stockholm University. Her research focuses on crisis management, communication and journalism. She has published in journals such as *Journalism*, *Journalism Practice*, *Risk Management*, *Convergence*, *Public Administration*, and *Journal of Contingencies and Crisis Management*. She is currently Assistant Professor at CRISMART and researcher at the Department of Communication and Media, Lund University.

**Andrew Seaberg** is an associate in the Investment Management Group of the law firm Drinker Biddle & Reath in Philadelphia, Pennsylvania. Seaberg earned his J.D., magna cum laude, from the Temple University Beasley School of Law in 2009. He researched the media coverage of SARS while he was a graduate student in the S.I. Newhouse School of Public Communications at Syracuse University. He received his B.A., cum laude, with a major in government and a minor in sociology from Hamilton College in 2001.

**Simon Shen** is Associate Professor in the Department of Social Sciences, Hong Kong Institute of Education, Visiting Fellow of the Center of Northeast Asian Policy Studies of Brookings Institution, and Adjunct Associate Professor and Chief Coordinator of the Master of Global Political Economy Programme, The Chinese University of Hong Kong. He holds a PhD degree from University of Oxford and BA/MA degrees from Yale University. His research interests include Sino-American Relations, Contemporary Chinese Foreign Policy, Chinese Nationalism, Anti-Terrorism and Regional Security and External Relations of Hong Kong. He is the author of *Redefining Nationalism in Modern China: Sino-American Relations and the Emergence of Chinese Public Opinion in the Twenty First Century* (Palgrave Macmillan, 2007) and has published extensively in leading international journals including *China Quarterly, Asian Survey, Pacific Affairs, Pacific Review, Terrorism and Political Violence*, among others.

**Eric K. Stern** is Professor of Political Science/Crisis Management at the Swedish National Defense College in Stockholm as well as Director of the Swedish National Center for Crisis Management Research and Training (CRISMART). He holds a PhD from Stockholm University and a B.A. from Dartmouth College (USA). He has published extensively in the fields of crisis management, security studies, foreign policy analysis and political psychology. Among his monographs and edited volumes are *The Politics of Crisis Management: Leadership Under Pressure* (Cambridge University Press, 2005), which was the winner of the American Political Science Association's 2007 Herbert Simon Award, and *Beyond Groupthink: Political Group Dynamics and Foreign Policymaking* (University of Michigan Press, 1997). In addition to his scholarly work, he has collaborated closely with many government agencies and international organizations on a wide range of training, consulting and applied research projects.

**Christopher Stoney** is Associate Professor in the School of Public Policy and Administration, Carleton University in Ottawa where he teaches MA courses on federal and local government, public sector management, strategy, and urban sustainability. His research focuses on urban planning, emergency management, infrastructure, and mega-projects. His recent research (with professor emeritus Joe Scanlon) focuses on the handling of the dead in mass death incidents in Canada and internationally. Prior to taking up his position at Carleton, he held a position at the Tanaka Business School at Imperial College in London, UK.

**Lan Xue** is professor and Dean of School of Public Policy and Management (SPPM), Tsinghua University. His current research includes crisis management and science and technology policy. He coauthored *Crisis Management in China: the Challenge of Transition* (2003, Tsinghua University Press in Beijing). He has a Ph.D. in Engineering and Public Policy from Carnegie Mellon University and taught at the George Washington University before moving back to Tsinghua. He is a member of the Expert Committee for Emergency Management of the State Council of China and the founding director of the Center for Crisis Management Research at Tsinghua University.

**Grace Han Yao** holds a Master's Degree in Mass Communications/Media Studies from S. I. Newhouse School of Public Communications at Syracuse University and a Bachelor's Degree in Broadcast Journalism from School of Journalism at Fudan University. Currently, she is a research associate at Netpop Research, LLC, where she works on both customized and syndicated market research projects, with a primary focus on Internet population. Prior to joining Netpop Research, she worked as an account executive at Survey.com, a research assistant at Syracuse University, and a journalist at China Central Television (CCTV).

**Kaibin Zhong** is associate professor of public management at The Chinese Academy of Governance (CAG). He has a Ph.D. in public management from Tsinghua University. He is the author of *Crisis Decision-making: Explaining the SARS Crisis* (Beijing: The Chinese Academy of Governance Press, 2009). He also co-authored *Crisis Management in China: The Challenge of Transition* (Beijing: Tsinghua University Press, 2003). He was a visitor researcher at CRISMART Swedish National Defence College for working together on a project about SARS crisis management from December 2005 to February 2006. His research interests include crisis decision-making, risk communication, and social regulation.

**Qin Zhu** has a master's degree in public management from Tsinghua University and a bachelor's degree from Peking University. She currently works for the Emergency Management Office of the Beijing Municipal Government. Her current research includes risk assessment and crisis communication.

# Index

Made in the USA
Las Vegas, NV
12 November 2024

11367759R00163